CHALLENGES IN PANCREATIC PATHOLOGY

Edited by **Andrada Seicean**

Challenges in Pancreatic Pathology
http://dx.doi.org/10.5772/62754
Edited by Andrada Seicean

Contributors

Vincenzo Neri, George Van Buren, Christopher Riley, Nicole Villafane, Nikola Vladov, Ivelin Takorov, Tsonka Lukanova, Natalia Zambudio, Betsabé Reyes, Laureano Vázquez, Jonathan Lakey, Michael Alexander, Shiri Li, Antonio Flores, Paul De Vos, Huy Nguyen, Elliot Botvinick, Yoshinobu Sato, Alejandro Serrablo, Andraž Stožer, Jurij Dolenšek, Marjan Slak Rupnik, Viljem Pohorec, Roxana Sirli, Alina Popescu, Yuliya Krivova, Alexandra Proshchina, Valeriy Barabanov, Sergey Saveliev, Erkut Borazanci, Susan Haag

Published by InTech
Janeza Trdine 9, 51000 Rijeka, Croatia

Publishing Process Manager Iva Simcic
Technical Editor SPi Global
Cover InTech Design team

First published April, 2017
Printed in Croatia
Legal deposit, Croatia: National and University Library in Zagreb

Additional hard copies can be obtained from orders@intechopen.com

Challenges in Pancreatic Pathology, Edited by Andrada Seicean
p. cm.
Print ISBN 978-953-51-3115-1
Online ISBN 978-953-51-3116-8

For EU product safety concerns:
IN TECH d.o.o., Prolaz Marije Krucifikse Kozulić 3, 51000 Rijeka, Croatia,
info@intechopen.com or visit our website at intechopen.com.

Meet the editor

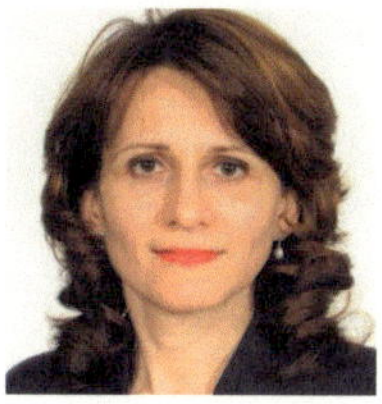

Dr. Andrada Seicean is a professor of Gastroenterology and Internal Medicine at the University of Medicine and Pharmacy, Cluj-Napoca, Romania, and holds a PhD in chronic pancreatitis, specializing in pancreatology and digestive endoscopy, mainly endosonography. She especially focused on the therapeutic endosonography fields, such as celiac plexus neurolysis and pancreatic pseudocyst drainage. Recently, her research has been on the contrast-enhanced endosonography-guided fine-needle aspiration in pancreatic pathology. Dr. Seicean published over 70 peer-reviewed scientific articles, 4 books, and more than 50 book chapters. She is an active member in many professional societies and has served as a reviewer for various scientific journals.

Contents

Preface

The assessment of the pancreas is a challenging problem because it is a "deep" organ that often presents difficulties in diagnosis and treatment. Despite many efforts in dealing with pancreatic diseases, the pathogenesis is not completely understood, the symptoms and imaging methods are unspecific, and the treatment possibilities are sometimes very limited.

The major purpose of this book is to offer the reader a better understanding of the challenging aspects in pancreatic pathology, starting with anatomy and following with the main pancreatic pathology.

The first section discusses the very close interaction between the nervous system and the endocrine cells within the pancreas, details about pancreas anatomy, and the physiology of the exocrine pancreas.

The second section reviews the surgical resection strategies in chronic pancreatitis.

The third section includes chapters concerning the cystic lesions of the pancreas, such as precancerous conditions, including the current opinion on intraductal papillary mucinous neoplasms and mucinous cystadenoma. The improvement of imaging, endoscopic modalities, and cyst fluid studies that allow the differential diagnosis of these lesions and the selection of high-risk factors for malignant progression are largely discussed.

The fourth section includes the majority of data in this book. Hereditary pancreatic cancer and the risk factors associated with pancreatic cancer development are presented extensively. The new method of contrast-enhanced ultrasound represents a valuable method for evaluation of the solid and liquid pancreatic lesions, and the selection of the subsequent imaging method needed is facilitated. New surgical methods for pancreatic resection and vascular resection represent challenging problems in the treatment of the pancreatic cancer, and they are also presented here.

The last section focuses on the discussion of the difficult issue of islet autotransplantation for the treatment of type I diabetes, related to the inflammatory response generated after transplant. The technologies to avoid immune rejection or immediate contact with cytotoxic inflammatory response are revealed in detail.

This book is meant to provide a thorough guide in pancreatology. The information offered will be useful for the clinicians, students, and patients, as well. The contributing authors to this volume are well-known scientists in the field of their expertise, and we are indebted to their efforts for dissemination of knowledge in pancreatology.

Andrada Seicean, MD, PhD
Professor of Gastroenterology and Internal Medicine
Regional Institute of Gastroenterology and Hepatology, Cluj-Napoca
University of Medicine and Pharmacy
Cluj-Napoca, Romania

Section 1

Normal Anatomy and Physiology of the Pancreas

Chapter 1

Neuro-Insular Complexes in the Human Pancreas

Yuliya S. Krivova, Alexandra E. Proshchina,
Valeriy M. Barabanov and Sergey V. Saveliev

Additional information is available at the end of the chapter

http://dx.doi.org/10.5772/65059

Abstract

It is well known that pancreatic islets are complex structures composed of endodermally derived endocrine cells, integrated with endothelial cells and other cells, originating from the mesoderm, and innervated by nerve fibers that have a neuroectodermal origin. In our studies, we focused on the interactions between the structures of the nervous system and endocrine cells, the so-called neuro-insular complexes, in the human pancreas. In this chapter, we present our results and literature data concerning the morphological organization of neuro-insular complexes in humans and other mammals. We also discuss the possible functional role of neuro-insular complexes, such as the involvement of the nervous system in the regulation and synchronization of islet hormone secretion and the morphogenetic plasticity of the endocrine pancreas in adults, as well as in the regulation of endocrine cell proliferation and maturation during prenatal development of the pancreas.

Keywords: pancreas, islets of Langerhans, neuro-insular complex, human development

1. Introduction

Pancreatic innervation is of interest due its role in the pathogenesis of some diseases, including chronic pancreatitis [1], pancreatic cancer [2] and type 1 diabetes [3–5]. The pancreas is well innervated by the autonomic nervous system [6–10]. In histological studies on the mammalian pancreas, the abundant innervation of the blood vessels, exocrine and endocrine part of the gland has been identified [11, 12]. Later, nerve endings were found around blood vessels, as well as pancreatic acinar, ductal and endocrine cells using immunohistochemistry and electron microscopy [13, 14]. Four types of plexuses (perivascular, periductal, periacinar and peri-insular) have been identified in the mouse pancreas [14]. Similar data were obtained in studies on the pancreas of the rat [15] and nutria [16].

Since the classical study by Claude Bernard, which showed that an injury to the floor of the fourth cerebral ventricle caused hyperglycemia, the involvement of the nervous system in the regulation of pancreatic endocrine function and metabolic control has been shown in many studies [17–19]. At the same time, the precise innervation patterns of islets were unknown, particularly in humans [9]. Single nerve cells and nerve ganglia, as myelinated and demyelinated nerve fibers, have been identified in the human pancreas [1, 20–22]. However, the literature data indicate poor innervation of adult human pancreatic islets in comparison with rodents [1, 9, 20, 23].

One of the most interesting features of the mammalian pancreas is that endocrine cells may form highly organized complexes with structures of the nervous system, so-called neuro-insular complexes (NIC). The structure of NIC in the human pancreas has not been studied in detail since their first description by Van Campenhout [24] and Simard [25].

In this chapter, we summarize the literature data and our previous results concerning the morphological organization of NIC in the human fetal and adult pancreas. We also discuss the possible role of the close integration between the nervous system and endocrine cells in the development of the endocrine pancreas.

2. Morphological organization of NIC in the mammalian pancreas

These structures consist of autonomic nerve cells, islet cells and nerve fibers in juxtaposition with each other, as described for the first time by Van Campenhout in studies on the histogenesis of islets in human, sheep and dog [24]. Later, Simard [25] confirmed the presence of such complexes in the human pancreas at different ages and termed these structures the neuro-insular complex (NIC) (cited from [26]).

In 1959, Fujita described two types of NIC, which he observed in the fetal and adult pancreas of the dog, cat and rabbit [26]. Some of the ganglia enclosed by the perineural sheath contained islet cells (β- or α-cells) forming NIC type I (NIC I). In NIC I, islet cells contact directly with nerve cells and no intercellular element can be recognized between these two cell types. In NIC type II (NIC II), islet cells lie on the surface of, or even in the midst of, the nerve bundle. However, the distinction between these two types of complexes is conditional because there is an intermediate type of complex in which a mass of islet cells associates with nerve cells in one part of the complex and with nerve fibers in another. Moreover, the ratio between nervous and endocrine elements in different complexes varies greatly [26]. As a variation of NIC I, complexes in which a single or a few nerve cells lying in a corner of a pancreatic islet were observed in the pancreas of the rabbit [26].

Consequently, the structure of the NIC has been intensively studied using histochemical, immunohistochemical methods and electron microscopy [13, 14, 27–31]. Analysis of the thin structure of NIC I and NIC II has shown that endocrine cells contact either directly with axons or with the processes of glial cells (Schwann cells or satellite cells) [27–29]. The gap between the plasmalemma of endocrine cells and glial cells is about 30 nm [28, 29]. Desmosome-like contacts and synaptic contacts between endocrine cells and glial cells or axons have occasionally been found by some authors [28]. As in histological studies, various morphological forms of the NIC were detected using electron microscopy. In many mammals, pancreatic islets are richly innervated by thin nerve fibers, which are located at the periphery of islets, forming peri-insular nerve plexuses; they occasionally pass through islets separately or along capillaries [14, 16, 27, 29, 32, 33]. The density of the peri-insular neural network varies between species [27]. It has also been shown that various transitional forms between the classical NIC II in which endocrine cells are located inside nerve bundles and innervated islets are present in the pancreas of the dog [27]. Similarly, various NIC I representing all transitional forms between pure islets with a single neuron and pure ganglia containing only a few endocrine cells have been detected in the pancreas of the cat [28]. Based on these findings, Böck [28] in 1986 introduced the classification of NIC reflecting a gradual transformation between pure neural and pure endocrine structures: 1. An autonomic ganglion with no endocrine cells; 2. NIC I: a) a few endocrine cells in the ganglion; b) a few ganglion cells in the islet; 3. NIC II: a) a single or few endocrine cells integrated with a bundle of nerve fibers; b) heavily innervated islet tissue; 4. A classical islet of Langerhans, either a) innervated or b) not innervated.

In addition to neurons and nerve fibers, glial cells immunopositive for S100 protein and glial fibrillary acidic protein (GFAP) have been detected at the periphery of islets in many mammals [3, 13, 14, 32, 34]. These cells have a triangular or spindle-like shape and possess long, thin leaf-like processes which cover endocrine cells, separating them from the connective tissue and from the acini.

Thus, the NIC are highly organized structures composed of endocrine cells, neurons, nerve fibers and glial cells (Schwann cells or satellite cells). The morphological organization of NIC varies considerably depending on the types of cells forming the complex and their ratios.

3. Structure of NIC in human pancreas

According to the literature, few nerve fibers are found in pancreatic islets in adult humans [1, 9, 20, 23]. However, the human pancreas receives extensive innervation, with peculiar growth dynamics during prenatal development [21]. In our previous study, rich innervation of human fetal islets was reported, and both NIC I and NIC II were detected [22].

As mentioned above, the structure of NIC in the human pancreas has not been studied in detail since their first description by Van Campenhout [24] and Simard [25]. In our studies, we investigated the structure of NIC in the human pancreas using immunohistochemistry [22, 35]. We analyzed pancreatic autopsies from 46 fetuses (from the 10th to 40th gestational week (g.w.)), 2 children (3 months old and 3 years old) and 15 adults (24–91 years old). The gestational age of fetuses was determined as the time since the last menstrual period on the basis of the measured crown-rump length and biparietal diameter by ultrasonography. Fetal pancreatic autopsies were divided into four groups, according to the classification of the fetal period [36]:

pre-fetal period (10–12 g.w.), early fetal period (13–20 g.w.), middle fetal period (21–28 g.w.) and late fetal period (29–40 g.w.).

To identify structures of the nervous system, we used various neural markers, such as neural cell adhesion molecule (NCAM), peripherin, neuron-specific class III β-tubulin, synaptosomal-associated protein of 25 kDa (SNAP-25), S100 protein and neuron-specific enolase (NSE) [22, 35]. Both types of NIC representing groups of islet cells integrated with ganglionic neurons (NIC I) or with nerve bundles (NIC II) were detected in the fetal pancreas from 14th g.w. onwards [22, 35]. In the pre-fetal period (10–13 g.w.), only contacts between single endocrine cells or small groups and thin nerve fibers were detected [35], and classical NIC I and NIC II were not found.

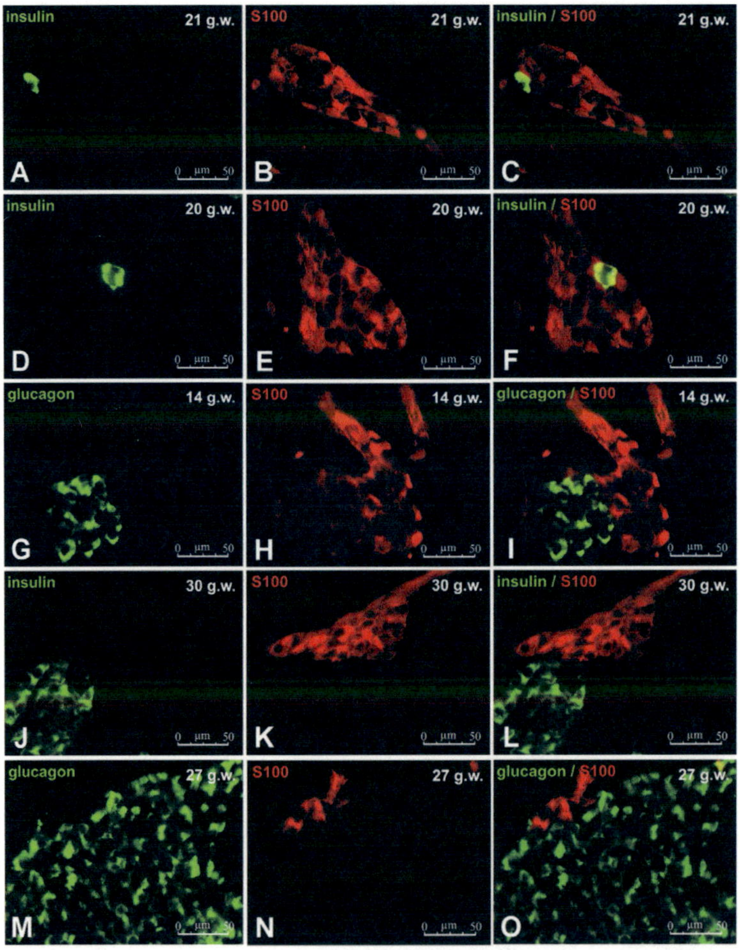

Figure 1. Various forms of NIC I in the human fetal pancreas: single (A–C) or few (D–F) β-cells in the ganglion; pancreatic islets associated with the ganglia (G–L) and few S100-positive cells in the large islet (M–O). Immunofluorescent labeling with antibodies to insulin or glucagon (green) and S100 protein (red).

http://dx.doi.org/10.5772/65059

To identify various subtypes of NIC in the human pancreas we used double immunohistochemical labeling with antibodies to neural makers (S100 protein or NSE) and endocrine hormones (insulin or glucagon) [35]. During prenatal development, i.e. from the 14th to 40th g.w., NIC I was present in the following forms: single (**Figure 1 A–C**) or few (**Figure 1 D–F**) endocrine cells located among ganglionic cells, pancreatic ganglia associated with islets (**Figure 1 G–L**) and few ganglionic cells located at the periphery of islets (**Figure 1 M-O**). We also detected various forms of NIC II: single or few endocrine cells in nerve bundles (**Figure 2 A–C**), pancreatic islets associated with nerve bundles (**Figure 2 D–F**), thin nerve fibers in close proximity to single endocrine cells or small groups and to islets (**Figure 2 G–L**).

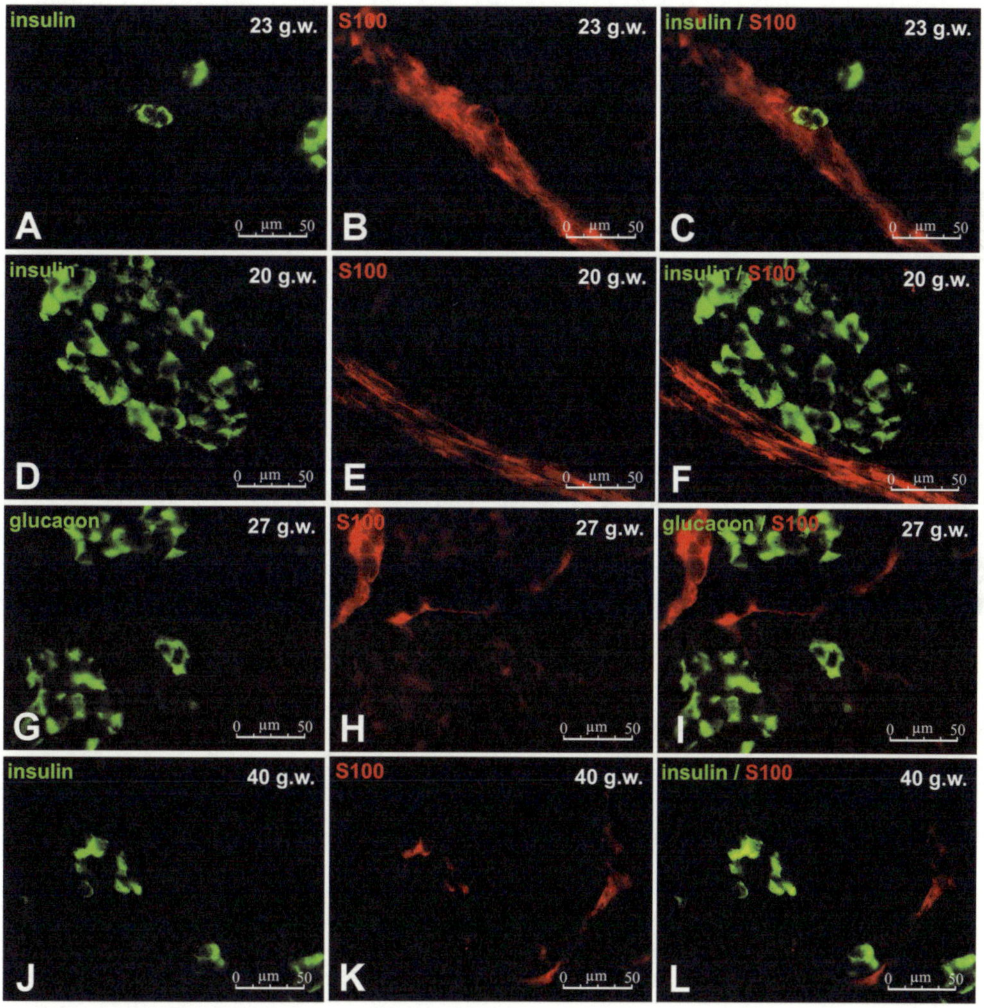

Figure 2. Various forms of NIC II in the human fetal pancreas: two β-cells in the nerve bundle (A–C); pancreatic islet associated with the nerve bundle (D–F) and thin nerve fibers in close proximity to the islets and single endocrine cells (G–L). Immunofluorescent labeling with antibodies to insulin or glucagon (green) and S100 protein (red).

Thus, the various forms of NIC that we observed in the human fetal pancreas are similar in their morphological organization to the NIC, which were found in the fetal and adult pancreas of other mammals [26–29].

The amount of NIC gradually decreases at birth. In the pancreas of children and adults, NIC are less abundant than in the fetal pancreas [22]. Our quantitative data indicate that the largest number of NIC I was observed in the early and middle fetal periods, during the active morphogenesis of pancreatic islets, whereas at birth (in the late fetal period) and in the adult, NIC II became more prevalent [35]. It should also be noted that NIC I and NIC II in which a single or few endocrine cells were located inside ganglia or in nerve bundles were found only in the fetal pancreas. We did not find these types of NIC in the adult pancreas, probably due to an insufficient number of fields of observation. Therefore, we could not exclude that these types of NIC can be present in the adult pancreas, but they are rare. NIC I in which pancreatic islets were associated with ganglia were more numerous in the fetal pancreas and were occasionally found in the pancreas of children [22] and adults [35]. Among the NIC II, at all investigated stages of development, as well as in children and adults, interactions between thin nerve fibers and endocrine cells located separately or inside the islets prevailed [35].

To identify whether glial (Schwann) cells cover the periphery of islets in humans, as in other mammals, we used immunohistochemical labeling with antibodies against S100 protein and GFAP as well as electron microscopy. We found small S100-positive cells with thin processes at the periphery of some islets in humans [37, 38]. The same small oval, triangular or elongated cells with long thin processes were observed in the fetal pancreas using electron microscopy [38]. The processes of these cells were often cover or surround nerve fibers passing into islets [38]. In contrast to mice and rats [3, 13], these cells were immunonegative to GFAP. However, according to their ultrastructural characteristics and integration with nerve fibers, these small S100-positive cells with thin processes that we detected in the human pancreas correspond to the glial (Schwann) cells observed at the periphery of islets in other mammals [3, 13, 14, 34]. It should be noted that, in humans, S100-positive glial cells are present only in some islets in small numbers and their processes do not cover endocrine cells, as has been described in other mammals [3, 13, 14, 32, 34].

Taken together, our findings indicate that, in the human pancreas, NIC are more abundant and variable in their morphological organization in the prenatal period, i.e. during the active morphogenesis of pancreatic islets. Based on these findings, we suggest that the nervous system may be involved in the development of the human endocrine pancreas. In the next part of this chapter, we discuss the existing points of view on the possible functional role of NIC.

4. Functional role of NIC

Since the description of NIC, researchers have been interested in questions about the functional role of NIC and the mechanisms of their formation. These two interrelated problems remain unresolved today. The idea of a regulatory role of the nervous system in endocrine secretion is commonly accepted now [8]. The pancreas is innervated by sympathetic and parasympathetic nerve fibers [8, 39]. Moreover, in the pancreatic islets of humans and rodents, there are the afferent (sensory) nerve fibers [7, 40, 41]. Many studies have demonstrated a role for the nervous system in the regulation and synchronization of hormone secretion from endocrine cells [7, 8, 17–19, 42, 43]. Stimulation of sympathetic nerves increases the release of glucagon and reduces the release of insulin and somatostatin [10, 41, 44]. Parasympathetic stimulation increases the release of insulin, glucagon, somatostatin and pancreatic polypeptides in various species [7, 8, 10, 44, 45]. Sensory nerves are also involved in the regulation of hormone secretion by pancreatic endocrine cells. The chemical destruction of sensory nerves (capsaicin treatment) in mice increases insulin secretion in response to glucose, compared to control. Consequently, sensory fibers may exert an inhibitory effect on insulin secretion [46].

Both the parasympathetic and sympathetic nervous systems impact the postnatal development of the endocrine pancreas and pancreatic plasticity in adult animals [17, 43]. For example, a decrease in the proliferation of β-cells has been detected in mice and rats after vagotomy [47, 48].

However, the concept of the regulatory role of the nervous system in the control of hormone secretion and endocrine cell proliferation does not explain the presence of endocrine cells inside ganglia or in nerve bundles. Simard [25] proposed that these endocrine cells may secrete hormones directly into nervous tissue. However, histological and cytological analysis performed by Fujita [26] has shown that endocrine cells in the NIC are similar in their mode of secretion to endocrine cells located in pancreatic islets, because their secretory granules accumulate on the side of the cell facing the capillaries.

In the second half of the twentieth century, there were two widespread concepts: APUD (amine precursor uptake and decarboxylation) [49, 50] and "paraneuron" [51]. It is well known that endocrine cells of the pancreas and neural cells express many common proteins, such as S100, glutamic acid decarboxylase (GAD), NSE, NPY and so on [3, 52–54], and have similarities in their developmental control mechanisms (for review, see [55, 56]). Similarities between endocrine cells and neurons are also confirmed by phylogenetic data. Endocrine cells (insulin-, glucagon-, somatostatin- and PP-secreting) were found in the brain in some invertebrates and lower vertebrates [57]. In the "APUD" and "paraneuron" concepts, these similarities were explained by the common embryonic origin of pancreatic endocrine cells and neurons from the neuroectoderm [49–51]. It has also been proposed that pancreatic islets can be regarded as modified ganglia because of the gradation between pure ganglia, mixed forms representing NIC, and pure islets [29]. This hypothesis was disproved in a series of classic experiments with quail-chick chimeras and in cell culture studies in which the endodermal origin of endocrine cells was established [58–60].

Today, it is well known that pancreatic endocrine cells differentiate from epithelial progenitors. In human fetal pancreas, epithelial ductal cells express numerous transcriptional factors that regulate endocrine cell differentiation [61–63], and differentiating endocrine cells transiently retain epithelial markers and are often associated with the ductal epithelium [61, 62]. The structures of the nervous system originate from the neuroectoderm [64]. The data concerning the mechanisms of the formation of NIC are very limited. Studies on rodents (mice and rats) have demonstrated that the innervation of islets develops in the early postnatal period [31,

65]. In other mammals (cats, dogs and rabbits) [26] including humans, NIC have been detected in the pancreas during prenatal development. The morphogenetic mechanisms underlying the integration between structures of the nervous system and endocrine cells remain unclear.

In his work, Van Campenhout [24] found that all primary islets (Laguesse islets) form NIC; he first suggested that the nervous system may be involved in the development of the endocrine pancreas. He proposed that NIC form through the budding of islet cells from the primitive ducts followed by their migration into adjacent neural tissue and that the differentiation of islet cells may occur under the influence of nervous components of these complexes (cited from [26]). Consequently, it was shown that both NIC and non-innervated islets can be detected in the fetal pancreas. In our studies, we also found NIC and non-innervated islets in the human fetal and adult pancreas [22, 35].

Nonetheless, genetic studies on mice have confirmed that the nervous system may regulate the differentiation of endocrine cells. In mice deficient for Phox2b or Foxd3 gene expression ($Phox2b^{-/-}$ or $Foxd3^{-/-}$), neural crest cells and their derivatives are absent in the pancreas. It was shown that, in such mutant embryos, the total β-cell mass and β-cell proliferation had increased [66]. Furthermore, β-cells in the mutant embryos were immature, since the expression levels of MafA and Pdx1 mRNA in β-cells were decreased, and insulin granules had abnormal morphology and were decreased in number [67]. Taken together, these data demonstrate that signals from the neural crest negatively regulate β-cell proliferation and positively regulate β-cell maturation [66, 67]. Moreover, in the developing mouse pancreas, neural crest cells and their derivatives are located in close proximity to endocrine β- and α-cells, suggesting that the regulation of β-cell mass and their maturation may occur through juxtacrine and paracrine signals from the nervous system [67, 68]. Similar results, demonstrating that co-culturing pancreatic islets with neural crest stem cells promotes the regeneration of functional β-cells, were observed in vitro [69].

A recent study has also shown an important role of sympathetic innervation in the establishment of pancreatic islet architecture and functional maturation during development. The absence of sympathetic innervation during development resulted in altered islet architecture, reduced insulin secretion and impaired glucose tolerance in adult mice [70].

Several studies have demonstrated that the structures of the nervous system interact with endocrine cells through the homophilic binding of cell adhesion molecules (NCAM and SynCAM), which are expressed on the surface of pancreatic endocrine cells and neural crest-derived cells in both rodents [68, 71] and humans [72]. Contacts between forming islets and NCAM-positive nerve fibers have been observed in the human fetal pancreas [72]. Therefore, it has been proposed that autonomic nerves may facilitate the outpouching of endocrine cell clusters to form islets through the homophilic binding of CD56 (NCAM) molecules on both of these tissues [72].

In our studies, we have demonstrated close integration between the structures of the nervous system and endocrine cells in the human pancreas, which was more frequently observed during prenatal development. We suggest that such integration may be necessary for the development of the endocrine pancreas in humans [22, 35]. It is possible that the nervous system may regulate endocrine cell mass and their maturation, as has been shown in mice. It is also possible that the contacts with structures of the nervous system may be necessary for the migration of epithelial progenitors into forming islets. In this case, different types of NIC may represent various stages of pancreatic islet morphogenesis.

5. Conclusions

In the pancreas of many mammals, including humans, endocrine islet cells are closely integrated with the structures of the nervous system into NIC. The morphological organization of such complexes varies considerably depending on the type of cells forming the complex and their ratios. According to the most current data, the nervous system is involved in the regulation and synchronization of islet hormone secretion and the morphogenetic plasticity of the endocrine pancreas in adults. During the prenatal development of the pancreas, the nervous system regulates endocrine cell proliferation and maturation and is involved in the establishment of islet architecture. In humans, NIC are more abundant and variable in their structure during prenatal development. This fact may serve as morphological evidence of the involvement of the nervous system in the morphogenesis of the human endocrine pancreas.

Author details

Yuliya S. Krivova*, Alexandra E. Proshchina, Valeriy M. Barabanov and Sergey V. Saveliev

*Address all correspondence to: homulkina@gmail.com

Laboratory of nervous system development, Research Institute of Human Morphology, Moscow, Russia

References

[1] Fink T, Di Sebastiano P, Bochlerj M, Beger HG, Weihe E. Growth-associated protein-43 and protein gene-product 9,5 innervation in human pancreas: changes in chronic pancreatitis. Neuroscience. 1994;63(1):249-266. DOI: 10.1016/0306-4522(94)90020-5

[2] Demir IE, Friess H, Ceyhan GO. Nerve-cancer interactions in the stromal biology of pancreatic cancer. Front Physiol. 2012;3:91. DOI: 10.3389/fphys.2012.00097. eCollection 2012.

[3] Winer S, Tsui H, Lau A, Song A, Li X, Cheung RK et al. Autoimmune islet destruction in spontaneous type 1 diabetes is not beta-cell exclusive. Nat Med. 2003;9(2):198-205. DOI: 10.1038/nm818

[4] Tsui H, Winer S, Chan Y, Truong D, Tang L, Yantha J et al. Islet glia, neurons, and beta cells. Ann NY Acad Sci. 2008;1150(1):32-42. DOI: 10.1196/annals.1447.033

[5] Mundinger TO, Mei Q, Foulis AK, Fligner CL, Hull RL, Taborsky GJ. Human type 1 diabetes is characterized by an early, marked, sustained and islet-selective loss of sympathetic nerves. Diabetes. 2016; 65(8):2322–2330. DOI: 10.2337/db16-0284

[6] Lindsay TH, Halvorson KG, Peters CM, Ghilardi JR, Kuskowsk MA, Wong GY et al. A quantitative analysis of the sensory and sympathetic innervation of the mouse pancreas. Neuroscience. 2006;137(4):1417-1426. DOI: 10.1016/j.neuroscience.2005.10.055

[7] Ahren B. Autonomic regulation of islet hormone secretion – implications for health and disease. Diabetologia. 2000;43(4):393-410. DOI: 10.1007/s001250051322

[8] Ahrén B. Islet nerves in focus—defining their neurobiological and clinical role. Diabetologia. 2012; 55(12):3152-3154. DOI: 10.1007/s00125-012-2727-6

[9] Rodriguez-Diaz R, Abdulreda MH, Formoso AL, Gans I, Ricordi C, Berggren PO et al. Innervation patterns of autonomic axons in the human endocrine pancreas. Cell Metab. 2011;14(1):45-54. DOI: 10.1016/j.cmet.2011.05.008

[10] Dolenšek J, Rupnik MS, Stožer A. Structural similarities and differences between the human and the mouse pancreas. Islets. 2015;7(1):e1024405. DOI: 10.1080/19382014.2015.1024405

[11] Richins CA. The innervation of the pancreas. J Comp Neurol. 1945;83(3):223-236. DOI: 10.1002/cne.900830303

[12] Coupland RE. The innervation of pancreas of the rat, cat and rabbit as revealed by the cholinesterase technique. J Anat. 1958;92(1):143-149.

[13] Sunami E, Kanazawa H, Hashizume H, Takeda M, Hatakeyama K, Ushiki T. Morphological characteristics of Schwann cells in the islets of Langerhans of the murine pancreas. Arch Histol Cytol. 2001;64(2):191-201. DOI: 10.1679/aohc.64.191

[14] Ushiki T, Watanabe S. Distribution and ultrastructure of the autonomic nerves in the mouse pancreas. Microsc Res Tech. 1997;37(5-6):399-406. DOI: 10.1002/(SICI)1097-0029(19970601)37:5/6<399::AID-JEMT4>3.0.CO;2-9

[15] Chumasov EI, Petrova ES, Korzhevskii DE. Distribution and structural organization of the autonomic nervous apparatus in the rat pancreas (an immunohistochemical study). Neurosci Behav Physiol. 2012;42(8):781-788. DOI: 10.1007/s11055-012-9635-6

[16] Krivova IuS, Barabanov VM, Savel'eva ES, Savel'ev SV. Neuroendocrine complexes in the pancreas of nutria (*Myocastor coypus*) (an immunohistochemical study) [Article in Russian]. Morfologiia. 2009;135(3):59-62.

[17] Thorens B. Neural regulation of pancreatic islet cell mass and function. Diabetes Obes Metab 2014;16(S1):87-95. DOI: 10.1111/dom.12346

[18] Roh E, Song DK, Kim M . Emerging role of the brain in the homeostatic regulation of energy and glucose metabolism. Exp Mol Med. 2016;48(3):e216. DOI: 10.1038/emm.2016.4

[19] Rosario W, Singh I, Wautlet A, Patterson C, Flak J, Becker TC et al. The brain to pancreatic islet neuronal map reveals differential glucose regulation from distinct hypothalamic regions. Diabetes. 2016. Forthcoming. DOI: 10.2337/db15-0629

[20] Castorina S, Romeo R, Marcello MF. Immunohistochemical study of intrinsic innervation in the human pancreas. Boll Soc Ital Biol Sper. 1996;72(1-2):1–7.

[21] Amella C, Cappello F, Kahl P, Fritsch H, Lozanoff S, Sergi C. Spatial and temporal dynamics of innervation during the development of fetal human pancreas. Neuroscience. 2008;154(4):1477-1487. DOI: 10.1016/j.neuroscience.2008.04.050

[22] Krivova YS, Proshchina AE, Barabanov VM, Saveliev SV. Development of the islets of Langerhans in the human fetal pancreas. In: Satou A, Nakamura H, editors. Pancreas: Anatomy, Diseases and Health Implications. NY:Nova Science Publishers; 2012. p. 53-88.

[23] Pour PM, Saruc M. The pattern of neural elements in the islets of normal and diseased pancreas and in isolated islets. JOP. 2011;12(4):395-403.

[24] Van Campenhout E. Contributions a l'etude de l'histogenese du pancreas, chez quelques mammiferes. Les complexes sympathico-insulaires. [Contributions to the study of the histogenesis of the pancreas in some mammals. The sympathico-insular complex]. Arch Biol. 1927;37:121-171.

[25] Simard LC. Les complecses neuro-insulaires. [The neuro-insular complex]. Arch Anat Micr. 1937;33:49-64.

[26] Fujita T. Histological studies on the neuro-insular complex in the pancreas of some mammals. Z Zselloforsch. 1959;50(1):94-109. DOI: 10.1007/bf00342656

[27] Kobayashi S, Fujita T. Fine structure of mammalian and avian pancreatic islets with a special reference to D-cells and nervous elements. Z Zellforsch Mikrosk Anat. 1969;100(3):340-363. DOI: 10.1007/bf00571491

[28] Böck P. Fine structure of the neuro-insular complex type II in the cat. Arch Histol Jpn. 1986;49(2):189-197. DOI: 10.1679/aohc.49.189

[29] Serizawa Y, Kobayashi S, Fujita T. Neuro-insular complex type I in the mouse. Reevaluation of the pancreatic islet as a modified ganglion. Arch Histol Jpn. 1979;42(3): 389-394. DOI: 10.1679/aohc1950.42.389

[30] Persson-Sjögren S, Zashihin A, Forsgren S. Nerve cells associated with the endocrine pancreas in young mice: an ultrastructural analysis of the neuroinsular complex type I. Histochem J. 2001;33(6):373-378.

[31] Burris R, Hebrok M. Pancreatic innervation in mouse development and β-cell regeneration. Neuroscience. 2007;150(3):592-602. DOI: 10.1016/j.neuroscience.2007.09.079

[32] Tang SC, Peng SJ, Chien HJ. Imaging of the islet neural network. Diabetes Obes Metab 2014;16(S1):77-86. DOI: 10.1111/dom.12342

[33] Chien HJ, Peng SJ, Hua TE, Kuo CH, Juang JH, Tang SC. 3-D imaging of islets in obesity: formation of the islet-duct complex and neurovascular remodeling in young hyperphagic mice. Int J Obes. 2015;40(4):685-697. DOI: 10.1038/ijo.2015.224

[34] Donev S. Ultrastructural evidence for presence of a glial sheath investing the islets of Langerhans in the pancreas of mammals. Cell Tissue Res. 1984;237(2):343-348. DOI: 10.1007/bf00217154

[35] Proshchina AE, Krivova YS, Barabanov VM, Saveliev SV. Ontogeny of neuro-insular complexes and islets innervation in the human pancreas. Front Endocrinol. 2014;5:57. DOI: 10.3389/fendo.2014.00057

[36] Milvanov AP, Saveliev SV. Rational periodization of prenatal human development and methodical aspects of embryology. In: Milovanov AP, Saveliev SV, editors. Prenatal Human Development. Moscow: MDV; 2006. p. 21-32.

[37] Proschina AE, Krivova YS, Barabanov VM, Saveliev SV. Distribution of S100-positive cells in islets of Langerhans of the fetal and adult human pancreas. Sovrem Technol Med. 2015;7(3):61-66. DOI: 10.17691/stm2015.7.3.08

[38] Krivova YS, Proshchina AE, Chernikov VP, Barabanov VM, Savel'ev SV. Immunohistochemical analysis and electron microscopy of glial cells in the pancreas of fetuses and children. Bull Exp Biol Med. 2015;159(5):666-669. DOI: 10.1007/s10517-015-3043-1. Epub 2015 Oct 13.

[39] Love JA, Yi E, Smith TG. Autonomic pathways regulating pancreatic exocrine secretion. Auton Neurosci. 2007;133(1):19-34. DOI: 10.1016/j.autneu.2006.10.001

[40] Salvioli B, Bovara M, Barbara G, De Ponti F, Stanghellini V, Tonini M et al. Neurology and neuropathology of the pancreatic innervation. JOP. 2002;3(2):26-33.

[41] Gilon P, Henquin JC. Mechanism and physiological significance of the cholinergic control of pancreatic b-cell function. Endocr Rev. 2001;22(5):565-604. DOI: 10.1210/er.22.5.565

[42] Buijs RM, Chun SJ, Niijima A, Romijn HJ, Nagai K. Parasympathetic and sympathetic control of the pancreas: a role for the suprachiasmatic nucleus and other hypothalamic centers that are involved in the regulation of food intake. J Comp Neurol. 2001;431(4):405-423. DOI: 10.1002/1096-9861(20010319)431:4<405::aid-cne1079>3.0.co;2-d

[43] Kiba T. Relationships between the autonomic nervous system and the pancreas including regulation of regeneration and apoptosis: recent developments. Pancreas. 2004;29(2):e51-e58. DOI: 10.1097/00006676-200408000-00019

[44] Rodriguez-Diaz R, Caicedo A. Novel approaches to studying the role of innervation in the biology of pancreatic islets. Endocrinol Metab Clin North Am. 2013;42(1):39-56. DOI: 10.1016/j.ecl.2012.11.001

[45] Eberhard D, Lammert E. The pancreatic beta-cell in the islet and organ community. Curr Opin Genet Dev. 2009;19(5):469-475. DOI: 10.1016/j.gde.2009.07.003

[46] Karlsson S, Scheurink AJ, Steffens AB, Ahrén B. Involvement of capsaicin-sensitive nerves in regulation of insulin secretion and glucose tolerance in conscious mice. Am J Physiol. 1994;267(4 Pt2):R1071-R1077.

[47] Edvell A, Lindstrom P. Vagotomy in young obese hyperglycemic mice: effects on syndrome development and islet proliferation. Am J Physiol 1998;274(6 Pt1):E1034-E1039.

[48] Lausier J, Diaz WC, Roskens V, Larock K, Herzer K, Fong CG et al. Vagal control of pancreatic beta-cell proliferation. Am J Physiol Endocrinol Metab. 2010;299(5):E786-E793. DOI: 10.1152/ajpendo.00202.2010

[49] Pearse AGE. Neurotransmission and the APUD concept. In: Coupland RE, Fujita T, editors. Chromaffin, Enterochromaffin and Related Cells. Amsterdam: Elsevier; 1976. p. 147-154.

[50] Pearse AG, Polak JM. Neural crest origin of the endocrine polypeptide (APUD) cells of the gastrointestinal tract and pancreas. Gut. 1971;12(10):783-788. DOI: 10.1136/gut.12.10.783

[51] Fujita T. The gastro-enteric endocrine cell and its paraneuronic nature. In: Coupland RE, Fujita T, editors. Chromaffin, Enterochromaffin and Related Cells. Amsterdam: Elsevier; 1976. p. 191-208.

[52] Kim J, Richter W, Aanstoot HJ, Shi Y, Fu Q, Rajotte R et al. Differential expression of GAD65 and GAD67 in human, rat, and mouse pancreatic islets. Diabetes. 1993;42(12):1799-1808. DOI: 10.2337/diabetes.42.12.1799

[53] Teitelman G, Alpert S, Polak JM, Martinez A, Hanahan D. Precursor cells of mouse endocrine pancreas coexpress insulin, glucagon and the neuronal proteins tyrosine hydroxylase and neuropeptide Y, but not pancreatic polypeptide. Development. 1993;118(4):1031-1039.

[54] Von Dorsche HH, Falt K, Hahn HJ, Reiher H. Neuron-specific enolase (NSE) as a neuroendocrine cell marker in the human fetal pancreas. Acta Histochem. 1989;85(2):227-228. DOI: 10.1016/s0065-1281(89)80073-x

[55] Edlund H. Developmental biology of the pancreas. Diabetes. 2001;50(S1):S5-S9. DOI: 10.2337/diabetes.50.2007.s5

[56] Bonal C, Herrera PL. Genes controlling pancreas ontogeny. Int J Dev Biol. 2008;52(7):823-835. DOI: 10.1387/ijdb.072444cb

[57] Falkmer S. Comparative morphology of pancreatic islets in animals. In: Volk BW, Arquilla EP, editors. The Diabetic Pancreas. 2nd ed. New York: Plenum; 1985. p. 17-52. DOI: 10.1007/978-1-4757-0348-1_2

[58] Andrew A. An experimental investigation into the possible neural crest origin of pancreatic APUD (islet) cells. J Embryol Exp Morphol. 1976;35(3):577-593.

[59] Fontaine J, Le Douarin NM. Analysis of endoderm formation in the avian blastoderm by the use of quail-chick chimaeras. The problem of the neuroectodermal origin of the cells of the APUD series. J Embryol Exp Morphol. 1977;41:209-222.

[60] Pictet RL, Rall LB, Phelps P, Rutter WJ. The neural crest and the origin of the insulin-producing and other gastrointestinal hormone-producing cells. Science. 1976;191 (4223): 191-192. DOI: 10.1126/science.1108195

[61] Piper K, Brickwood S, Turnpenny LW, Cameron IT, Ball SG, Wilson DI et al. Beta cell differentiation during early human pancreas development. J Endocrinol. 2004;181(1): 11-23. DOI: 10.1677/joe.0.1810011

[62] Lyttle BM, Li J, Krishnamurthy M, Fellows F, Wheeler MB, Goodyer CG et al. Transcription factor expression in the developing human fetal endocrine pancreas. Diabetologia. 2008;51(7):1169-1180. DOI: 10.1007/s00125-008-1006-z

[63] Jeon J, Correa-Medina M, Ricordi C, Edlund H, Diez JA. Endocrine cell clustering during human pancreas development. J Histochem Cytochem. 2009;57(9):811-824. DOI: 10.1369/jhc.2009.953307

[64] Young HM, Newgreen D. Enteric neural crest derived cells: origin, identification, migration, and differentiation. Anat Rec. 2001;262(1):1-15. DOI: 10.1002/1097-0185 (20010 101)262:1<1::aid-ar1006>3.0.co;2-2

[65] Cabrera-Vasquez S, Navarro-Tableros V, Sanchez-Soto C, Gutierrez-Ospina G, Hiriart M. Remodelling sympathetic innervation in rat pancreatic islets ontogeny. BMC Dev Biol. 2009;9(1):34. DOI: 10.1186/1471-213x-9-34

[66] Nekrep N, Wang J, Miyatsuka T, German MS. Signals from the neural crest regulate beta-cell mass in the pancreas. Development. 2008;135(12):2151-2160. DOI: 10.1242/dev.015859

[67] Plank JL, Mundell NA, Frist AY, LeGrone AW, Kim T, Musser MA et al. Influence and timing of arrival of murine neural crest on pancreatic beta cell development and maturation. Dev Biol. 2011;349(2):321-330.DOI: 10.1016/j.ydbio.2010.11.013

[68] Shimada K, Tachibana T, Fujimoto K, Sasaki T, Okabe M. Temporal and spatial cellular distribution of neural crest derivatives and alpha cells during islet development. Acta Histochem Cytochem. 2012;45(1):65-75. DOI: 10.1267/ahc.11052

[69] Olerud J, Kanaykina N, Vasylovska S, King D, Sandberg M, Jansson L et al. Neural crest stem cells increase beta cell proliferation and improve islet function in co-transplanted

murine pancreatic islets. Diabetologia. 2009;52(12):2594-2601. DOI: 10.1007/s00125-009-1544-z

[70] Borden P, Houtz J, Leach SD, Kuruvilla R. Sympathetic innervation during development is necessary for pancreatic islet architecture and functional maturation. Cell Rep. 2013;4(2):287-301. DOI: 10.1016/j.celrep.2013.06.019

[71] Esni F, Taljedal IB, Perl AK, Cremer H, Christofori G, Semb H. Neural cell adhesion molecule (N-CAM) is requires for islet cell type segregation and normal ultrastructure in pancreatic islets. J Cell Biol. 1999;144(2):325-337. DOI: 10.1083/jcb.144.2.325

[72] Fujisawa M, Notohara K, Tsukayama C, Mizuno R, Okada S. CD-56 positive cells with or without synaptophysin expression are recognized in the pancreatic duct epithelium: a study with adult and fetal tissues and specimens from chronic pancreatitis. Acta Med Okayama. 2003;57(6):279-284.

Chapter 2

Pancreas Physiology

Jurij Dolenšek , Viljem Pohorec ,

Marjan Slak Rupnik and Andraž Stožer

Additional information is available at the end of the chapter

http://dx.doi.org/10.5772/65895

Abstract

In the exocrine pancreas, the relationship between structure and function, as well as between normal and pathological functioning, can be easily understood if presented in a systematic and logical manner. In this chapter, we explain pancreas physiology. We start by explaining the embryological and ontogenetic development of the pancreas and describe the basic anatomical characteristics of the mature gland, i.e. the macro- and microscopic structure, its vascular supply and innervation. These form the foundation necessary to understand the mechanisms of acinar and ductal cell secretion and their regulation, which are covered in the middle part, with an emphasis on the ionic part of the pancreatic juice. In the last part, we focus on the enzymatic part of the pancreatic juice and its role in digestion of all main groups of energy-rich nutrients, i.e. carbohydrates, proteins and lipids. Two main sources of additional information will help the reader grasp the main concepts in pancreas physiology: figures summarize and combine various concepts encountered in the main text, and clinical boxes contain examples of how a given piece of knowledge can be relevant to understand some diseases.

Keywords: pancreas, exocrine, development, embryology, anatomy, vascularization, innervation, physiology, pathophysiology, acinar, ductal, cell, molecular, mechanism, regulation, digestion, secretion, nutrient

1. Introduction

The main aim of this review of pancreas physiology is to facilitate the understanding of other chapters of this book. It is divided into three main sections that deal with the development and the functional anatomy of the pancreas, with the two-compartment model of exocrine pancreas and the regulation of exocrine secretion and with the role pancreas plays in intestinal digestion of nutrients. Together, these topics shall provide a solid ground to understand etiopathophysiology of the most common pancreatic diseases, their symptoms and crucial clinical characteristics, as well as some key diagnostic and therapeutic principles.

2. Functional anatomy of the pancreas

This chapter is a brief review of human pancreas development and anatomy, with a special emphasis on the exocrine pancreas from both a physiological and a clinical point of view. In other words, this chapter presents developmental and structural basis to understanding pancreas physiology, its blood and lymphatic vasculature, innervation and the integrative regulation of its function, as well as the clinical symptoms and patterns of spreading in cases of malignancy.

2.1. Embryological and ontogenetic development of the pancreas

All parenchymal cell types of the pancreas (acinar, ductal and endocrine cells) are derived from primitive endodermal cells of the foregut [1, 2]. In humans, between the 26th and 28th day of gestation, two endodermal diverticula evaginate from the duodenum, thus forming the dorsal and the ventral pancreatic anlage [3–6]. The dorsal pancreatic bud lies in the dorsal mesentery opposite and above the liver bud. The ventral pancreatic bud develops in the ventral mesentery below the liver bud and connects with the bile duct. During further development, both the ventral bud and the bile duct rotate clockwise, as viewed in the craniocaudal direction, until they reach the dorsal pancreatic bud. Parenchyma of the two buds merges during the 7th week of gestation. The ventral pancreas gives rise to the ventral or lower part of the head of the pancreas that involves also the processus uncinatus, whereas the dorsal pancreas gives rise to the rest of the future pancreas, i.e. the dorsal or upper part of the head, the neck, the body and the tail [7]. Together with parenchyma, the ducts of the primitive pancreas also merge. Ducts of the ventral pancreas and the proximal part of the dorsal pancreas give rise to the main pancreatic duct (of Wirsung). The distal part of the duct of the dorsal pancreas may either obliterate or give rise to the accessory pancreatic duct (of Santorini). In the latter case, the accessory duct drains into the duodenum in the smaller papilla of Santorini that is located orally relative to the larger papilla of Vater [6].

During endoscopic retrograde cholangiopancreatography (ERCP), in approximately 3% of people the so-called anomalous pancreaticobiliary junction (APBJ) can be found. In this variation, the pancreatic duct joins the bile duct a few centimetres proximally from the duodenal wall. Due to a reflux and stasis of a mixture of bile and pancreatic juice in the bile duct and gallbladder, the incidence of gallbladder and bile duct carcinoma is increased in these people [8, 9]. In addition to APBJ, a number of other conditions result from defects in the embryological development of the pancreas, such as the annular pancreas and pancreas divisum, that are reviewed elsewhere [8]. The dual embryological origin of the pancreas also reflects in the smaller size and a tighter arrangement of the lobules in the ventral pancreas (lower head and the uncinate process), as well as a different cellular make-up of islets of Langerhans and vascular supply (see below) [10].

In newborns, the total weight of pancreas is around 3 g and the volume of the exocrine pancreas increases approximately linearly to 20 years of age [11–13]. During the period of 20–60 years of age, the volume remains stable and then decreases beyond 60 years of age [11] (**Figure 1**).

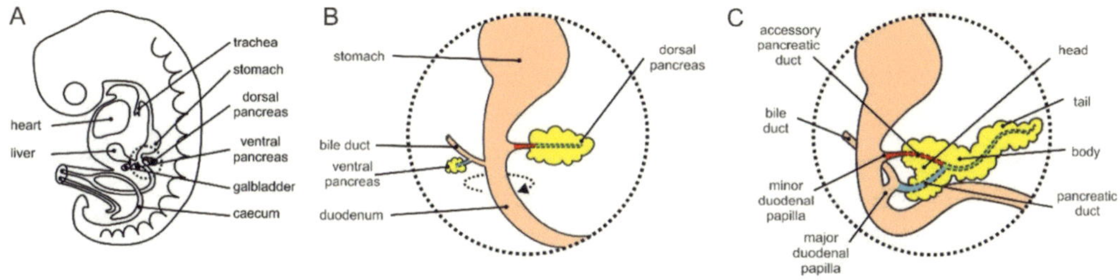

Figure 1. Embryonic development of the pancreas. (A) The position of the pancreatic buds in an embryo at the 5th week of development. (B) During development, the ventral pancreatic diverticulum rotates clockwise to reach its dorsal counterpart. (C) The ventral and dorsal bud as well as their duct merges during development of the gland.

2.2. Macro- and microscopic anatomy of the pancreas

The human pancreas is a large solitary retroperitoneal organ with well-defined outer borders located at the level of the L1 and L2 vertebrae. The gland is 14–18 cm long, 2–9 cm wide and 2–3 cm thick, weighing 50–125 g [11, 14–17]. It is surrounded by a fibrous capsule from which connective tissue septa extend into the gland dividing its parenchyma into distinct lobes and lobules. In contrast to the outer borders, there are no clear-cut macroscopic borders between the major parts in which the pancreas is usually divided for descriptive purposes: the head, the body and the tail. Generally, the left border of the superior mesenteric vein (SMV) is regarded as the border between the C-shaped head aligned with the upper duodenum on the right and the body located underneath the stomach and extending roughly horizontally in the medial plane on the left. The mid-point of the body and tail combined is then arbitrarily defined as the border between the body and the tail, with the tail usually ranging 1.5–3.5 cm in length [14, 17, 18]. Some authors define a fourth and a fifth part, the inferomedial uncinate process that lies beneath the SMV and the superior mesenteric artery (SMA), and the isthmus or neck, which is an approximately 2 cm wide part of the pancreas situated anterior to the SMA and the point where the SMV and the splenic vein (SV) join to form the portal vein [14–17].

Together with the mesenchyma, the exocrine part of the parenchyma amounts to 96–99% of the total pancreas volume (TPV) [14–16]. Each lobe contains several smaller lobes called lobules. In humans, the lobules are 1–10 mm in diameter [19]. The borders between adjacent lobules are incomplete and thus the whole parenchyma is a continuous unit [20]. Each morphologically recognizable lobule is also a single-functional glandular unit draining into a single duct. In turn, each lobule is supplied by 2–9 arterioles, thus each glandular lobule comprises a few so-called vascular or primary lobules, each of which, by definition, receives a single artery [20]. The remaining 1–4% of TPV contributes the endocrine parenchyma in the form of approximately a million islets of Langerhans, each of which measures around 100 μm and contains approximately a thousand endocrine cells of at least five different types [14].

From a pathophysiological point of view, as a basic microcirculatory unit the primary lobules resemble the liver units of Rappaport, in that different types of ischemic injuries involve different parts of primary lobules. In more proximal obstruction of a pancreatic artery (due to vasoconstriction in shock, for instance), the most peripheral parts of the primary lobule undergo necrosis, whereas in more distal obstruction (due to blockage of a terminal arteriole in malignant hypertension for instance) the most central parts of a lobule undergo necrosis [19, 21].

Finally, each lobule is composed of acini that are dome-shaped clusters of pyramid-shaped acinar cells. Exocrine secretions from apical poles of acinar cells flow into the lumen of the so-called intercalate duct. Intercalated ducts drain into intra-lobular ducts, these in turn into larger inter-lobular ducts and these finally converge into the main pancreatic duct. The main pancreatic duct empties into the duodenum together with the common bile duct. The end parts of both ducts constitute the so-called hepatopancreatic ampulla (of Vater). The ampulla communicates with the duodenal lumen via the major duodenal papilla (of Vater). The pancreas may have one accessory duct (of Santorini) that leads into the duodenum independently from the main duct and about 2 cm ventroproximally to it [8, 20, 22, 23]. Smooth muscle fibres in the wall of the distal part of the common bile duct, the main pancreatic duct and the papilla form a sphincter (of Oddi) [24], whether or not the smooth muscle fibres in the wall of the distal accessory duct form a functional sphincter remains a matter of debate [23].

Impaction of a gall stone in the ampulla is a specific cause of pancreatitis. Somewhat complimentary to the situation in APBJ, Opie proposed that the impaction creates a common channel between the pancreatic and the common bile duct and that the entry of bile into the pancreatic excretory system triggers the inflammation in pancreatitis [25].

2.3. Vascular supply of the pancreas

The regional blood flow to the pancreas approximates 1% of the cardiac output, 90% of which is directed to the exocrine part [26]. The arterial supply is derived from the celiac artery and the SMA [15, 27–30]. The neck, body and the tail of the pancreas (i.e. the major part of the dorsal pancreas) are irrigated by pancreatic branches of the splenic artery (SA) and by the dorsal pancreatic artery (DPA) that branches off near the origin of celiac, hepatic or splenic artery. DPA separates into two main branches: the right branch anastomoses with the anterior superior pancreaticoduodenal artery (PDA, see below) and the left branch gives rise to the transverse pancreatic artery (TPA, also termed the inferior pancreatic artery). TPA runs at the inferior border of the body and tail, usually anastomosing with the pancreatica magna artery, which is the largest pancreatic branch of the splenic artery [30, 31]. The head and the uncinate process are supplied by an anterior and a posterior arcade [32–35]. The anterior arcade is

http://dx.doi.org/10.5772/65895

formed by the anterior superior PDA, and the posterior arcade is formed by the posterior superior PDA [33]. The anterior and posterior superior PDA anastomoses with the anterior and posterior inferior PDA, respectively, both stem from the SMA [34, 35]. The uncinate process and the lower head of the pancreas (i.e. the ventral pancreas) are thus supplied by the SMA.

The venous drainage is anatomically less constant and roughly follows the arterial pattern. The splenic vein collects blood from the neck, the body and the tail via multiple small braches [17, 29]. The blood from the head of the pancreas is drained via two arcades. The anterior venous arcade is formed by the anterior superior and inferior pancreaticoduodenal veins (PDV) draining into the superior mesenteric vein. The posterior arcade consists of the posterior superior and inferior PDV. The posterior inferior PDV drains blood into the superior mesenteric vein, whereas the posterior superior PDV drains directly into the portal vein [15, 28, 29]. A number of anastomoses connect the veins and are typically more irregular than arterial anastomoses [15].

The smallest intra-lobular vessels are collectively termed the microvasculature of the pancreas [36]. A physiologically important relationship exists between the endocrine and exocrine tissue at the level of the microvasculature. In the human pancreas, the majority of islets of Langerhans are situated within exocrine lobules and the islet capillaries lead blood to a second capillary network surrounding acini. This arrangement of the two capillary networks in series is named the insulo-acinar portal system and forms an important basis for endocrine influences upon the exocrine pancreas [37–41]. The venous blood from inter-lobular islets flows directly into the inter-lobular veins and this type of flow is named the insulo-venous system. Noteworthy, from both the insulo-venous and -acinar system, the venous blood is ultimately passed to the portal vein [27, 42] (**Figure 2**).

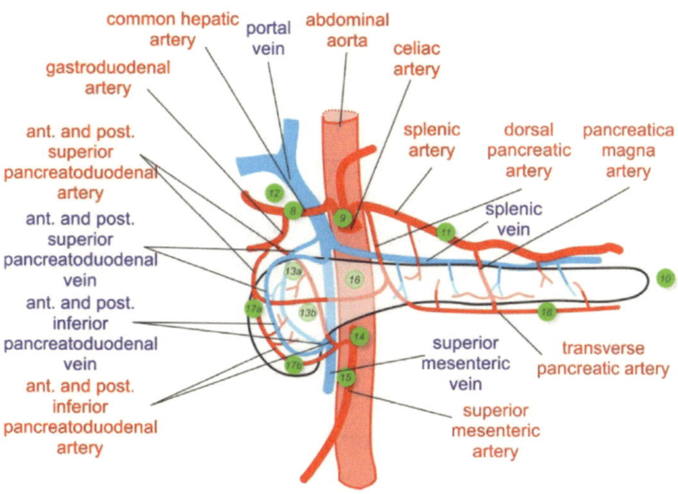

Figure 2. Blood vessels and lymph nodes of the pancreas. The main arteries (red) and veins (blue) supplying pancreas, as well as the main lymph nodes (green), indexed according to the numerical system (see text for details).

The lymphatic system of the pancreas is usually divided into an internal and an external system [43]. The former has been described to some extent only in rodents and is reviewed in detail elsewhere [14, 43]. In brief, the internal lymphatic system arises in the form of blind-beginning intra-lobular vessels distributed in intra-lobular septa, close by smallest blood vessels and ducts, but at a certain distance from acinar cells, with every lobule possessing many such vessels [43, 44]. Intra-lobular vessels drain into inter-lobular vessels running close by inter-lobular blood vessels and ducts in inter-lobular septa. The largest inter-lobular vessels, also called collecting vessels, reach the surface of the gland and drain into the external system [43].

An insufficient removal of extracellular fluid and pancreatic enzymes by the lymphatic overflow system from the interstitium may play an etiological role in pancreatitis. The interstitium and the lymphatic vessels are involved in the inflammatory damage and fibrosis, further hampering the lymphatic drainage and initiating a vicious cycle [43, 44].

The external system consists of large surface lymphatic vessels and regional lymph nodes. Due to the clinical importance of the external system, especially in carcinoma, it has been studied extensively in humans [17, 43, 45–50]. The external lymphatic vessels can be grouped into roughly seven different groups, each of which is associated with a corresponding group of blood vessels. The superior vessels close by the splenic artery and the inferior vessels close by the TPA drain the tail and the left part of the body. The anterosuperior, posterosuperior, anteroinferior and posteroinferior pancreaticoduodenal vessels (close by the arteries of the same name), as well as the gastroduodenal vessels, drain the head of the pancreas and the right part of the body. In general, authors also agree on the anatomical position of the lymph nodes to which the aforementioned vessels drain and on which nodes are most commonly affected in carcinoma of different parts of the pancreas. In contrast, there is much confusion with regard to the nomenclature of the nodes, with a descriptive [17, 46, 51] and a numerical system [49, 52]. In brief, the main groups (with their notation according to the numerical system in parentheses) that collect lymph from the tail and the body are the splenic and gastrosplenic nodes that lie within and superior to the splenic hilum (10), as well as the suprapancreatic (11) and infrapancreatic (18) nodes that lie close by the splenic and inferior pancreatic artery, respectively. The main groups that collect lymph from the head are the hepatic (8) and hepatoduodenal (12), as well as the superior anterior (17a), superior posterior (13a), inferior anterior (17b) and inferior posterior (13b) pancreaticoduodenal nodes. In addition to these nodes that encircle the pancreas, the paraaortic (16), celiac (9), superior mesenteric (14) and the middle colic nodes (15) lie close by the abdominal aorta and its trunks [43, 53]. The nodes tightly surrounding the pancreas and the nodes around the aorta probably do not correspond to first and second barriers of spread, respectively, since they both receive lymph directly from the pancreas as well as from other nodes [43]. Nodes indexed by numbers 1–7 probably do not drain the pancreas [53]. Noteworthy, the centrifugal path from the aforementioned nodes is via cisterna chyli and the thoracic duct [15].

Lymph node involvement is associated with a poor prognosis and is present in approximately four out of five patients with pancreatic cancer [17, 53]. The largely asymptomatic nature of cancer growth, with jaundice, duodenal obstruction and pain as the most common symptoms appearing late in the course of the disease, probably contributes to the fact that the tumours are detected at an advanced stage. Due to the numerous anastomoses between lymphatic vessels and the fact that obstruction of lymphatic vessels brought about by cancer growth and spread may further alter the already unpredictable routes of drainage, it is extremely difficult to exactly predict the spreading pattern of pancreatic cancer [17, 43, 49]. Tumours originating in the tail and the body most frequently spread to nodes 8, 11, 16 and 18 and only nodes 17 have not been involved in any of the cases [53, 54]. Tumours from the head of the pancreas most frequently spread to nodes 13, 17, 14 and 16, with only nodes 10 and 15 being spared in all cases [49, 50, 53]. It seems that the dual embryological origin of pancreas also influences the spreading pattern of cancer of the head. Tumours from the lower (ventral) head spread to nodes around the SMA (14), in contrast tumours from the upper (dorsal) head spread to nodes around the common hepatic artery (8) and in the hepatoduodenal ligament (12), which is in accordance with the arterial supply (see above) [55].

2.4. Innervation of the pancreas

The pancreas is innervated by sympathetic, parasympathetic and afferent nerve fibres that enter and exit the pancreas together with vessels and follow them also within the pancreatic tissue [36, 56–59]. The somata of preganglionic sympathetic neurons innervating the pancreas reside in the lateral horn of the C8-L3 spinal cord segments and project to paravertebral sympathetic ganglia. Alternatively, some axons do not terminate at synapses within the paravertebral ganglia but continue within splanchnic nerves to synapse within the celiac ganglia and the superior mesenteric ganglion [36, 56, 57]. The tail and the body of the pancreas are supplied by nerve fibres that originate in the celiac plexus and follow the splenic artery and TPA [60]. The majority of nerve fibres to the pancreas supply the head [61]. They originate in the anterior and posterior hepatic plexus. The fibres that enter the uncinate process originate in the superior mesenteric ganglion [60].

As already mentioned, lymph node involvement is one of the most important prognostic factors in pancreaticobiliary tract carcinomas. In general, lymph node metastasis is established by lymphatic invasion; however, tumour cells were shown to be able to spread into the hilum of lymph nodes via neural invasion. The knowledge of patterns of neural architecture may improve curative procedures [62]. Moreover, embryological development of the pancreas served as a useful template for patterns of extrapancreatic nerve plexus invasion of pancreatic head carcinoma [63].

The efferent autonomous nerves in the pancreas have release sites that are not in close contact with cells and thus probably influence many targets at a time [58, 64]. In the exocrine pancreas, the sympathetic terminals contact predominantly the intra-pancreatic ganglia, blood vessels and ducts. Stimulation of sympathetic fibres indirectly inhibits the exocrine secretion by inhibiting intra-pancreatic ganglia and by decreasing supply of fluid via vasoconstriction [36].

The somata of the parasympathetic preganglionic neurons reside in the dorsal motor nucleus of vagus and the nucleus ambiguus [36, 56]. The majority of their axons join the vagus and some the splanchnic nerves and reach the neural plexuses around arteries where they intermingle with sympathetic fibres [61]. The preganglionic parasympathetic neurons finally reach intra-pancreatic ganglia together with vessels supplying them [36, 56]. The parasympathetic ganglia that reside within the inter-lobular septa, lobules and also close to islets receive input not only from parasympathetic preganglionic fibres, but also from other pancreatic ganglia, sympathetic fibres (see above), the myenteric plexus, as well as the sensory fibres (see below) [36]. Postganglionic fibres innervate acinar and ductal epithelial cells, ductal smooth muscle cells and vascular plexuses, as well as other ganglia. These fibres mediate parasympathetic stimulation of secretion from acinar and ductal cells, constriction of ducts, as well as an increase in fluid supply by vasodilation [36, 61].

In the pancreas, sympathetic and parasympathetic afferent fibres can also be found. They contain substance P (SP) or calcitonin gene-related product (CGRP) as neurotransmitters. Sympathetic afferents that innervate both the exocrine and the endocrine tissue join the sympathetic splanchnic nerves and transmit noci- and mechano-receptive sensory information to somata within the dorsal root ganglia and further on to preganglionic sympathetic neurons in the lateral horn of the spinal medulla and probably higher centres [36].

Pancreatic sympathetic innervation is altered in chronic pancreatitis and pancreatic cancer and may contribute to the neuropathic pain and visceral neuropathy in these states [65, 66]. Dorsal root ganglion sympathetic afferent neurons send collaterals to efferent ganglia, representing a neuroanatomical substrate for intrapancreatic monosynaptic vegetative reflexes. For example, SP and CGRP released at intra-pancreatic ganglia inhibit exocrine secretion. Intra-pancreatic ganglia are also contacted by vagal afferents [36].

Somata of vagal afferent neurons reside within the nodose ganglia. They innervate the blood vessels, ducts, acini and islets. However, their centripetal pathways are not well known [36].

3. Integrative physiology of the exocrine pancreas

In this chapter we elucidate the mechanisms by which the exocrine pancreas secretes pancreatic ductal fluid and digestive enzymes under physiological conditions, the regulatory mechanisms that govern its function, and describe the response of pancreatic secretion to a meal. Moreover, this chapter offers some insight into the pathophysiological background of pancreatic diseases related to exocrine pancreas secretion.

3.1. Composition of pancreatic fluid

In humans, the secretion of a neutral, isotonic, Na^+, Cl^- and H^+-rich fluid, active digestive proteins, as well as zymogens by the pancreatic acinar cells, and of an alkaline, isotonic and HCO_3^--rich fluid by the pancreatic ductal cell yields between 1 and 2.5 L of pancreatic fluid per day, which contains around 20 g of digestive enzymes [67–69]. More than 20 different enzymes are secreted by the acinar cells [70], and some of them are precursor enzymes, such as trypsinogen and chymotrypsinogen. The enzymes released from the acinar cells in an active form are lipases, colipases, A-amylases, collagenases, elastases, ribonucleases and phospholipases A [70, 71].

Human pancreatic fluid contains up to 150 mmol/L of HCO_3^-. Its concentration increases with pancreatic fluid flow rate, and reaches its peak at 30–50% of maximal flow [72, 73]. The Cl^- concentration relates inversely with the pancreatic fluid flow rate and maintains an isotonic osmolality with respect to HCO_3^-. The composition of cations remains fairly constant, irrespective of pancreatic fluid flow rate, with 140 mmol/L Na^+, and 10–15 mmol/L K^+. The sum of HCO_3^- and Cl^- concentration closely matches the sum of Na^+ and K^+ concentration. Electrolytes, such as Ca^{2+}, Mg^{2+}, Zn^{2+}, PO_4^{3-} and SO_4^{2-}, are also present, but at minimal concentrations [74–76].

3.2. Regulation of acinar cell secretion

Secretion of digestive enzymes from acinar cells is primarily mediated by acetylcholine (ACh) release from vagal nerve endings and by the intestinal hormone, cholecystokinin (CCK). In addition to its primary role in ductal secretion (see below), the hormone secretin also influences acinar cell function, as does the vasoactive intestinal peptide (VIP) [77, 78].

The pancreas is innervated by postganglionic nerves, which receive input from the preganglionic motor neurons that stem from the dorsal motor nucleus of the vagus (DMV) [79]. ACh mediates its effects on acinar cell secretion via M1 and M3 muscarinic receptors [80], with M3 muscarinic receptors playing a predominant role [81]. The pancreas is also innervated by sensory vagal afferents, which project to the solitary nucleus, where information is integrated and relayed to the preganglionic motor neurons of the DMV, and the two together constitute the so-called dorsal vagal complex [79]. M1 and M3 muscarinic receptors are linked to the Gq/11 family of G-proteins and cause hydrolysis of phosphatidylinositol 4,5-bisphosphate (PIP_2) by phospholipase C, yielding inositol 1,4,5,-trisphosphate (1,4,5-IP_3) and 1,2-diacylglycerol (DAG) [82–84]. DAG goes on to phosphorylate various proteins via protein kinase C activation, while IP_3 mobilizes Ca^{2+} from internal stores to stimulate amylase secretion [82, 85].

Digestive elements of fats and proteins, such as fatty acids with acyl chains longer than 12 carbon atoms, and amino acids, phenylalanine and tryptophan, are prime secretagogues for CCK secretion by the intestinal I cells. Carbohydrates, on the other hand, do not exhibit particular potency. The mechanisms of CCK action on pancreatic acinar cells seem to exhibit species-specificity [86]. It was thought that the main, if not exclusive, influence of CCK on human acinar cells was mediated via interaction with cholinergic nerves by presynaptic modulation of vagal output [80]. It has been recently shown, however, that CCK can activate human pancreatic acinar cell secretion both directly [87] and indirectly through CCK-A receptors on vagal afferents [77, 79]. Mechanisms of CCK-relayed digestive enzyme secretion have not yet been fully clarified [87]. The CCK-B subtype of CCK receptors seems to be the predominant form in the human pancreas, while the presence of the CCK-A subtype has been difficult to demonstrate [88]. Similar to the M1 and M3 muscarinic receptors, CCK-B receptors are coupled to the Gq/11 family of G-proteins, and follow a similar signalling pathway to elevate intracellular calcium [83].

An alternative pathway of pancreatic acinar fluid and protein secretion is mediated by secretin and vasoactive intestinal peptide (VIP). By stimulating their respective Gα G-protein-coupled receptors an increase in cAMP is observed, which in turn increases PKA activity, leading to secretion [78, 89].

3.3. Molecular mechanisms of acinar cell secretion

In response to stimulation with ACh and CCK, acinar cells secrete an isotonic, plasma-like, protein-rich fluid containing Na^+, Cl^- and H^+, which is later modified by the ductal cells to form the final fluid [69, 70, 74]. Both secretagogues stimulate mechanisms that cause Ca^{2+} oscillations in the cytosol of acinar cells, which is a signalling mechanism for both fluid and enzyme secretions [90–92].

The fluid secretion of acinar cells is a result of ion transport across the basolateral and apical membranes, as well as paracellular transport mechanisms [90–92]. The driving force for acinar cell fluid secretion stems from the Na^+/K^+-ATPase located on the basolateral membrane and from the trans-cellular ion gradient it creates. The $Na^+/K^+/2Cl^-$ co-transporter NKCC1 on the basal side is responsible for approximately 70% of the Cl^- uptake for subsequent secretion by the pancreatic gland. The Ca^{2+}- and voltage-activated K^+ maxi-K channel on the basolateral membrane and others set the acinar cell membrane potential close to the K^+ diffusion potential. The membrane potential, in turn, serves as the electromotive force for Cl^- exit at the apical membrane. Along with the above-mentioned basolateral transport proteins, the Na^+/H^+ exchanger NHE1 and the AE2 isoform of the Cl^-/HCO_3^- exchanger family also play a role in basolateral Cl^- uptake. Both NKCC1 and NHE1 also provide Na^+ for the Na^+/K^+-ATPase and regulate intracellular pH, keeping it at about pH = 7.2 [90, 93]. Luminal secretion of Cl^- occurs via a voltage- and Ca^{2+}-activated Cl^- channel TMEM16A/Ano1. As Cl^- flows through the cell into the lumen of the acinus, Na^+ follows via the paracellular pathway. The subsequent osmotically driven water flow is mediated by aquaporin AQP1 [70, 74, 93].

Digestive enzymes are stored in zymogene granules at the apical membrane of acinar cells and are released by way of exocytosis. Fusion of granules with the apical plasma membrane releases their contents into the acinar lumen and later on into the small intestine [94]. As with fluid and electrolyte secretion from pancreatic acinar cells, Ca^{2+} ions are the key messenger in triggering and controlling a series of events termed stimulus-secretion coupling, i.e. pathways that regulate digestive enzyme secretion from acinar cells. Upon stimulation with secretagogues, a spike in intracellular Ca^{2+}, released from intracellular Ca^{2+} stores, causes fusion of zymogen granules with the plasma membrane [94, 95]. Physiological stimulants can evoke various intracellular Ca^{2+} patterns: (i) global Ca^{2+} oscillations, (ii) Ca^{2+} waves that flow across the cell and (iii) local calcium spikes [96]. Local apical Ca^{2+} spikes, which occur with lower levels of stimulation, as well as global Ca^{2+} spikes will increase the permeability of Ca^{2+}-dependent Cl^- channels, resulting in fluid secretion. It seems, however, that physiological stimulation yields zymogene granule fusion only when a global Ca^{2+} spike is observed [95].

http://dx.doi.org/10.5772/65895

In acute pancreatitis, a condition, which most frequently occurs due to alcohol abuse and biliary disease, the pro-enzymes stored in acinar cells become activated prematurely, causing autodigestion with inflammation and necrosis of the pancreatic tissue. Under normal conditions, intracellular Ca^{2+} is a key secondary messenger in pancreatic acinar cell secretion. Recently, however, a body of evidence suggests Ca^{2+} is a key initiator of pancreatitis. Noxious stimuli, such as alcohol, long-chain fatty acids and bile acids, provoke extensive Ca^{2+} release from intracellular stores, causing a prolonged and global Ca^{2+} elevation. This kind of abnormal calcium signalling in turn activates trypsinogen that causes pancreatic autodigestion [97–99].

3.4. Regulation of ductal cell secretion

Secretory control of pancreatic ductal cells exhibits great complexity as it involves a variety of receptors on both the basolateral and apical membranes. Activation of these receptors can be a stimulatory or an inhibitory factor in HCO_3^- and fluid secretion [67].

The most important secretagogue for HCO_3^- secretion from pancreatic ductal cells is the peptide hormone secretin [78]. The primary stimulus for secretin release from the neuroendocrine S cells in the proximal duodenum is intra-duodenal pH below 2–4.5, which occurs upon entry of acidic chyme from the stomach. Fatty acids and bile salts are also stimuli for secretin release [78, 100–102]. Upon activation of the secretin receptor on the basolateral side, which is coupled to adenylyl cyclase, increase and accumulation of cAMP are observed. cAMP activates PKA, which in turn phosphorylates the CF transmembrane conductance regulator (CFTR) in the apical membrane of ductal cells [101] and the basolateral Na^+-HCO_3^- co-transporter NBCe1-B [74]. Possible alternative routes of cAMP/PKA pathway activation are the release of VIP from vagal nerve terminals, with subsequent VIP receptor VPAC1 activation and beta-adrenergic receptor activation [103]. Vagal nerve fibres release VIP together with the main neurotransmitter ACh. Ductal cells express M2 and M3 muscarinic receptors located on the basolateral membrane [104]. Stimulation with ACh and CCK causes an increase in intracellular Ca^{2+} concentration by stimulating G-protein coupled receptors that activate the phospholipase C pathway, which activates the calcium-activating chloride channels and possibly also the apical Cl^-/HCO_3^- exchanger, triggering ductal secretion [67, 105]. The effect of cholecystokinin (CCK) in humans is that of a potentiator of secretin effects on ductal HCO_3^- and fluid output. The enhancing effects of secretin most likely occur by stimulation of vagal afferent fibres [68]. This indicates a synergistic relationship between the Ca^{2+} and cAMP pathways [74]. Ductal cells also express several types of purinergic receptors and intra-luminal application of ATP and UTP results in enhanced HCO_3^- secretion [73, 106]. Luminal ATP causes stimulation of HCO_3^- and pancreatic fluid which quantitatively approaches 75% of maximal secretin stimulation. In contrast, on the basolateral side, ATP inhibits both spontaneous and secretin-evoked secretion by as much as 50% [107].

Substance P, 5-HT, AVP, and the afore-mentioned basolateral ATP fall in the category of potential inhibitory factors in pancreatic HCO_3^- secretion. Although molecular mechanisms of inhibition are not yet fully understood, their role is most likely curtailment of luminal hydrostatic pressure, which precludes enzyme leakage into the pancreatic parenchyma and discontinuation of secretion after a meal [67].

3.5. Molecular mechanisms of ductal cell secretion

One of the earlier models of ductal cell HCO_3^- secretion proposed by Ashton, Argent and Green presupposes intracellular generation of HCO_3^- from CO_2, and hydration by carbonic anhydrase. The dissociated proton is transported by a Na^+/H^+ exchanger, located on the basolateral membrane, and the HCO_3^- ions are transported into the lumen by a HCO_3^-/Cl^- exchanger that is driven by the luminal Cl^- availability. The luminal Cl^- gradient is maintained by a cAMP-activated Cl^- channel, regulated by secretin. Since the exit of HCO_3^- in this model is electrogenic, it is accompanied by outflow of K^+ ions through the cAMP activated maxi-K channels. This model, while providing an explanation for much of what is observed in pancreatic duct cell secretion in many species, is however, limited to a maximum luminal HCO_3^- concentration of about 70 mmol/L. Human pancreatic duct cells, on the other hand, create a luminal HCO_3^- concentration as high as 140 mmol/L and above [67, 68, 108, 109].

In attempts to bring the mechanisms that account for such a high HCO_3^- secretion to light, several models have been proposed [110, 111]. As new information about the identity and properties of ion transporters and channels as well as cellular mechanisms of their action were discovered, a revised two-step model as described below has been suggested.

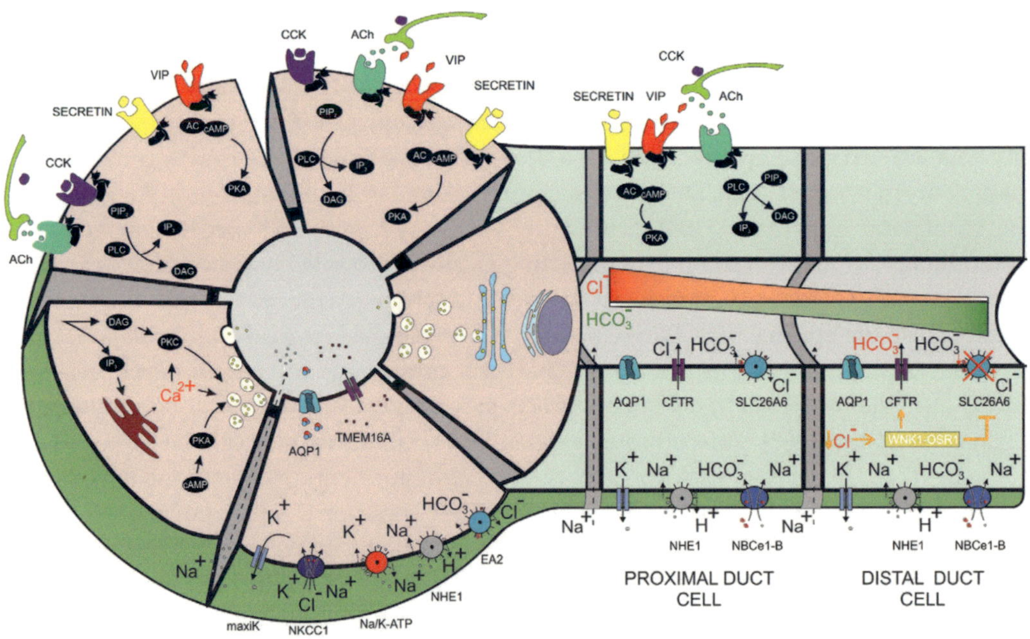

Figure 3. Regulation and molecular mechanisms of secretion in pancreatic acinar and ductal cells. Depiction of molecular mechanisms of pancreatic secretion in the lower half of the image and regulation of pancreatic secretion in the upper half of the image and changes in luminal Cl^-, and HCO_3^- concentrations in the lumen (see text for details).

In the proximal duct, HCO_3^- is actively transported and accumulated in the cytosol of ductal cells by a $1Na^+$-$2HCO_3^-$ co-transporter NBCe1-B on the basolateral membrane, which is driven by the Na^+ gradient. Secretion of HCO_3^- on the luminal side occurs by way of a $1Cl^-/2HCO_3^-$ exchanger SLC26A6, while the CFTR provides a recycling path for Cl^- ions. HCO_3^- secretion drives the translocation of Na^+ ions to the lumen by a paracellular pathway. These two processes create a driving force for water efflux by AQP1 [74]. The proximal duct absorbs a part of the Cl^- and secretes up to 100 mmol/L of HCO_3^- and provides much of the aqueous part of the pancreatic fluid. By the time the fluid reaches the distal segments of the duct, the lumen is Cl^- depleted to approximately 30 mmol/L and due to the active CFTR, the intracellular Cl^- concentration drops to 10 mmol/L or less. Low concentration of Cl^- activates the WNK1-OSR1/SPAK pathway, which results in two events. First, the permeability of CFTR changes in favour of HCO_3^-, making CFTR a route for HCO_3^- secretion. Second, the SLC26A6 is inhibited, which favours HCO_3^- accumulation in the lumen since its active state would most likely result in reabsorption, not secretion as in the proximal lumen [67, 74, 93, 112, 113] (**Figure 3**).

A mutation in the CFTR encoding gene that codes for the chloride and bicarbonate channel involved in pancreatic ductal cell fluid secretion results in a disease called cystic fibrosis, where anomalous fluid secretion results in dysfunction in several organ systems such as the lung, gastrointestinal tract, liver, male reproductive tract and pancreas. Reduced or even absent CFTR function causes a change in ductal fluid composition – decreased pH and fluid volume, and hyper-concentration of fluid components – that is thought to lead to obstruction. As the disease progresses, acinus plugging and dilation provoke epithelial injury and destruction, with inflammation, calcium deposits and fibrosis. These pathological processes lead to indigestion and malnutrition [114, 115].

3.6. Meal-response of pancreatic secretion and the inter-digestive phase

The basal pancreatic exocrine secretion rate reaches approximately 20% of the maximum capacity for enzyme secretion in humans. This basal secretion could be explained by an intrinsic characteristic of the pancreas, stimulation of the gland by low levels of CCK or secretin, or by ACh release [88]. Inhibition of ACh and CCK input reduces pancreatic enzyme secretion by about 50% [116].

The basal pancreatic duct HCO_3^- secretion amounts to only 1–2% in comparison with secretion stimulated with exogenous secretin. Since secretin is the primary regulator of HCO_3^- secretion, basal HCO_3^- mainly parallels plasma secretin levels, along with cholinergic input [88].

In the long term, this is, however, not the full extent of regulation. Inter-digestive pancreatic exocrine function is cyclically coupled with fasting motility phases termed the inter-digestive migratory motor complex (MMC), although they do follow different trends for overall daytime and night time secretory and motor activity [117, 118]. Upon ingestion of a meal, this behaviour is interrupted within minutes. Postprandial enzyme secretion reaches peak levels within the first hour and decreases followed by a stable phase of secretion, only to return to inter-digestive levels in 3–4 h [119].

The meal response of pancreatic secretion can be divided into four phases, i.e. cephalic, gastric, intestinal and inter-digestive phases. The names correspond to the origin of the predominant form of pancreatic secretion control. There is however significant overlap and integration between these regulatory mechanisms in response to a meal. Average pancreatic secretion stimulated by a meal amounts to about 50–60% of the maximum output of the gland [120–122].

The cephalic phase contributes approximately 25% of the meal-response secretion. It is caused by input of visual, olfactory, gustatory and tactile (mastication) sensory modalities. Sham feeding (a process, in which people are allowed to see, smell, taste but not swallow the food) causes pancreatic secretion that is rich in enzymes but low in concentration and volume of HCO_3^- [88]. It amounts to a response that is up to 50% of maximum secretory capacity. The main mediator of the cephalic phase is the vagus nerve with ACh as the dominant neurotransmitter [123].

The gastric phase accounts for about 10% of the meal-response secretion and starts with arrival of food into the stomach. It is regulated by enteropancreatic, vagovagal reflexes, which are stimulated by gastric distension [121].

The majority of the meal-response pancreatic secretion occurs in the intestinal phase. The secretory output amounts to 50–60% of maximal capacity [120]. It starts as the acidic chyme from the stomach, passes into the intestine, where components of the chyme, HCl, bile and bile salts elicit hormonal and neural responses. Hormonal influence on pancreatic secretion in the intestinal phase is mainly the result of CCK and secretin and the amplification of the secretory response by neural influences of the enteropancreatic reflex [121]. Passing of stomach contents into the intestine lowers the luminal pH, which is a signal for the duodenal S cells to release secretin. It, in turn, functions as the main secretagogue for HCO_3^- secretion from the ductal cells and also as an enhancer of enzyme secretion from the acinar cells [77, 102].

4. Role of the exocrine pancreas in digestion

Pancreas plays a crucial role in digestion. Its exocrine part secretes enzymes that are involved in digestion of carbohydrates, proteins and lipids. In this section, we will briefly review the digestive processes in general, and specifically point out the contribution of the pancreatic juice.

4.1. Assimilation of carbohydrates

In the western diet, the mean daily intake of carbohydrates is about 300 g that yield about 1200 kcal in metabolism [124]. Starch, the plant storage polysaccharide, constitutes by far the largest percentage of the carbohydrate intake (70%). About 30% of starch is composed of amylose (a straight polymer of glucose), the remainder of amylopectin (a branched polymer of glucose) [125, 126]. These different constituents of starch require different enzymes for their cleavage. Further 20% of carbohydrates in the food contribute refined sugars (e.g. sucrose, fructose and glucose) and approximately 10% the disaccharide lactose from various sources [127].

http://dx.doi.org/10.5772/65895

Digestion of carbohydrates takes place in two subsequent steps that are separated spatially: (i) digestion in the lumen and (ii) at the enterocyte brush border. Acinar cells of salivary glands (parotid, sublingual and submandibular) and of exocrine pancreas all produce and secrete the closely related enzyme α-amylase [128, 129]. α-amylase is secreted in an active form and has an optimal pH for enzymatic activity at pH = 7.0 [130]. It is an endo-enzyme that cleaves internal α-1,4 glycosidic bonds, but not α-1,6 bonds, terminal α-1,4 bonds, or α-1,4 bonds that are next to the branches in the molecular structure [131]. Amylopectin is thus cleaved to maltose and α-limit dextrins, whereas amylose is cleaved to maltose and maltotriose. The reactions seem to yield also a small percentage of free glucose [131].

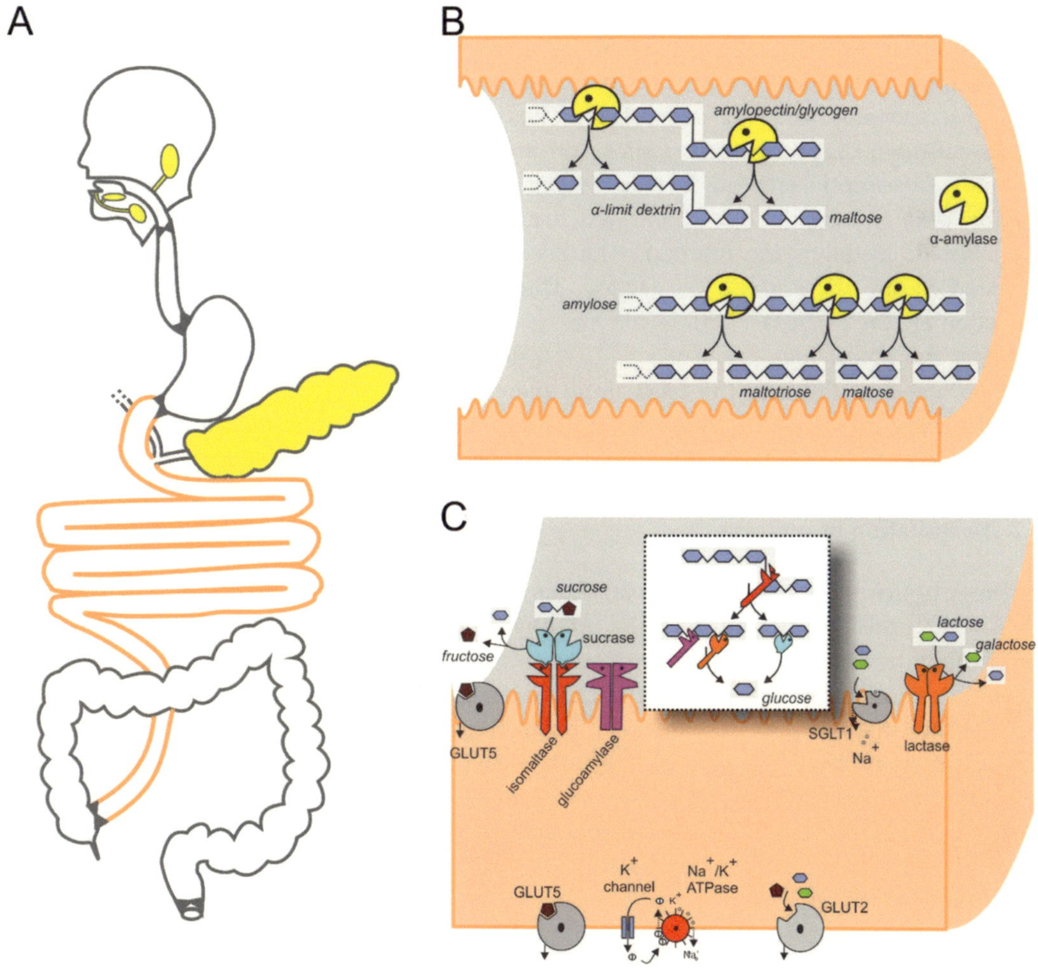

Figure 4. Assimilation of carbohydrates. (A) A schematic representation of the gastrointestinal tract. The origin of digestive enzymes is depicted in yellow and the location of carbohydrate absorption in beige. (B) The luminal phase of digestion critically depends on α-amylase. (C) The brush border phase involves enzymes embedded in the apical membrane of enterocytes. Monosaccharides are then transported across the epithelium by transport proteins in the apical and the basolateral enterocyte membrane.

The digestion of carbohydrates starts with intra-luminal digestion in the oral cavity. This appears not to have an important physiological role, since the salivary α-amylases are mostly inactivated in the acid milieu of the gastric lumen [130]. The activity of salivary α-amylases is partly rescued by occupying the active site of the enzyme with the substrate [132]. The digestion continues in the duodenum with the activity of pancreatic α-amylase, which has a rather neutral pH optimum, brought about by alkalinization of acidic chyme from the stomach by duodenal bicarbonate secretion. Contribution of the salivary amylase in starch degradation remains controversial and may become quantitatively more important when mastication time is prolonged [129, 133].

Following the intra-luminal digestion, membrane-bound enzymes of the enterocyte brush border degrade oligosaccharides produced by the luminal digestion to monosaccharides that are then absorbed into enterocytes [134]. The apical membrane of enterocyte brush border contains four major enzymes that act on the luminal side: (i) lactase, (ii) glucoamylase (maltase), (iii) isomaltase and (iv) sucrase [135]. The latter two are located on the same polypeptide chain with two distinctive active sites and are often referred to as the sucrase-isomaltase complex. An essential enzyme for starch digestion is the isomaltase, which is the only enzyme capable of degrading the α-1,6 bond, whereas the other (sucrase, glucoamylase and lactase) are involved in degrading internal α-1,4 bonds. The disaccharides sucrose and lactose are digested by the sucrase and the lactase. The final products of luminal and brush border digestion are the monosaccharides glucose, galactose and fructose, which are then absorbed through the apical membrane via SGLT-1 (glucose and galactose) and GLUT5 (fructose) transporters and through the basolateral membrane via GLUT2 [136–138]. Additionally, GLUT5 transporter in the basolateral membrane may serve as an alternative exit route for fructose (**Figure 4**).

4.2. Assimilation of proteins

Intake of proteins in the western diet amounts to approximately 70–100 g/day, which accounts for 300–400 kcal [124]. In contrast to the carbohydrates, protein digestion starts in the stomach, as virtually no significant proteolytic enzymes are found in saliva. The chief (zymogenic, peptic) cells of the gastric glands synthesize and secrete the pro-enzyme pepsinogen, the inactive precursor of pepsin, which is a proteolytic enzyme specifically suited to act in the acidic gastric milieu [139]. At $pH < 5$ in the gastric lumen, pepsinogen is spontaneously converted into the active form, pepsin, by cleavage of an N-terminal peptide. At pH values >5.0 and >7.5 pepsin inactivates reversibly and irreversibly, respectively [140]. Pepsin has its pH optimum at pH = 1.5–2.5. Pepsin functions as an endopeptidase, yielding oligopeptides and amino acids [141, 142].

Bulk proteolysis occurs in the small intestine. The pancreatic acinar cells secrete into the duodenum five major proteolytic proenzymes: trypsin, chymotrypsin, elastase and carboxypeptidase A and B [143–145]. First, the proenzyme trypsinogen is activated by the membrane-bound enterokinase to its active form trypsin [146]. The specific expression of enterokinase serves to limit proteolysis to the lumen of the small intestine. Trypsin, in turn, activates additional trypsin molecules and also converts the other four proenzymes, i.e. chymotrypsinogen, proelastase, as well as procarboxypeptidase A and B to their active forms. Carboxypeptidase A and B are ectopeptidases and cleave amino acids at the C-terminus, whereas trypsin, chymotrypsin, and elastase are endopeptidases that cleave polypeptides at specific sites resulting in 2–6 amino acid oligopeptides [144]. The oligopeptides from the lumen are further cleaved by both brush border-bound and intracellular cytosolic peptidases [134].

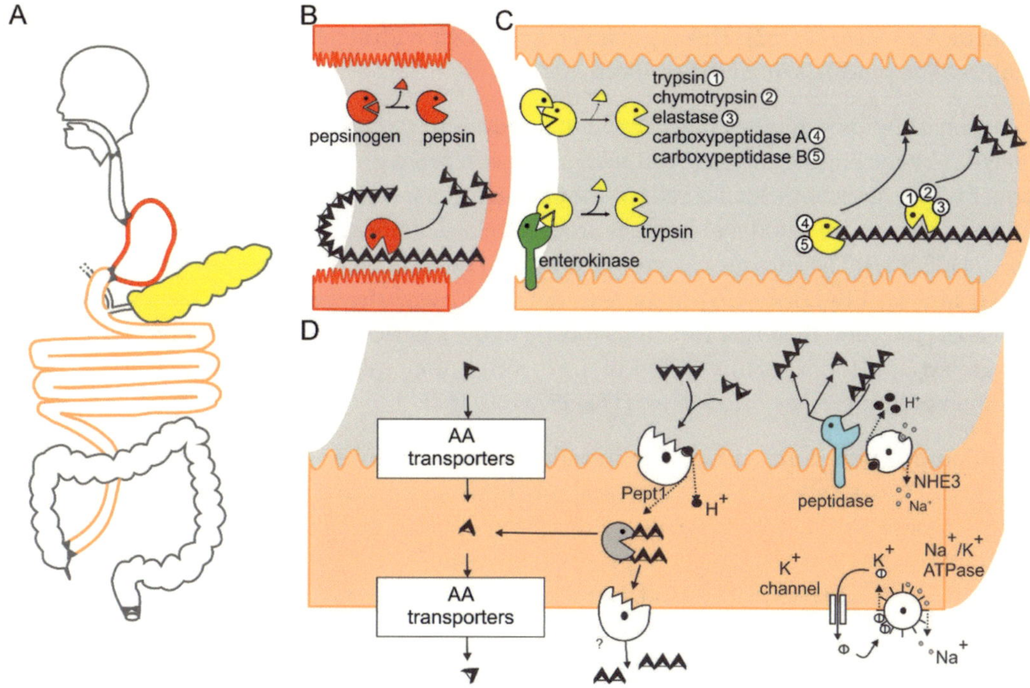

Figure 5. Protein assimilation. (A) A schematic representation of the gastrointestinal tract. Red denotes the start of digestion in the stomach, whereas beige indicates the site of digestion by pancreatic enzymes (indicated in yellow) as well as absorption. (B) Gastric luminal digestion of proteins by pepsin. (C) Intestinal luminal digestion of proteins by trypsin, chymotrypsin, elastase and carboxypeptidase A and B. (D) Brush-border assimilation of proteins involves membrane-bound peptidases, as well as peptone and amino acid (AA) transport mechanisms.

The absorption of oligopeptides and free amino acids differs. The oligopeptides are absorbed through the apical membrane with the PepT1, a H^+/oligopeptide co-transporter driven by an H^+ gradient generated by the NHE3 (Na/H exchanger type 3) [147, 148]. The amino acid absorption at the apical and basolateral membrane involves at least seven and five different transport systems, respectively; however, a detailed description of these systems is beyond the scope of this chapter [149, 150] (**Figure 5**).

4.3. Assimilation of lipids

In the western diet, 60–100 g of lipids are ingested daily, which account for about 500–900 kcal [124]. Most of the ingested lipids are in the form of triacylglycerol (TAG, 90–95%), the rest are in the form of phospholipids (PL, 5%) and cholesterol (C, < 0,5%).

Enzymes for digestion of lipids act in the watery environment of intestinal lumen, and due to their hydrophilic character, they act on the surface of ingested lipids organized in amphiphilic droplets. In the process of emulsification, larger droplets are broken into smaller ones, thereby increasing surface to volume ratio, and, consequently, enzyme efficacy [151]. Emulsification starts with food preparation, and continues in the mouth with mastication and in the gastric and intestinal lumen with churning of the ingested food. Lipid droplets organize such that the core is composed of hydrophobic TAG, whereas amphiphilic PL, C and free fatty acids (FFA) are on the surface [152, 153]. This organization, together with some proteins and carbohydrates stabilizes the products of emulsification.

Digestion of lipids exhibits a large functional redundancy [154]. It starts in the gastric lumen catalysed by the lingual and gastric lipase, together termed pre-duodenal lipase [155, 156]. The former is synthesized by acinar cells of the salivary glands and the latter by gastric chief cells. pH optimum for pre-duodenal lipase is around pH = 4, quite appropriate for the acidic gastric milieu [155, 157]. The enzyme cleaves the first ester bond in the TAG producing diacylglycerol (DAG) and an FFA [158, 159]. It is resistant to cleavage by pepsin but not by pancreatic proteases [156], and therefore functions mostly in the gastric lumen where it digests up to 15% of ingested lipids in a healthy individual. However, they might contribute to some extent to digestion of lipids in the duodenum [151, 157, 160, 161].

Digestion of lipids continues in the intestinal lumen by three major enzymes secreted by pancreatic acinar cells: the (i) pancreatic, (ii) nonspecific (carboxylic ester) lipase and (iii) phospholipase A_2. The pancreatic lipase is active in the presence of a colipase (which is in turn activated by trypsin), in an alkaline pH, in the presence of Ca^{2+} and bile salts [162, 163]. The pancreatic lipase cleaves the first and the third ester bond in TAGs yielding 2-monoacylglycerol (MAG) and FFAs [159, 164]. Phospholipase A_2 acts on the second ester bond in glycerophospholipids, giving rise to lysophospholipid (LPL) and FFAs [162]. It is secreted in an inactive form and requires for its activity an alkaline pH and bile salts. The specificity of the nonspecific lipase is low, notably, and it is able to cleave cholesterol esters and MAG [162]. The quantitative contribution of the nonspecific lipase is relatively low compared with the pancreatic lipase. During infancy, the pancreatic lipase related protein 2 contributes to digestion of lipids [165].

The luminal enzyme activity outlined above, in conjunction with an ever-ongoing emulsification, results in a multi-lamellar envelope developing around the droplet, and consisting of FFAs, bile acids, C, MAG and LPLs [166–168]. The multi-lamellar envelope bursts from the droplets in the form of vesicles that are eventually transformed to mixed micelles (especially under the influence of bile salts) that then finally serve as the main vehicle for absorption of lipids. FFAs enter the enterocyte by (i) collision with the plasmalemma and crossing of the plasmalemma by the flip-flop mechanism, or (ii) by diffusion of non-ionic fatty acids or (iii) by carrier-mediated transport. The latter probably involves the fatty acid binding protein (FABP), the fatty acid transporter protein type 4 (FATP4) and CD36 [169, 170]. MAG, LPLs and C probably enter the enterocyte by means of transport proteins or by simple diffusion. Finally, the FFAs, MAG, LPLs and C are re-esterified within the enterocyte, together with apolipoproteins assembled into chylomicrons, exocytosed into the extracellular space on the basolateral side of the plasma membrane, and reach the systemic circulation via the lymphatic circulation.

http://dx.doi.org/10.5772/65895

In contrast, monosaccharides and amino acids reach the systemic circulation via the portal vein [151, 171] (**Figure 6**).

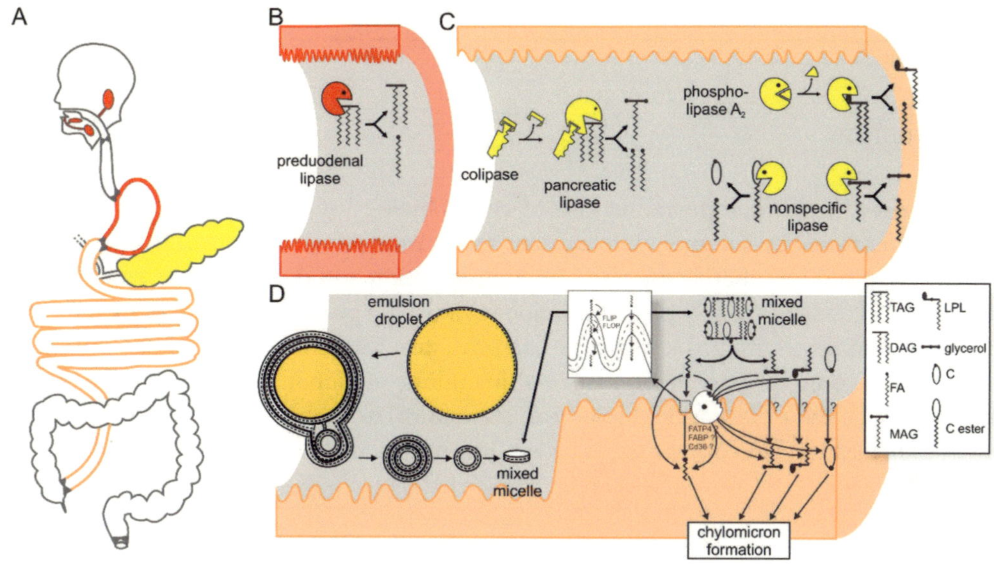

Figure 6. Assimilation of lipids. (A) A schematic representation of the gastrointestinal tract. Digestion starts in the mouth and gastric lumen (red) catalysed by activity of preduodenal lipases. The exocrine pancreas secretes lipolytic enzymes (yellow) that act in the lumen of the small intestine (beige). (B) Gastric luminal digestion of lipids by preduodenal lipase. (C) Intestinal luminal digestion of lipids by pancreatic lipase, phospholipase A_2 and nonspecific lipase. And (D) mixed micelles are formed in the lumen of the small intestine. These act as vehicles for absorption of FFAs, MAG, LPLs and C into enterocytes.

Exocrine pancreatic insufficiency (EPI) due to chronic pancreatitis or cystic fibrosis will eventually result in digestive malfunctioning [172]. However, because of the redundancy of the digestive processes described above, the effect is noticed rather late in the course of the disease [173]. In fact, malabsorption will not present itself until the exocrine pancreas function falls to <10% [174]. Among all the ingested nutrients, assimilation of lipids is most dependent on normal pancreas function. This seems unexpected due to a large redundancy of the lipid digestion, in fact the pre-duodenal lipase output may even increase in the EPI [175] and the pre-duodenal lipases can rescue up to 80% of fat digestion [176, 177]. However, as the destruction of the pancreas progresses, the ductal cells fail to neutralize acidic gastric juice leading to intra-intestinal acidification resulting in bile salt precipitation [175]. Bile salts are necessary for the mixed micelle formation, and this strongly hampers assimilation of lipids. Protein and carbohydrate digestion may have greater digestion potential during EPI due to the fact that the digestion is also initiated independently of pancreas, and continued by the brush-border peptidases and oligosaccharidases that are pancreas-independent. An analogue of the brush-border enzymes is missing in the digestion of lipids; therefore, it is not surprising that in EPI, lipid malabsorption is the most overwhelming problem causing many of the clinical symptoms and signs, leading to weight loss, steatorrhea, abdominal discomfort and a deficit in the lipid-soluble vitamins (A, D, E, K) [178, 179]. The digestive function can largely be rescued and nutrient malabsorption ameliorated by pancreatic enzyme replacement therapy (PERT), a therapy that involves oral administration of enzyme mixtures consisting of lipases, amylases and proteases [179–181].

5. Conclusions

Despite the ever-growing reductionist record on cell biology of constitutive parts of pancreas (exocrine, ductal and endocrine), whole organ integrative physiology detailing organ development, blood and lymphatic vascularization, innervation and direct links to pancreatic role in intestinal digestion, is rarely part of a single review. The present chapter goes even further and gives examples where this knowledge can provide a basis to understand etiopathophysiology of most common pancreatic diseases, including malignancy. We created a series of images to merge the different cell biological, anatomical and physiological layers to explain modern pancreas function and possible causes for dysfunction.

Author details

Jurij Dolenšek[1], Viljem Pohorec[1], Marjan Slak Rupnik[1,2] and Andraž Stožer[1*]

*Address all correspondence to: andraz.stozer@um.si

1 Institute of Physiology, Faculty of Medicine, University of Maribor, Maribor, Slovenia

2 Center for Physiology and Pharmacology, Medical University Vienna, Vienna, Austria

References

[1] Peters J, Jürgensen A, Klöppel G. Ontogeny, differentiation and growth of the endocrine pancreas. *Virchows Arch*. 2000;436(6):527–538. http://www.ncbi.nlm.nih.gov/pubmed/10917166.

[2] Edlund H. Developmental biology of the pancreas. *Diabetes*. 2001;50(Suppl 1):S5–S9. http://www.ncbi.nlm.nih.gov/pubmed/11272202.

[3] Deltour L, Leduque P, Paldi A, Ripoche MA, Dubois P, Jami J. Polyclonal origin of pancreatic islets in aggregation mouse chimaeras. *Development*. 1991;112(4):1115–1121. http://www.ncbi.nlm.nih.gov/pubmed/1682130.

[4] Teitelman G, Alpert S, Polak JM, Martinez A, Hanahan D. Precursor cells of mouse endocrine pancreas coexpress insulin, glucagon and the neuronal proteins tyrosine

http://dx.doi.org/10.5772/65895

hydroxylase and neuropeptide Y, but not pancreatic polypeptide. *Development*. 1993;118(4):1031–1039. http://www.ncbi.nlm.nih.gov/pubmed/7903631.

[5] Habener JF, Kemp DM, Thomas MK. Minireview: transcriptional regulation in pancreatic development. *Endocrinology*. 2005;146(3):1025–1034. doi:10.1210/en.2004-1576.

[6] Böck P, Abdel-Moneim M, Egerbacher M. Development of pancreas. *Microsc Res Tech*. 1997;37(5–6):374–383. doi:10.1002/(SICI)1097-0029(19970601)37:5/6<374::AID-JEMT2>3.0.CO;2-E.

[7] In't Veld P, Marichal M. Microscopic anatomy of the human islet of Langerhans. *Adv Exp Med Biol*. 2010;654:1–19. doi:10.1007/978-90-481-3271-3_1.

[8] Tadokoro H, Takase M, Nobukawa B. Development and congenital anomalies of the pancreas. *Anat Res Int*. 2011;2011:351217. doi:10.1155/2011/351217.

[9] Tadokoro H, Takase M, Nobukawa B. Unusual fusion between ventral and dorsal primordia causes anomalous pancreaticobiliary junction. *Pathol Int*. 2008;58(8):498–502. doi:10.1111/j.1440-1827.2008.02263.x.

[10] Fiocca R, Sessa F, Tenti P, et al. Pancreatic polypeptide (PP) cells in the PP-rich lobe of the human pancreas are identified ultrastructurally and immunocytochemically as F cells. *Histochemistry*. 1983;77(4):511–523. http://www.ncbi.nlm.nih.gov/pubmed/6345484.

[11] Saisho Y, Butler AE, Meier JJ, et al. Pancreas volumes in humans from birth to age one hundred taking into account sex, obesity, and presence of type-2 diabetes. *Clin Anat*. 2007;20(8):933–942. doi:10.1002/ca.20543.

[12] Meier JJ, Butler AE, Saisho Y, et al. Beta-cell replication is the primary mechanism subserving the postnatal expansion of beta-cell mass in humans. *Diabetes*. 2008;57(6): 1584–1594. doi:10.2337/db07-1369.

[13] Rahier J, Wallon J, Henquin JC. Cell populations in the endocrine pancreas of human neonates and infants. *Diabetologia*. 1981;20(5):540–546. http://www.ncbi.nlm.nih.gov/pubmed/6116638. Accessed August 4, 2016.

[14] Dolenšek J, Rupnik MS, Stožer A. Structural similarities and differences between the human and the mouse pancreas. *Islets*. 2015;7(1):e1024405. doi:10.1080/19382014.2015.1024405.

[15] Bockman DE. Anatomy of the pancreas. In: Go VLW, DiMagno EP, Gardner JD, Lebenthal E, Reber HA, Scheele GA, eds. *The Pancreas: Biology, Pathobiology, and Disease*. 2nd edition. New York: Raven Press; 1993:1–8.

[16] Rahier J, Goebbels RM, Henquin JC. Cellular composition of the human diabetic pancreas. *Diabetologia*. 1983;24(5):366–371. http://www.ncbi.nlm.nih.gov/pubmed/6347784.

[17] Cesmebasi A, Malefant J, Patel SD, et al. The surgical anatomy of the lymphatic system of the pancreas. *Clin Anat*. 2015;28(4):527–537. doi:10.1002/ca.22461.

[18] Suda K, Nobukawa B, Takase M, Hayashi T. Pancreatic segmentation on an embryological and anatomical basis. *J Hepatobiliary Pancreat Surg*. 2006;13(2):146–148. doi:10.1007/s00534-005-1039-3.

[19] Yaginuma N, Takahashi T, Saito K, Kyoguku M. The microvasculature of the human pancreas and its relation to Langerhans islets and lobules. *Pathol Res Pract*. 1986;181(1):77–84. doi:10.1016/S0344-0338(86)80191-1.

[20] Watanabe T, Yaegashi H, Koizumi M, Toyota T, Takahashi T. The lobular architecture of the normal human pancreas: a computer-assisted three-dimensional reconstruction study. *Pancreas*. 1997;15(1):48–52. http://www.ncbi.nlm.nih.gov/pubmed/9211492.

[21] Takahashi T, Yaginuma N. Ischemic injury of the human pancreas. Its basic patterns correlated with the pancreatic microvasculature. *Pathol Res Pract*. 1985;179(6):645–651. doi:10.1016/S0344-0338(85)80211-9.

[22] Reichert M, Rustgi AK. Pancreatic ductal cells in development, regeneration, and neoplasia. *J Clin Invest*. 2011;121(12):4572–4578. doi:10.1172/JCI57131.

[23] Suda K. Histopathology of the minor duodenal papilla. *Dig Surg*. 2010;27(2):137–139. doi:10.1159/000286920.

[24] Bosch A, Peña LR. The sphincter of oddi. *Dig Dis Sci*. 2007;52(5):1211–1218. doi:10.1007/s10620-006-9171-8.

[25] Opie EL, Meakins JC. Data concerning the etiology and pathology of hemorrhagic necrosis of the pancreas (acute hemorrhagic pancreatitis). *J Exp Med*. 1909;11(4):561–578. http://www.ncbi.nlm.nih.gov/pubmed/19867267.

[26] Lewis MP, Reber HA, Ashley SW. Pancreatic blood flow and its role in the pathophysiology of pancreatitis. *J Surg Res*. 1998;75(1):81–89. doi:10.1006/jsre.1998.5268.

[27] Wharton GK. The blood supply of the pancreas, with special reference to that of the islands of Langerhans. *Anat Rec*. 1932;53(1):55–81. doi:10.1002/ar.1090530108.

[28] Mikami Y, Otsuka A, Unno M. Surgical vascular anatomy and histology. In: *Diseases of the Pancreas*. Berlin, Heidelberg: Springer Berlin Heidelberg; 2008:19–28. doi:10.1007/978-3-540-28656-1_3.

[29] Meyers MA, Charnsangavej C, Oliphant M. Patterns of spread of disease from the pancreas. In: *Meyers' Dynamic Radiology of the Abdomen*. New York, NY: Springer New York; 2010:259–274. doi:10.1007/978-1-4419-5939-3_10.

[30] Woodburne RT, Olsen LL. The arteries of the pancreas. *Anat Rec*. 1951;111(2):255–270. http://www.ncbi.nlm.nih.gov/pubmed/14894836.

[31] Bertelli E, Di Gregorio F, Mosca S, Bastianini A. The arterial blood supply of the pancreas: a review. V. The dorsal pancreatic artery. An anatomic review and a radiologic

study. *Surg Radiol Anat*. 1998;20(6):445–452. http://www.ncbi.nlm.nih.gov/pubmed/9932331.

[32] Bertelli E, Di Gregorio F, Bertelli L, Mosca S. The arterial blood supply of the pancreas: a review. I. The superior pancreaticoduodenal and the anterior superior pancreaticoduodenal arteries. An anatomical and radiological study. *Surg Radiol Anat*. 1995;17(2): 97–106, 1–3. http://www.ncbi.nlm.nih.gov/pubmed/7482159.

[33] Bertelli E, Di Gregorio F, Bertelli L, Civeli L, Mosca S. The arterial blood supply of the pancreas: a review. II. The posterior superior pancreaticoduodenal artery. An anatomical and radiological study. *Surg Radiol Anat*. 1996;18(1):1–9. http://www.ncbi.nlm.nih.gov/pubmed/8685804.

[34] Bertelli E, Di Gregorio F, Bertelli L, Civeli L, Mosca S. The arterial blood supply of the pancreas: a review. III. The inferior pancreaticoduodenal artery. An anatomical review and a radiological study. *Surg Radiol Anat*. 1996;18(2):67–74. http://www.ncbi.nlm.nih.gov/pubmed/8782310.

[35] Bertelli E, Di Gregorio F, Bertelli L, Orazioli D, Bastianini A. The arterial blood supply of the pancreas: a review. IV. The anterior inferior and posterior pancreaticoduodenal aa., and minor sources of blood supply for the head of the pancreas. An anatomical review and radiologic study. *Surg Radiol Anat*. 1997;19(4):203–212. http://www.ncbi.nlm.nih.gov/pubmed/9381324.

[36] Love JA, Yi E, Smith TG. Autonomic pathways regulating pancreatic exocrine secretion. *Auton Neurosci*. 2007;133(1):19–34. doi:10.1016/j.autneu.2006.10.001.

[37] Murakami T, Hitomi S, Ohtsuka A, Taguchi T, Fujita T. Pancreatic insulo-acinar portal systems in humans, rats, and some other mammals: scanning electron microscopy of vascular casts. *Microsc Res Tech*. 1997;37(5–6):478–488. doi:10.1002/(SICI)1097-0029(19970601)37:5/6<478::AID-JEMT10>3.0.CO;2-N.

[38] Murakami T, Fujita T, Taguchi T, Nonaka Y, Orita K. The blood vascular bed of the human pancreas, with special reference to the insulo-acinar portal system. Scanning electron microscopy of corrosion casts. *Arch Histol Cytol*. 1992;55(4):381–395. http://www.ncbi.nlm.nih.gov/pubmed/1482603.

[39] Merkwitz C, Blaschuk OW, Schulz A, et al. The ductal origin of structural and functional heterogeneity between pancreatic islets. *Prog Histochem Cytochem*. 2013;48(3):103–140. doi:10.1016/j.proghi.2013.09.001.

[40] Czakó L, Hegyi P, Rakonczay Z, Wittmann T, Otsuki M. Interactions between the endocrine and exocrine pancreas and their clinical relevance. *Pancreatology*. 2009;9(4): 351–359. doi:10.1159/000181169.

[41] Henderson JR, Daniel PM, Fraser PA. The pancreas as a single organ: the influence of the endocrine upon the exocrine part of the gland. *Gut*. 1981;22(2):158–167. http://www.ncbi.nlm.nih.gov/pubmed/6111521.

[42] Brunicardi FC, Stagner J, Bonner-Weir S, et al. Microcirculation of the islets of Langerhans. Long beach veterans administration regional medical education center symposium. *Diabetes*. 1996;45(4):385-–392. http://www.ncbi.nlm.nih.gov/pubmed/8603757.

[43] O'Morchoe CC. Lymphatic system of the pancreas. *Microsc Res Tech*. 1977;37(5–6):456–477. doi:10.1002/(SICI)1097-0029(19970601)37:5/6<456::AID-JEMT9>3.0.CO;2-B.

[44] Regoli M, Bertelli E, Orazioli D, Fonzi L, Bastianini A. Pancreatic lymphatic system in rodents. *Anat Rec*. 2001;263(2):155–160. http://www.ncbi.nlm.nih.gov/pubmed/11360232.

[45] Hoggan G, Hoggan FE. The lymphatics of the pancreas. *J Anat Physiol*. 1881;15(Pt 4):474.1–495. http://www.ncbi.nlm.nih.gov/pubmed/17231401.

[46] Cubilla AL, Fortner J, Fitzgerald PJ. Lymph node involvement in carcinoma of the head of the pancreas area. *Cancer*. 1978;41(3):880–887. http://www.ncbi.nlm.nih.gov/pubmed/638975.

[47] Deki H, Sato T. An anatomic study of the peripancreatic lymphatics. *Surg Radiol Anat*. 1988;10(2):121–135. http://www.ncbi.nlm.nih.gov/pubmed/3135617.

[48] Donatini B, Hidden G. Routes of lymphatic drainage from the pancreas: a suggested segmentation. *Surg Radiol Anat*. 1992;14(1):35–42. http://www.ncbi.nlm.nih.gov/pubmed/1589845.

[49] Kayahara M, Nagakawa T, Kobayashi H, et al. Lymphatic flow in carcinoma of the head of the pancreas. *Cancer*. 1992;70(8):2061–2066. http://www.ncbi.nlm.nih.gov/pubmed/1327485.

[50] Nagakawa T, Kobayashi H, Ueno K, Ohta T, Kayahara M, Miyazaki I. Clinical study of lymphatic flow to the paraaortic lymph nodes in carcinoma of the head of the pancreas. *Cancer*. 1994;73(4):1155–1162. http://www.ncbi.nlm.nih.gov/pubmed/8313317.

[51] Pissas A. Anatomoclinical and anatomosurgical essay on the lymphatic circulation of the pancreas. *Anat Clin*. 1984;6(4):255–280. http://www.ncbi.nlm.nih.gov/pubmed/6395876.

[52] Nagakawa T, Kobayashi H, Ueno K, et al. The pattern of lymph node involvement in carcinoma of the head of the pancreas. A histologic study of the surgical findings in patients undergoing extensive nodal dissections. *Int J Pancreatol*. 1993;13(1):15–22. doi:10.1007/BF02795195.

[53] Kayahara M, Nagakawa T, Ohta T, et al. Analysis of paraaortic lymph node involvement in pancreatic carcinoma: a significant indication for surgery? *Cancer*. 1999;85(3):583–590. http://www.ncbi.nlm.nih.gov/pubmed/10091731.

[54] Kayahara M, Nagakawa T, Futagami F, Kitagawa H, Ohta T, Miyazaki I. Lymphatic flow and neural plexus invasion associated with carcinoma of the body and tail of the

pancreas. *Cancer*. 1996;78(12):2485–2491. http://www.ncbi.nlm.nih.gov/pubmed/8952555.

[55] Kitagawa H, Ohta T, Makino I, et al. Carcinomas of the ventral and dorsal pancreas exhibit different patterns of lymphatic spread. *Front Biosci*. 2008;13:2728–2735. http://www.ncbi.nlm.nih.gov/pubmed/17981748.

[56] Ahrén B. Autonomic regulation of islet hormone secretion—implications for health and disease. *Diabetologia*. 2000;43(4):393–410. doi:10.1007/s001250051322.

[57] Gilon P, Henquin JC. Mechanisms and physiological significance of the cholinergic control of pancreatic beta-cell function. *Endocr Rev*. 2001;22(5):565–604. doi:10.1210/edrv.22.5.0440.

[58] Rodriguez-Diaz R, Caicedo A. Novel approaches to studying the role of innervation in the biology of pancreatic islets. *Endocrinol Metab Clin North Am*. 2013;42(1):39–56. doi:10.1016/j.ecl.2012.11.001.

[59] Lindsay TH, Halvorson KG, Peters CM, et al. A quantitative analysis of the sensory and sympathetic innervation of the mouse pancreas. *Neuroscience*. 2006;137(4):1417–1426. doi:10.1016/j.neuroscience.2005.10.055.

[60] Yi S-Q, Miwa K, Ohta T, et al. Innervation of the pancreas from the perspective of perineural invasion of pancreatic cancer. *Pancreas*. 2003;27(3):225–229. http://www.ncbi.nlm.nih.gov/pubmed/14508126.

[61] Tiscornia OM. The neural control of exocrine and endocrine pancreas. *Am J Gastroenterol*. 1977;67(6):541–560. http://www.ncbi.nlm.nih.gov/pubmed/20775.

[62] Kayahara M, Nakagawara H, Kitagawa H, Ohta T. The nature of neural invasion by pancreatic cancer. *Pancreas*. 2007;35(3):218–223. doi:10.1097/mpa.0b013e3180619677.

[63] Makino I, Kitagawa H, Ohta T, et al. Nerve plexus invasion in pancreatic cancer: spread patterns on histopathologic and embryological analyses. *Pancreas*. 2008;37(4):358–365. http://www.ncbi.nlm.nih.gov/pubmed/18972625.

[64] Ushiki T, Watanabe S. Distribution and ultrastructure of the autonomic nerves in the mouse pancreas. *Microsc Res Tech*. 1997;37(5–6):399–406. doi:10.1002/(SICI)1097-0029(19970601)37:5/6<399::AID-JEMT4>3.0.CO;2-9.

[65] Ceyhan GO, Demir IE, Rauch U, et al. Pancreatic neuropathy results in "neural remodeling" and altered pancreatic innervation in chronic pancreatitis and pancreatic cancer. *Am J Gastroenterol*. 2009;104(10):2555–2565. doi:10.1038/ajg.2009.380.

[66] Salvioli B, Bovara M, Barbara G, et al. Neurology and neuropathology of the pancreatic innervation. *JOP*. 2002;3(2):26–33. http://www.ncbi.nlm.nih.gov/pubmed/11884764.

[67] Argent BE, Gray MA, Steward MC, Case RM. Cell physiology of pancreatic ducts. In: Johnson LR, ed. *Physiology of the Gastrointestinal Tract*. 5th edition. New York: Academic Press; 2012:1399–1423. doi:10.1016/B978-0-12-382026-6.00051-8.

[68] Lee MG, Muallem S. Physiology of duct cell secretion. In: *The Pancreas: An Integrated Textbook of Basic Science, Medicine, and Surgery*. 2nd edition. Oxford: Wiley-Blackwell; 2009:78–90. doi:10.1002/9781444300123.ch7.

[69] Hegyi P, Maléth J, Venglovecz V, Rakonczay Z. Pancreatic ductal bicarbonate secretion: challenge of the acinar Acid load. *Front Physiol*. 2011;2(July):36. doi:10.3389/fphys.2011.00036.

[70] Hegyi P, Petersen OH. The exocrine pancreas: the acinar-ductal tango in physiology and pathophysiology. *Rev Physiol Biochem Pharmacol*. 2013;165(April):1–30. doi:10.1007/112_2013_14.

[71] Petersen OH. Physiology of acinar cell secretion. In: *The Pancreas*. Oxford, UK: Blackwell Publishing Ltd.; 2009:69–77. doi:10.1002/9781444300123.ch6.

[72] Domschke S, Domschke W, Rösch W, Konturek SJ, Wünsch E, Demling L. Bicarbonate and cyclic AMP content of pure human pancreatic juice in response to graded doses of synthetic secretin. *Gastroenterology*. 1976;70(4):533–536. doi:10.1016/S0016-5085(76)80491-X.

[73] Ishiguro H, Yamamoto A, Nakakuki M, et al. Physiology and pathophysiology of bicarbonate secretion by pancreatic duct epithelium. *Nagoya J Med Sci*. 2012;74(1–2):1–18. http://www.ncbi.nlm.nih.gov/pubmed/22515107.

[74] Lee MG, Ohana E, Park HW, Yang D, Muallem S. Molecular mechanism of pancreatic and salivary gland fluid and HCO_3 secretion. *Physiol Rev*. 2012;92(1):39–74. doi:10.1152/physrev.00011.2011.

[75] Denyer ME, Cotton PB. Pure pancreatic juice studies in normal subjects and patients with chronic pancreatitis. *Gut*. 1979;20(2):89–97. http://www.ncbi.nlm.nih.gov/pubmed/428831.

[76] Bro-Rasmussen F, Killmann SA, Thaysen JH. The composition of pancreatic juice as compared to sweat, parotid saliva and tears. *Acta Physiol Scand*. 1956;37(2–3):97–113. doi:10.1111/j.1748-1716.1956.tb01346.x.

[77] Williams JA. Regulation of pancreatic acinar cell function. *Curr Opin Gastroenterol*. 2006;22(5):498–504. doi:10.1097/01.mog.0000239863.96833.c0.

[78] Leung PS. The renin-angiotensin system: current research progress in: *The Pancreas*. Vol. 690. Dordrecht: Springer Netherlands; 2010. doi:10.1007/978-90-481-9060-7.

[79] Chandra R, Liddle RA. Recent advances in pancreatic endocrine and exocrine secretion. *Curr Opin Gastroenterol*. 2011;27(5):439–443. doi:10.1097/MOG.0b013e328349e2e1.

[80] Singer MV, Niebergall-Roth E. Secretion from acinar cells of the exocrine pancreas: role of enteropancreatic reflexes and cholecystokinin. *Cell Biol Int*. 2009;33(1):1–9. doi:10.1016/j.cellbi.2008.09.008.

[81] Nakamura K, Hamada K, Terauchi A, et al. Distinct roles of M1 and M3 muscarinic acetylcholine receptors controlling oscillatory and non-oscillatory $[Ca^{2+}]^{i}$ increase. *Cell Calcium*. 2013;54(2):111–119. doi:10.1016/j.ceca.2013.05.004.

[82] Noble F, Roques BP. CCK-B receptor: chemistry, molecular biology, biochemistry and pharmacology. *Prog Neurobiol*. 1999;58(4):349–379. doi:10.1016/S0301-0082(98)00090-2.

[83] Williams JA. Intracellular signaling mechanisms activated by cholecystokinin-regulating synthesis and secretion of digestive enzymes in pancreatic acinar cells. *Annu Rev Physiol*. 2001;63(1):77–97. doi:10.1146/annurev.physiol.63.1.77.

[84] Shah N, Khurana S, Cheng K, Raufman J-P. Muscarinic receptors and ligands in cancer. *Am J Physiol Cell Physiol*. 2009;296(2):C221–C232. doi:10.1152/ajpcell.00514.2008.

[85] Mikoshiba K. Role of IP3 receptor signaling in cell functions and diseases. *Adv Biol Regul*. 2015;57:217–227. doi:10.1016/j.jbior.2014.10.001.

[86] Wang BJ, Cui ZJ. How does cholecystokinin stimulate exocrine pancreatic secretion? From birds, rodents, to humans. *Am J Physiol Regul Integr Comp Physiol*. 2007;292(2): R666–R678. doi:10.1152/ajpregu.00131.2006.

[87] Murphy JA, Criddle DN, Sherwood M, et al. Direct activation of cytosolic Ca^{2+} signaling and enzyme secretion by cholecystokinin in human pancreatic acinar cells. *Gastroenterology*. 2008;135(2):632–641. doi:10.1053/j.gastro.2008.05.026.

[88] Liddle RA. Regulation of pancreatic secretion. In: *Physiology of the Gastrointestinal Tract*. Elsevier London; 2012:1425–1460. doi:10.1016/B978-0-12-382026-6.00052-X.

[89] Chandra R, Liddle R a. Recent advances in the regulation of pancreatic secretion. *Curr Opin Gastroenterol*. 2014;30(5):490–494. doi:10.1097/MOG.0000000000000099.

[90] Petersen OH. Ca^{2+} signalling and Ca^{2+}-activated ion channels in exocrine acinar cells. *Cell Calcium*. 2005;38(3–4):171–200. doi:10.1016/j.ceca.2005.06.024.

[91] Cancela JM. Specific Ca^{2+} signaling evoked by cholecystokinin and acetylcholine: the roles of NAADP, cADPR, and IP3. *Annu Rev Physiol*. 2001;63(1):99–117. doi:10.1146/annurev.physiol.63.1.99.

[92] Yule DI, Lawrie AM, Gallacher DV. Acetylcholine and cholecystokinin induce different patterns of oscillating calcium signals in pancreatic acinar cells. *Cell Calcium*. 1991;12(2–3):145–151. doi:10.1016/0143-4160(91)90016-8.

[93] Hong JH, Park S, Shcheynikov N, Muallem S. Mechanism and synergism in epithelial fluid and electrolyte secretion. *Pflügers Arch Eur J Physiol*. 2014;466(8):1487–1499. doi:10.1007/s00424-013-1390-1.

[94] Weiss FU, Halangk W, Lerch MM. New advances in pancreatic cell physiology and pathophysiology. *Best Pract Res Clin Gastroenterol*. 2008;22(1):3–15. doi:10.1016/j.bpg.2007.10.017.

[95] Low JT, Shukla A, Thorn P. Pancreatic acinar cell: new insights into the control of secretion. *Int J Biochem Cell Biol*. 2010;42(10):1586–1589. doi:10.1016/j.biocel.2010.07.006.

[96] Thorn P, Lawrie AM, Smith PM, Gallacher DV, Petersen OH. Ca^{2+} oscillations in pancreatic acinar cells: spatiotemporal relationships and functional implications. *Cell Calcium*. 1993;14(10):746–757. <Go to ISI>://A1993MH25500008.

[97] Gerasimenko JV, Gerasimenko OV, Petersen OH. The role of Ca^{2+} in the pathophysiology of pancreatitis. *J Physiol*. 2014;592(2):269–280. doi:10.1113/jphysiol.2013.261784.

[98] Lerch MM, Gorelick FS. Models of acute and chronic pancreatitis. *Gastroenterology*. 2013;144(6):1180–1193. doi:10.1053/j.gastro.2012.12.043.

[99] Li J, Zhou R, Zhang J, Li Z-F. Calcium signaling of pancreatic acinar cells in the pathogenesis of pancreatitis. *World J Gastroenterol*. 2014;20(43):16146–16152. doi: 10.3748/wjg.v20.i43.16146.

[100] Schaffalitzky de Muckadell OB, Fahrenkrug J, Nielsen J, Westphall I, Worning H. Meal-stimulated secretin release in man: effect of acid and bile. *Scand J Gastroenterol*. 1981;16(8):981–988. doi:10.3109/00365528109181015.

[101] Pallagi P, Hegyi P, Rakonczay Z. The Physiology and pathophysiology of pancreatic ductal secretion: the background for clinicians. *Pancreas*. 2015;44(8):1211–1233. doi: 10.1097/MPA.0000000000000421.

[102] Soleimani M. Impaired pancreatic ductal bicarbonate secretion in cystic fibrosis. *J Pancreas*. 2001;2(4):237–242. doi:v02i04a18 [pii].

[103] Evans RL, Perrott MN, Lau KR, Case RM. Elevation of intracellular cAMP by noradrenaline and vasoactive intestinal peptide in striated ducts isolated from the rabbit mandibular salivary gland. *Arch Oral Biol*. 1996;41(7):689–694. doi:10.1016/S0003-9969(96)00028-3.

[104] Szalmay G, Varga G, Kajiyama F, et al. Bicarbonate and fluid secretion evoked by cholecystokinin, bombesin and acetylcholine in isolated guinea-pig pancreatic ducts. *J Physiol*. 2001;535(Pt 3):795–807. doi:10.1111/j.1469-7793.2001.00795.x.

[105] Jung J, Lee MG. Role of calcium signaling in epithelial bicarbonate secretion. *Cell Calcium*. 2014;55(6):376–384. doi:10.1016/j.ceca.2014.02.002.

[106] Luo X, Zheng W, Yan M, Lee MG, Muallem S. Multiple functional P2X and P2Y receptors in the luminal and basolateral membranes of pancreatic duct cells. *Am J Physiol*. 1999;277(2 Pt 1):C205–C215. http://ajpcell.physiology.org/content/277/2/C205.abstract.

[107] Ishiguro H, Naruse S, Kitagawa M, Hayakawa T, Case RM, Steward MC. Luminal ATP stimulates fluid and HCO_3^- secretion in guinea-pig pancreatic duct. *J Physiol*. 1999;519(Pt 22):551–558. doi:10.1111/j.1469-7793.1999.0551m.x.

[108] Ashton N, Argent BE, Green R. Characteristics of fluid secretion from isolated rat pancreatic ducts stimulated with secretin and bombesin. *J Physiol*. 1991;435:533–546. http://www.ncbi.nlm.nih.gov/pubmed/1770448.

[109] Whitcomb DC, Ermentrout GB. A mathematical model of the pancreatic duct cell generating high bicarbonate concentrations in pancreatic juice. *Pancreas*. 2004;29(2): e30–e40. doi:10.1097/00006676-200408000-00016.

[110] Steward MC, Ishiguro H, Case RM. Mechanisms of bicarbonate secretion in the pancreatic duct. *Annu Rev Physiol*. 2005;67(1):377–409. doi:10.1146/annurev.physiol. 67.031103.153247.

[111] Ko SBH, Zeng W, Dorwart MR, et al. Gating of CFTR by the STAS domain of SLC26 transporters. *Nat Cell Biol*. 2004;6(4):343–350. doi:10.1038/ncb1115.

[112] Steward MC, Ishiguro H. Molecular and cellular regulation of pancreatic duct cell function. *Curr Opin Gastroenterol*. 2009;25(5):447–453. doi:10.1097/MOG.0b013e32 832e06ce.

[113] Park HW, Nam JH, Kim JY, et al. Dynamic regulation of CFTR bicarbonate permeability by $[Cl^-]^i$ and its role in pancreatic bicarbonate secretion. *Gastroenterology*. 2010;139(2): 620–631. doi:10.1053/j.gastro.2010.04.004.

[114] Gibson-Corley KN, Meyerholz DK, Engelhardt JF. Pancreatic pathophysiology in cystic fibrosis. *J Pathol*. 2016;238(2):311–320. doi:10.1002/path.4634.

[115] Wilschanski M, Novak I. The cystic fibrosis of exocrine pancreas. *Cold Spring Harb Perspect Med*. 2013;3(5):1–17. doi:10.1101/cshperspect.a009746.

[116] Adler G, Reinshagen M, Koop I, et al. Differential effects of atropine and a cholecystokinin receptor antagonist on pancreatic secretion. *Gastroenterology*. 1989;96(4):1158–1164. http://www.ncbi.nlm.nih.gov/pubmed/2647576.

[117] Keller J, Gröger G, Cherian L, Günther B, Layer P. Circadian coupling between pancreatic secretion and intestinal motility in humans. *Am J Physiol Gastrointest Liver Physiol*. 2001;280(2):G273–G278. http://ajpgi.physiology.org/content/280/2/G273.short.

[118] Vantrappen GR, Peeters TL, Janssens J. The secretory component of the interdigestive migrating motor complex in man. *Scand J Gastroenterol*. 1979;14(6):663–667. doi: 10.3109/00365527909181934.

[119] Keller J, Layer P. Human pancreatic exocrine response to nutrients in health and disease. *Gut*. 2005;54(Suppl 6):vi1-vi28. doi:10.1136/gut.2005.065946.

[120] Adler G. Regulation of human pancreatic secretion. *Digestion*. 1997;58(Suppl 1):39–41. http://www.ncbi.nlm.nih.gov/pubmed/9225089.

[121] Morisset J. Control of pancreatic secretion in humans. *Adv Med Sci*. 2010;55(1):1–15. doi: 10.2478/v10039-010-0013-8.

[122] Beglinger C, Fried M, Whitehouse I, Jansen JB, Lamers CB, Gyr K. Pancreatic enzyme response to a liquid meal and to hormonal stimulation. Correlation with plasma secretin and cholecystokinin levels. *J Clin Invest*. 1985;75(5):1471–1476. doi:10.1172/JCI111850.

[123] Anagnostides A, Chadwick VS, Selden AC, Maton PN. Sham feeding and pancreatic secretion. Evidence for direct vagal stimulation of enzyme output. *Gastroenterology*. 1984;87(1):109–114. http://www.ncbi.nlm.nih.gov/pubmed/6724252.

[124] Panel on Macreonutrients. *Dietary Reference Intakes for Energy, Carbohydrate, Fiber, Fat, Fatty Acids, Cholesterol, Protein, and Amino Acids (Macronutrients)*. Washington, D.C.: National Academies Press; 2005. doi:10.17226/10490.

[125] Shi Y-C, Capitani T, Trzasko P, Jeffcoat R. Molecular structure of a low-amylopectin starch and other high-amylose maize starches. *J Cereal Sci*. 1998;27(3):289–299. doi: 10.1006/jcrs.1997.9998.

[126] Tester RF, Karkalas J, Qi X. Starch—composition, fine structure and architecture. *J Cereal Sci*. 2004;39(2):151–165. doi:10.1016/j.jcs.2003.12.001.

[127] Cordain L, Eaton SB, Sebastian A, et al. Origins and evolution of the Western diet: health implications for the 21st century. *Am J Clin Nutr*. 2005;81(2):341–354. http://www.ncbi.nlm.nih.gov/pubmed/15699220.

[128] Horii A, Emi M, Tomita N, et al. Primary structure of human pancreatic alpha-amylase gene: its comparison with human salivary alpha-amylase gene. *Gene*. 1987;60(1):57–64. http://www.ncbi.nlm.nih.gov/pubmed/2450054.

[129] Butterworth PJ, Warren FJ, Ellis PR. Human α-amylase and starch digestion: an interesting marriage. *Starch-Stärke*. 2011;63(7):395–405. doi:10.1002/star.201000150.

[130] Sky-Peck HH, Thuvasethakul P. Human pancreatic alpha-amylase. II. Effects of pH, substrate and ions on the activity of the enzyme. *Ann Clin Lab Sci*. 1977;7(4):310–317. http://www.ncbi.nlm.nih.gov/pubmed/20029.

[131] Aaberg B, Albaum HG, Arnold A. Aufbau, Speicherung, Mobilisierung und Umbildung der Kohlenhydrate = Formation, storage, mobilization and transformation of carbohydrates. In: *Handbuch Der Pflanzenphysiologie Encyclopedia of Plant Physiology*. 6th edition. Berlin; 1958:1444.

[132] Rosenblum JL, Irwin CL, Alpers DH. Starch and glucose oligosaccharides protect salivary-type amylase activity at acid pH. *Am J Physiol*. 1988;254(5 Pt 1):G775–G780. http://www.ncbi.nlm.nih.gov/pubmed/2452576.

[133] Lebenthal E. Role of salivary amylase in gastric and intestinal digestion of starch. *Dig Dis Sci*. 1987;32(10):1155–1157. http://www.ncbi.nlm.nih.gov/pubmed/2443325.

[134] Hooton D, Lentle R, Monro J, Wickham M, Simpson R. The secretion and action of brush border enzymes in the mammalian small intestine. *Rev Physiol Biochem Pharmacol*. 2015;168:59–118. doi:10.1007/112_2015_24.

[135] Van Beers EH, Büller HA, Grand RJ, Einerhand AW, Dekker J. Intestinal brush border glycohydrolases: structure, function, and development. *Crit Rev Biochem Mol Biol*. 1995;30(3):197–262. doi:10.3109/10409239509085143.

[136] Wright EM, Martín MG, Turk E. Intestinal absorption in health and disease—sugars. *Best Pract Res Clin Gastroenterol*. 2003;17(6):943–956. http://www.ncbi.nlm.nih.gov/pubmed/14642859.

[137] Wright EM, Hirayama BA, Loo DF. Active sugar transport in health and disease. *J Intern Med*. 2007;261(1):32–43. doi:10.1111/j.1365-2796.2006.01746.x.

[138] Wright EM, Loo DDF, Hirayama BA. Biology of human sodium glucose transporters. *Physiol Rev*. 2011;91(2):733–794. doi:10.1152/physrev.00055.2009.

[139] Fruton JS. A history of pepsin and related enzymes. *Q Rev Biol*. 2002;77(2):127–147. http://www.ncbi.nlm.nih.gov/pubmed/12089768.

[140] Piper DW, Fenton BH. pH stability and activity curves of pepsin with special reference to their clinical importance. *Gut*. 1965;6(5):506–508. http://www.ncbi.nlm.nih.gov/pubmed/4158734.

[141] Fruton JS. Specificity and mechanism of pepsin action on synthetic substrates. *Adv Exp Med Biol*. 1977;95:131–140. http://www.ncbi.nlm.nih.gov/pubmed/339686.

[142] Powers JC, Harley AD, Myers DV. Subsite specificity of porcine pepsin. *Adv Exp Med Biol*. 1977;95:141–157. http://www.ncbi.nlm.nih.gov/pubmed/339687.

[143] Geokas MC, McKenna RD, Beck IT. Elastase in normal canine pancreas. *Can J Biochem*. 1967;45(6):999–1002. http://www.ncbi.nlm.nih.gov/pubmed/6034709.

[144] Beck IT. The role of pancreatic enzymes in digestion. *Am J Clin Nutr*. 1973;26(3):311–325. http://www.ncbi.nlm.nih.gov/pubmed/4347665.

[145] Neurath H. Proteolytic enzymes past and present: the second golden era. Recollections, special section in honor of Max Perutz. *Protein Sci*. 1994;3(10):1734–1739. doi:10.1002/pro.5560031013.

[146] Hadorn B. Pancreatic proteinases; their activation and the disturbances of this mechanism in man. *Med Clin North Am*. 1974;58(6):1319–1331. http://www.ncbi.nlm.nih.gov/pubmed/4610296.

[147] Daniel H. Molecular and integrative physiology of intestinal peptide transport. *Annu Rev Physiol*. 2004;66:361–384. doi:10.1146/annurev.physiol.66.032102.144149.

[148] Daniel H, Kottra G. The proton oligopeptide cotransporter family SLC15 in physiology and pharmacology. *Pflügers Arch Eur J Physiol.* 2004;447(5):610–618. doi:10.1007/s00424-003-1101-4.

[149] Bröer S. Amino acid transport across mammalian intestinal and renal epithelia. *Physiol Rev.* 2008;88(1):249–286. doi:10.1152/physrev.00018.2006.

[150] Bröer S. Apical transporters for neutral amino acids: physiology and pathophysiology. *Physiology (Bethesda).* 2008;23:95–103. doi:10.1152/physiol.00045.2007.

[151] Mu H, Høy C-E. The digestion of dietary triacylglycerols. *Prog Lipid Res.* 2004;43(2):105–133. http://www.ncbi.nlm.nih.gov/pubmed/14654090.

[152] Linthorst JM, Bennett Clark S, Holt PR. Triglyceride emulsification by amphipaths present in the intestinal lumen during digestion of fat. *J Colloid Interface Sci.* 1977;60(1):1–10. doi:10.1016/0021-9797(77)90250-8.

[153] Lairon D, Nalbone G, Lafont H, et al. Possible roles of bile lipids and colipase in lipase adsorption. *Biochemistry.* 1978;17(24):5263–5269. http://www.ncbi.nlm.nih.gov/pubmed/728399.

[154] Carrière F, Grandval P, Gregory PC, et al. Does the pancreas really produce much more lipase than required for fat digestion? *JOP.* 2005;6(3):206–215. http://www.ncbi.nlm.nih.gov/pubmed/15883471.

[155] Hamosh M, Scow RO. Lingual lipase and its role in the digestion of dietary lipid. *J Clin Invest.* 1973;52(1):88–95. doi:10.1172/JCI107177.

[156] Fink CS, Hamosh P, Hamosh M. Fat digestion in the stomach: stability of lingual lipase in the gastric environment. *Pediatr Res.* 1984;18(3):248–254. doi:10.1203/00006450-198403000-00006.

[157] DeNigris SJ, Hamosh M, Kasbekar DK, Fink CS, Lee TC, Hamosh P. Secretion of human gastric lipase from dispersed gastric glands. *Biochim Biophys Acta.* 1985;836(1):67–72. http://www.ncbi.nlm.nih.gov/pubmed/4027260.

[158] Gargouri Y, Moreau H, Verger R. Gastric lipases: biochemical and physiological studies. *Biochim Biophys Acta.* 1989;1006(3):255–271. http://www.ncbi.nlm.nih.gov/pubmed/2688745.

[159] Canaan S, Roussel A, Verger R, Cambillau C. Gastric lipase: crystal structure and activity. *Biochim Biophys Acta.* 1999;1441(2–3):197–204. http://www.ncbi.nlm.nih.gov/pubmed/10570247.

[160] Gargouri Y, Pieroni G, Rivière C, et al. Importance of human gastric lipase for intestinal lipolysis: an in vitro study. *Biochim Biophys Acta.* 1986;879(3):419–423. http://www.ncbi.nlm.nih.gov/pubmed/3778930.

[161] Carriere F, Barrowman JA, Verger R, Laugier R. Secretion and contribution to lipolysis of gastric and pancreatic lipases during a test meal in humans. *Gastroenterology.* 1993;105(3):876–888. http://www.ncbi.nlm.nih.gov/pubmed/8359655.

[162] Borgström B. Fat digestion and absorption. In: *Intestinal Absorption*. Boston, MA: Springer US; 1974:555–620. doi:10.1007/978-1-4684-3336-4_1.

[163] Lowe ME. Structure and function of pancreatic lipase and colipase. *Annu Rev Nutr*. 1997;17:141–158. doi:10.1146/annurev.nutr.17.1.141.

[164] Mattson FH, Volpenheim RA. The digestion and absorption of triglycerides. *J Biol Chem*. 1964;239:2772–2777. http://www.ncbi.nlm.nih.gov/pubmed/14216426.

[165] Lowe ME. Properties and function of pancreatic lipase related protein 2. *Biochimie*. 2000;82(11):997–1004. http://www.ncbi.nlm.nih.gov/pubmed/11099796.

[166] Patton JS, Carey MC. Watching fat digestion. *Science*. 1979;204(4389):145–148. http://www.ncbi.nlm.nih.gov/pubmed/432636.

[167] Carey MC, Small DM, Bliss CM. Lipid digestion and absorption. *Annu Rev Physiol*. 1983;45:651–677. doi:10.1146/annurev.ph.45.030183.003251.

[168] Hernell O, Staggers JE, Carey MC. Physical-chemical behavior of dietary and biliary lipids during intestinal digestion and absorption. 2. Phase analysis and aggregation states of luminal lipids during duodenal fat digestion in healthy adult human beings. *Biochemistry*. 1990;29(8):2041–2056. http://www.ncbi.nlm.nih.gov/pubmed/2328238.

[169] Mansbach CM, and Abumrad NA. Enterocyte Fatty Acid Handling Proteins and Chylomicron Formation. In: Johnson LR, ed. Physiology of the Gastrointestinal Tract. 5th edition. New York: Academic 30 Press; 2012:1399–1423. doi:10.1016/B978-0-12-382026-6.00051-8.

[170] Niot I, Poirier H, Tran TTT, Besnard P. Intestinal absorption of long-chain fatty acids: evidence and uncertainties. *Prog Lipid Res*. 2009;48(2):101–115. http://www.ncbi.nlm.nih.gov/pubmed/19280719.

[171] Ratnayake WMN, Galli C. Fat and fatty acid terminology, methods of analysis and fat digestion and metabolism: a background review paper. *Ann Nutr Metab*. 2009;55(1–3):8–43. doi:10.1159/000228994.

[172] Berry AJ. Pancreatic enzyme replacement therapy during pancreatic insufficiency. *Nutr Clin Pract*. 2014;29(3):312–321. doi:10.1177/0884533614527773.

[173] Domínguez-Muñoz JE. Pancreatic exocrine insufficiency: diagnosis and treatment. *J Gastroenterol Hepatol*. 2011;26(Suppl 2):12–16. doi:10.1111/j.1440-1746.2010.06600.x.

[174] DiMagno EP, Go VL, Summerskill WH. Relations between pancreatic enzyme ouputs and malabsorption in severe pancreatic insufficiency. *N Engl J Med*. 1973;288(16):813–815. doi:10.1056/NEJM197304192881603.

[175] Carrière F, Grandval P, Renou C, et al. Quantitative study of digestive enzyme secretion and gastrointestinal lipolysis in chronic pancreatitis. *Clin Gastroenterol Hepatol*. 2005;3(1):28–38. http://www.ncbi.nlm.nih.gov/pubmed/15645402.

[176] Ross CA. Fat absorption studies in the diagnosis and treatment of pancreatic fibrosis. *Arch Dis Child.* 1955;30(152):316–321. http://www.ncbi.nlm.nih.gov/pubmed/13249617.

[177] Fredrikzon B, Bläckberg L. Lingual lipase: an important lipase in the digestion of dietary lipids in cystic fibrosis? *Pediatr Res.* 1980;14(12):1387–1390. doi:10.1203/00006450-198012000-00026.

[178] Pezzilli R. Chronic pancreatitis: maldigestion, intestinal ecology and intestinal inflammation. *World J Gastroenterol.* 2009;15(14):1673–1676. http://www.ncbi.nlm.nih.gov/pubmed/19360910.

[179] Fieker A, Philpott J, Armand M. Enzyme replacement therapy for pancreatic insufficiency: present and future. *Clin Exp Gastroenterol.* 2011;4:55–73. doi:10.2147/CEG.S17634.

[180] Ferrone M, Raimondo M, Scolapio JS. Pancreatic enzyme pharmacotherapy. *Pharmacotherapy.* 2007;27(6):910–920. doi:10.1592/phco.27.6.910.

[181] Sikkens ECM, Cahen DL, Kuipers EJ, Bruno MJ. Pancreatic enzyme replacement therapy in chronic pancreatitis. *Best Pract Res Clin Gastroenterol.* 2010;24(3):337–347. doi:10.1016/j.bpg.2010.03.006.

Section 2

Chronic Pancreatitis

Chapter 3

Surgical Indications and Techniques to Treat the Pain in Chronic Pancreatitis

Alejandro Serrablo, Mario Serradilla Martín,
Leyre Serrablo and Luis Tejedor

Additional information is available at the end of the chapter

http://dx.doi.org/10.5772/67032

Abstract

Chronic pancreatitis (CP) is a progressive inflammatory process, of the pancreatic gland and leads to damage and decrease in glandular tissue. Clinically, the pain is the most outstanding and incapacitating sign (95% of patients), as well as exocrine pancreatic insufficiency. The two main objectives in CP treatment are pain relief and complication management. Pain is the main surgical treatment indication. Patients with pancreatic duct dilation require surgical drainage, which provides an important pain relief (70–80%). Decompression (drainage), resection and neuroablation are the most commonly used surgical treatment options of CP. Derivative surgical procedures as Puestow-Gillesby or its modification, Partington-Rochelle, are the best options if the Wirsung duct is dilated, and Izbiki procedure if it is not. Resection is the choice when there is an important affectation of the head of pancreas with repercussion in bile duct or duodenum, as well as those patients with suspicion of carcinoma or in those ones who cannot be ruled a malignant tumour. The resection surgical procedures are Whipple, Traverso-Longmire, Frey (resective-derivative) and Beger (resective-derivative). To conclude, surgeon must know not only every surgical procedure indications but also be familiarised with all of them. The surgical procedure must be individualised to the patient and the disease stage.

Keywords: chronic pancreatitis, pain, surgical management

1. Introduction

Chronic pancreatitis (CP) is a progressive inflammatory process, which affects pancreatic gland and leads to damage and decrease in glandular tissue [1]. Clinically, the pain is the most outstanding and incapacitating sign (95% of patients), as well as exocrine pancreatic insufficiency. The most important pathologic finding in CP is the replacement of normal pancreatic tissue for irreversible fibrosis [2–6]. The CP incidence is between 2 and 200 per 100,000 persons and shows an increasing trend year by year. Historically, excess alcohol consumption plays the leading cause role in Western countries, accounting for 60% of CP cases, although tobacco consumption, usually joined to alcohol consumption, plays the most important role in pancreas cell injury [7].

On the basis of the histopathological changes in the pancreas, CP can be classified into three types: (1) chronic obstructive pancreatitis, (2) chronic calcifying pancreatitis (the most common type of CP, which includes alcoholic CP) and (3) chronic inflammatory pancreatitis, including CP resulting from chronic inflammation of the biliary tract and stenosis induced by scar formation [8, 9].

In principle, patients with CP need medical treatment for long periods of time or indefinitely, as long as the medical treatment relieves symptoms and patients do not develop any complication requiring surgery. Disabling pain, analgesic treatment refractory or cause opiate dependence, is the most frequent symptom sets the surgical indication. However, other well-established surgical prescriptions are the complications of adjacent organs such as bile duct or duodenum stenosis, associated pseudocysts with ductal anomalies, pancreatic fistulas, ascites, gastrointestinal bleeding from oesophageal varices secondary to segmental thrombosis of the splenic vein and portal hypertension or inability to differentiate whether a pancreatic mass is really a focal CP or a neoplasia [10–13].

Furthermore, several authors suggest the superiority of surgical therapy over endoscopic therapy for chronic pancreatitis and pancreatic duct obstruction. However, many papers have been published on the possibilities offered by interventional endoscopy nevertheless the endoscopic therapy only reach a rate of 32% in pain relief, the worse result than any surgery procedure [14–20].

The two main objectives in CP treatment are pain relief and complications management. An optimum treatment must provide social and occupational rehabilitation as well as no pain recurrence. The problem is that there is neither an exact or validated measure of pain control nor randomised clinical studies comparing surgery with conservative treatment to help establish the indication of surgery [10]. It is usually recommended to consider surgery when the patient needs major opioids for more than 3 months and in case of treatment side effects or lack of obvious benefit [21–24].

2. Indications of surgery

The most accepted surgical indications are as follows [23]:

1. Refractory abdominal pain
2. Local complications:

- Bile duct stricture causing cholestasis
- Severe duodenal stricture (<1 cm diameter)
- Persistent inflammatory mass in the head of the pancreas
- Pancreatic pseudocyst greater than 6 cm
- Pancreatic abscess
- Portal vein compression
- Gastric outflow obstruction
- Transverse colon stricture
- Pancreatico-enteric or pancreatico-pleural fistula

3. Pancreas divisum causing CP
4. Wirsung stricture with body and tail dilation
5. Suspicion of underlying malignant pancreatic lesion

Patients with pancreatic duct dilation require surgical drainage, which achieves pain relief in 70–80% of the cases [10]. Decompression (drainage), resection and neuroablation are the most commonly used surgical treatment options of CP [25–27]. If the pancreatic involvement involved the head or the tail of pancreas or if the Wirsung is dilated, a pancreatic resection of the head or the tail or a pancreatojejunostomy is required. Chronic inflammation in the head of pancreas leads to main bile duct stricture in 60%, to duodenal stricture in 36% and to portal hypertension in 17% of the patients. Surgical indication in this group of patients is evident; however, when the whole pancreas is damaged or the Wirsung duct is not dilated, the surgical indication is not so clear [28].

Derivative surgical procedures as the techniques described by Puestow, Gillesby or its modification, Partington-Rochelle, are the best options [29, 30]. The Wirsung duct should have enough diameters (6–8 mm) to perform a pancreatojejunal anastomosis. If the diameter is smaller, a longitudinal V resection of the anterior pancreas can be performed, followed by a pancreatojejunal anastomosis, as Izbiki published [31–34]. The main advantages of drainage procedures are their low morbidity and mortality rates, although up to 20–30% of the patients do not benefit of the surgical drainage and have persistent pain. We should select this group of patients and offer them a different treatment [31].

Resection is indicated when there is an important involvement of the pancreas head, a bile duct or duodenum obstruction and for those patients with suspicion of carcinoma or when a malignant tumour diagnosis cannot be discarded [35]. Resective surgical procedures are the techniques of Whipple, Traverso-Longmire, Frey (resective-derivative) and Beger (resective-derivative) [11–13, 26, 27, 35–37]. Beger and Frey procedures are both complex techniques with no differences in terms of pain relief and exocrine function preservation. The main drawback for these last techniques is the risk of tumour dissemination during surgery, as they are incomplete resection procedures and the risk of an underlying carcinoma is around 10% of the patients. Literature reports show a great variation in morbidity and mortality for each technique.

The surgeon should know every surgical procedure and its indications and be also familiarised with all of them. The surgical procedure should also be individualised to the patient and his stage of disease.

3. Surgical techniques

3.1. Decompression techniques

Wirsung duct originates in the pancreatic tail and crosses the gland midway between its superior and inferior borders, slightly posterior. Around 15–20 secondary ducts joint it in a perpendicular way. Main duct diameter ranges between 3.1 and 4.8 mm in the head, decreasing progressively to 0.9–2.4 mm in the tail. Accessory Santorini duct usually drains the anterosuperior part of the head and ends either in the duodenum through the minor papilla or in the main duct [38, 39].

Between 40 and 60% of patients with symptomatic chronic pancreatitis present ductal dilation, i.e. a ductal diameter >5 mm. Duct dilation may be due to a single stenosis, multiple stenosis, intraductal litiasis or a combination of stenosis and litiasis. Assuming that ductal dilation implies ductal hypertension and indeed pain, ductal decompression is the main surgical goal for these cases of CP [39]. These procedures should be done when Wirsung diameter is greater than 7–8 mm, but always in the absence of an inflammatory mass [40].

The first techniques described by DuVal and Zollinger in 1954 entailed the resection of the pancreatic tail and the anastomosis to a Roux-en-Y bowel loop [41, 42]. Obviously, this procedure is useful in the few patients with a single stenosis between the tail and the ampulla and is rarely used nowadays. Puestow and Gillesby reported in 1958 a technique providing a wider drainage. To the splenectomy and the resection of the tail, they added a longitudinal opening of the main duct and a latero-lateral pancreatojejunostomy. This technique is neither frequently used [29].

Two years later, Partington and Rochelle reported a procedure involving the longitudinal opening of the Wirsung duct but avoiding the resection of the pancreatic gland and the splenectomy. This technique is the most used as of today. It entails the opening of the duct from the tail to the head, stopping at 1 cm from the duodenal wall, the removal of all the existing calculi and the anastomosis to a Roux-en-Y bowel loop [30]. Although there is no consensus on the minimum diameter of the duct to indicate the procedure, most of the surgeons choose this technique for a size of the duct, when it is 7 mm or more. The procedure achieves relief of pain in 65–80% of patients, with a low mortality (less than 3%) and an acceptable morbidity (less than 20%) [25].

3.2. Resection techniques

Between 30 and 50% of the patients with CP develop inflammatory and fibrotic pancreatic masses. Many researchers refer the pain of the CP to the neural entrapment of the fibrotic pancreatic tissue and to the damage of the neural Schwann sheath by inflammatory cells.

This process may be limited to some parts of the gland and go along with or without ductal dilation [43–46]. When the CP presents with an inflammatory mass without ductal dilation or when drainage procedures had failed, surgical treatment is based on resection. Metabolic effects must be taken into account when pancreatic parenchyma is resected [47].

Depending on the affected area, resective procedures are pancreatoduodenectomy, duodenum-preserving head pancreatectomy, distal pancreatectomy, central pancreatectomy and total pancreatectomy.

3.2.1. Duodenopancreatectomy

The pancreatic head is the part of the gland more frequently affected by ductal changes and inflammatory masses and the site where biliary and duodenal complications arise. Many authors consider the pancreatic head as the "pacemaker" of the disease and emphasise its resection as the most important part of the treatment [48–52].

Whipple performed the first pancreatoduodenectomy in 1935 and the first one for CP in 1946 [12, 53, 54]. This procedure is the more commonly used for masses in the pancreatic head. Its main disadvantage is the removal of healthy organs: stomach, duodenum and bile duct. This is why Traverso and Longmire designed a modification in 1978, preserving pylorus (pylorus preserving pancreatoduodenectomy or PPPD) and thus avoiding the loss of gastric digestion and absorption functions, thereby decreasing the risk of postoperative malnutrition [11–13, 32, 33, 43, 44, 53–60].

Pancreatoduodenectomy, with or without pyloric preservation, relieves pain in more than 80% of the patients [48–52]. Mortality is less than 5% in high volume centres, but morbidity is around 40%, more frequently due to exocrine (23–95%) than endocrine (10–40%) insufficiency [50].

3.2.2. Duodenum-preserving head pancreatectomy

The procedure was described by Beger in the 1970s [13, 61]. Duodenum is of the outmost importance in the regulation of glycaemia and gastric emptying. This technique is considered a combined decompression-resection procedure. When a malignant neoplasm is ruled out, this is the procedure of choice, although it is also the most technically demanding. It includes the transection of the pancreatic neck above the portal vein, the resection of pancreatic head masses, the preservation of the posterior branch of the gastroduodenal artery to retain the blood supply of the duodenum and the preservation of the integrity of the lower end of the common bile duct to obtain a decompression effect in the common bile duct and duodenum. The proximal pancreatic duct is ligated and the distal end is used for pancreatojejunostomy. The same loop may be used for latero-lateral anastomoses to the proximal duct. Even in cases with biliary or duodenal stenosis due to entrapment by the tumour, this technique permits an adequate drainage without resecting bile duct or duodenum [61].

Pain is improved in 80–90% of the patients, with a low recurrence rate (8–11%) during follow up. Morbidity of this technique is between 15% and 55%. Mortality is exceedingly low (0.8%)

in Beger experience. This author reported that endocrine function kept unchanged in 82%, improved in 9% and worsened in 2% of the patients. Regarding exocrine function, around 65% of the patients needed some enzymatic supplements [55, 57, 58].

For those patients with a mass in the pancreatic head and ductal dilation, a combination of a latero-lateral pancreatojejunostomy with the enucleation of the pancreatic head was described by Frey in 1987. Like Beger's technique, it spares duodenum and bile duct but is technically less demanding since the posterior part of the head is preserved and the anastomosis is performed at the anterior aspect of the gland. This technique should not be used when there is a large mass in the head and no stenosis of the main duct [21, 22, 35–37, 57–59].

Recent reports comparing Frey's, Beger's and pancreatoduodenectomy resections (**Table 1**) showed that, if patients are correctly selected, any of the three techniques is able to improve symptoms in around 90% of the cases [32, 43, 45, 46, 58]. They were similarly useful in treating complications on neighbouring organs, bile duct and duodenum. The former two procedures resulted in better quality of life and earlier postoperative recovery and had a mortality rate lower than 3% in skilled hands. Morbidity was somewhat less frequent in Frey's than in Beger's technique, and in both two was quite lower than in pancreatoduodenectomy. Endocrine and exocrine activities are similarly affected by the all three.

Authors	Procedure	*N*	Surgical mortality (%)	Morbidity	Fistula (%)	Pain relief (%)
Koninger et al.	Beger/Frey	32/33	0/0	20/21	7/3	–/–
Buchler et al.	Beger/DP	20/20	0/0	15/20	0/5	94/77
Farkas et al.	Beger/DP	20/20	0/0	0/40	–/–	100/100
Izbicki et al.	Frey/DP	31/30	3/0	19/53	3/7	80/75
Izbicki et al	Beger/Frey	20/22	0/0	20/9	5/0	70/70
Klempa et al.	Beger/DP	22/21	1/0	54/51	0/5	100/70

Beger, Beger procedure; Frey, Frey procedure; DP, duodenopancreatectomy; *N*, number of patients included.

Table 1. Randomised control trials among different surgical techniques in abdominal pain relief (follow up, 1–4 years).

These techniques have been compared in several reports. A retrospective randomised controlled trial showed that the recurrence rate after Frey procedure (19%) was lower than that after Traverso-Longmire (53%). Another report showed lower recurrence rate for Frey procedure (22%) than for Beger's (32%). Endocrine insufficiency rate after 7 years was reported to be better for Frey procedure (86%) than for PPPD (96%), as well as after 8 years for Frey procedure (78%) compared with Beger procedure (88%).

Others techniques include Berne's modification, which preserves the neck of the gland and shows better results and less morbidity than PPPD and Beger's technique [55, 62]. Its goal is to avoid dissection in the portal region, sometimes affected by the inflammatory process. The recurrence rate is 20–23%. Izbicki modification of the Frey procedure, reported in 1998, consists in a wide V-shaped resection of the head and uncinate process. It is indicated in CP with a duct smaller than 3 mm. Imizumi modification of the Beger's technique is useful in patients with intrapancreatic biliary stenosis, achieving a relief of pain in 90% of the patients with little metabolic changes [61, 63].

3.2.3. Distal pancreatectomy

When CP affects mostly to the left part of the gland and the head is normal, the treatment is a distal pancreatectomy. Trendelenburg performed the first distal pancreatectomy for the treatment of a neoplasm in 1882. This procedure is indicated when there is a break in the duct or a suspicious humoral mass and the duct diameter is less than 5 mm [64, 65].

Two important technical issues regarding this surgical technique are spleen preservation and pancreatic remnant management. Spleen must be spared whenever possible, but not in cases of splenic thrombosis or of pancreatic pseudocyst adherent to the spleen or splenic hilum. Regarding the pancreatic remnant, a suture of the duct and the parenchyma can be done or, alternatively, it may be sutured to a Roux-en-Y loop after DuVal technique. In both instances, the main duct should be explored to rule out stenosis or litiasis.

The mortality of the procedure is around 5% and the morbidity is 20%. From 0 to 7% of the patients develop a pancreatic fistula [42, 66]. The greater drawback of this surgery is a failure rate of 17–74% (media 36%) in relieving symptoms, mainly pain, although these results may be due to a deficient selection of patients. On the other hand, metabolic derangement greatly depends on the amount of the resected glandular tissue, but malabsorption needing treatment appears in 25–30% and diabetes in 17–85% of the patients [64, 65].

3.2.4. Central resection

In a few patients, inflammatory changes sit at the pancreatic neck or slightly to its left. Sometimes, there is a sole ductal stenosis or a ductal litiasis between head and body of the pancreas. In these rare cases, neither deemed to drainage nor to head or distal resection, central resection with suture of both distal ends of the duct to a jejunal loop is the technique of choice.

Central resection shows notable success in dealing with pain and has low mortality and morbidity rates and mild deleterious effect on pancreatic functions [10, 59, 67–70] .

3.2.5. Total pancreatectomy

Priestley is credited with the first total pancreatectomy to treat a patient with hyperinsulinemia [47]. Around 20% of the patients treated with surgery for CP show unsatisfactory outcomes, although it is difficult to determine whether they are due to the natural progression of the disease or to surgical failure. It is also intricate to elucidate what amount of analgesic use is due to drug dependence and what to real pain. Moreover, the recurrence of the symptoms may be caused by a superimposed disease. Finally, a relapse in alcohol intake may further complicate this complex matter.

Total pancreatectomy is not necessarily the next step of the treatment for the reappearance of the symptoms. After a failed drainage technique, improving draining capacity through widening the pancreatojejunal anastomoses or partially resecting the pancreatic head may be adequate. If the new changes appear in the pancreatic tail, a distal pancreatectomy may be the solution.

The results after total pancreatectomy are not very fair, mainly because of endocrine and exocrine morbidity. Nevertheless, it is indicated for patients with failed surgical procedures who already present endocrine and exocrine insufficiency, for patients with diffuse CP with multiple litiasis in small ducts and gland insufficiency and, probably the most controversial indication, for patients with diffuse disease without changes of the duct who present with repeated bouts of pancreatitis and are unresponsive to conservative treatment [65, 71, 72].

After surgery, symptoms improve in 50% of the patients; mortality is 5–10% and morbidity is around 40%. The most serious complications are metabolic, hypoglycaemic shock above all [73].

4. Summary

There are several surgical techniques to treat CP, recommended when medical treatment is ineffective or appear complications that can be surgically corrected. Success of these treatments depends on the natural history of the disease, on the appropriate selection of the technique and on the objectives and expected results. Surgeons must be aware of their surgical expertise and of the rate of pain control, morbi-mortality, quality of life and functional changes of the chosen technique.

Recommendations	Evidence level	Recommendation grade
Surgery is effective in the treatment of pancreatic pain	1b	A
When there is a pseudocyst in patients with abdominal pain, it is recommended that therapeutic interventions include treatment of pseudocyst	3b	B
In patients with ductal dilatation and pain, surgery offers better results than endoscopic treatment	1a	A

Author details

Alejandro Serrablo[1,*], Mario Serradilla Martín[1], Leyre Serrablo[2] and Luis Tejedor[3]

*Address all correspondence to: ALMALEY@telefonica.net

1 Miguel Servet University Hospital, Zaragoza, Spain

2 Medicine School of Zaragoza University, Zaragoza, Spain

3 General Surgery of Punta Europa Hospital, Algeciras, Spain

References

[1] Banks PA. Epidemiology, natural history, and predictors of disease outcome in acute and chronic pancreatitis. Gastrointest Endosc. 2002;56Suppl:S226–30

[2] Yadav D, Timmons L, Benson JT, Dierkhising RA, Chari ST. Incidence, prevalence, and survival of chronic pancreatitis: a population-based study. Am J Gastroenterol. 2011;106:2192–9.

[3] Garg PK, Tandon RK. Survey on chronic pancreatitis in the Asia-Pacific region. J Gastroenterol Hepatol. 2004;19:998–1004.

[4] Tandon RK, Sato N, Garg PK. Chronic pancreatitis: Asia-Pacific consensus report. J Gastroenterol Hepatol. 2002;17:508–18.

[5] Bhardwaj P, Garg PK, Maulik SK, Saraya A, Tandon RK, Acharya SK. A randomized controlled trial of antioxidant supplementation for pain relief in patients with chronic pancreatitis. Gastroenterology. 2009;136:149–159.e2.

[6] Di Sebastiano P, di Mola FF, Büchler MW, Friess H. Pathogenesis of pain in chronic pancreatitis. Dig Dis. 2004;22:267–72.

[7] Liao Z, Jin G, Cai D, Sun X, Hu B, Wang X, et al. Guidelines: diagnosis and therapy for chronic pancreatitis. J Interv Gastroenterol. 2013;3:133–6.

[8] Bird GH, Irimia A, Ofek G, Kwong PD, Wilson IA, Walensky LD. Stapled HIV-1 peptides recapitulate antigenic structures and engage broadly neutralizing antibodies. Nat Struct Mol Biol. 2014;21:1058–67.

[9] Banks PA. Classification and diagnosis of chronic pancreatitis. J Gastroenterol. 2007;42 Suppl 17:148–51

[10] Warshaw AL, Rattner DW, Fernández-del Castillo C, Z'graggen K. Middle segment pancreatectomy: a novel technique for conserving pancreatic tissue. Arch Surg. 1998;133:327–31.

[11] Büchler MW, Friess H, Muller MW, Wheatley AM, Beger HG. Randomized trial of duodenum-preserving pancreatic head resection versus pylorus-preserving Whipple in chronic pancreatitis. Am J Surg. 1995;169:65–9.

[12] Traverso LW, Kozarek RA. The Whipple procedure for severe complications of chronic pancreatitis. Arch Surg. 1993;128:1047–53.

[13] Beger HG, Witte C, Krautzberger W, Bittner R. [Experiences with duodenum-sparing pancreas head resection in chronic pancreatitis]. Chirurg. 1980;51:303–7. German.

[14] Invalid reference.

[15] Cahen DL, Gouma DJ, Nio Y, Rauws EA, Boermeester MA, Busch OR, et al. Endoscopic versus surgical drainage of the pancreatic duct in chronic pancreatitis. N Engl J Med. 2007;356:676–84.

[16] Díte P, Ruzicka M, Zboril V, Novotný I. A prospective, randomized trial comparing endoscopic and surgical therapy for chronic pancreatitis. Endoscopy. 2003;35:553–8.

[17] Rösch T, Daniel S, Scholz M, Huibregtse K, Smits M, Schneider T, et al. Endoscopic treatment of chronic pancreatitis: a multicenter study of 1000 patients with long-term follow-up. Endoscopy. 2002;34:765–71.

[18] Deviere J, Bell Jr RH, Beger HG, Traverso LW. Treatment of chronic pancreatitis with endotherapy or surgery: critical review of randomized control trials. J Gastrointest Surg. 2008;12:640–4.

[19] Kahl S, Zimmermann S, Genz I, Glasbrenner B, Pross M, Schulz HU, et al. Risk factors for failure of endoscopic stenting of biliary strictures in chronic pancreatitis: a prospective follow-up study. Am J Gastroenterol. 2003;98:2448–53.

[20] Cahen DL, Gouma DJ, Laramee P, Nio Y, Rauws EA, Boermeester MA, et al. Long-term outcomes of endoscopic vs surgical drainage of the pancreatic duct in patients with chronic pancreatitis. Gastroenterology. 2011;141:1690–5.

[21] Vasile D, Ilco A, Popa D, Belega A, Pana S. The surgical treatment of chronic pancreatitis: a clinical series of 17 cases. Chirurgia (Bucur). 2013;108:794–9.

[22] Andersen DK, Frey CF. The evolution of the surgical treatment of chronic pancreatitis. Ann Surg. 2010;251:18–32.

[23] Forsmark CE. Management of chronic pancreatitis. Gastroenterology. 2013;144:1282–91.

[24] Yin Z, Sun J, Yin D, Wang J. Surgical treatment strategies in chronic pancreatitis: a meta-analysis. Arch Surg. 2012;147:961–8.

[25] Bachmann K, Kutup A, Mann O, Yekebas E, Izbicki JR. Surgical treatment in chronic pancreatitis timing and type of procedure. Best Pract Res Clin Gastroenterol. 2010;24:299–310.

[26] Traverso LW, Longmire Jr WP. Preservation of the pylorus in pancreaticoduodenectomy. Surg Gynecol Obstet. 1978;146:959–62.

[27] Traverso LW. The pylorus preserving Whipple procedure for the treatment of chronic pancreatitis. Swiss Surg. 2000;6:259–63.

[28] Strobel O, Büchler MW, Werner J. Surgical therapy of chronic pancreatitis: indications, techniques and results. Int J Surg. 2009;7:305–12.

[29] Puestow CB, Gillesby WJ. Retrograde surgical drainage of pancreas for chronic relapsing pancreatitis. AMA Arch Surg. 1958;76:898–907.

[30] Partington PF, Rochelle RE. Modified Puestow procedure for retrograde drainage of the pancreatic duct. Ann Surg. 1960;152:1037–43.

[31] Izbicki JR, Bloechle C, Broering DC, Kuechler T, Broelsch CE. Longitudinal V-shaped excision of the ventral pancreas for small duct disease in severe chronic pancreatitis: prospective evaluation of a new surgical procedure. Ann Surg. 1998;227:213–9.

[32] Izbicki JR, Bloechle C, Knoefel WT, Kuechler T, Binmoeller KF, Broelsch CE. Duodenum-preserving resection of the head of the pancreas in chronic pancreatitis: a prospective, randomized trial. Ann Surg. 1995;221:350–8.

[33] Izbicki JR, Bloechle C, Knoefel WT, Wilker DK, Dornschneider G, Seifert H, et al. Complications of adjacent organs in chronic pancreatitis managed by duodenum-preserving resection of the head of the pancreas. Br J Surg. 1994;81:1351–5.

[34] Izbicki JR, Bloechle C, Broering DC, Knoefel WT, Kuechler T, Broelsch CE. Extended drainage versus resection in surgery for chronic pancreatitis: a prospective randomized trial comparing the longitudinal pancreaticojejunostomy combined with local pancreatic head excision with the pylorus-preserving pancreatoduodenectomy. Ann Surg. 1998;228:771–9.

[35] Frey CF, Child CG, Fry W. Pancreatectomy for chronic pancreatitis. Ann Surg. 1976; 184:403–13.

[36] Frey CF, Smith GJ. Description and rationale of a new operation for chronic pancreatitis. Pancreas. 1987;2:701–7.

[37] Frey CF, Amikura K. Local resection of the head of the pancreas combined with longitudinal pancreaticojejunostomy in the management of patients with chronic pancreatitis. Ann Surg. 1994;220:492–507.

[38] Somala M, Fisher WE. Pancreatic Anatomy and Physiology. Ed: Zyromski NJ. Wolters Kluwer. 2015. Handbook of Hepato-Pancreato-Biliary Surgery, pp. 2–14. ISBN/ISSN 978 1451185010

[39] Kutup A, Vashist Y, Kaifi JT, Yekebas EF, Izbicki JR. For which type of chronic pancreatitis is the "Hamburg procedure" indicated? J Hepatobiliary Pancreat Sci. 2010;17:758–62.

[40] Friess H, Berberat PO, Wirtz M, Büchler MW. Surgical treatment and long-term follow-up in chronic pancreatitis. Eur J Gastroenterol Hepatol. 2002;14:971–7.

[41] Duval Jr MK. Caudal pancreatico-jejunostomy for chronic relapsing pancreatitis. Ann Surg. 1954;140:775–85.

[42] Rattner DW, Fernandez-del Castillo C, Warshaw AL. Pitfalls of distal pancreatectomy for relief of pain in chronic pancreatitis. Am J Surg. 1996;171:142–6.

[43] Klempa I, Spatny M, Menzel J, Baca I, Nustede R, Stockmann F, et al. [Pancreatic function and quality of life after resection of the head of the pancreas in chronic pancreatitis. A prospective, randomized comparative study after duodenum preserving resection of the head of the pancreas versus Whipple's operation]. Chirurg. 1995;66:350–9.

[44] Büchler MW, Friess H, Bittner R, Roscher R, Krautzberger W, Müller MW, et al. Duodenum-preserving pancreatic head resection: long-term results. J Gastrointest Surg. 1997;1:13–9.

[45] Büchler MW, Warshaw AL. Resection versus drainage in treatment of chronic pancreatitis. Gastroenterology. 2008;134:1605–7.

[46] Prinz RA, Greenlee HB. Pancreatic duct drainage in chronic pancreatitis. Hepatogastroenterology. 1990;37:295–300.

[47] Priestley JT, Comfort MW, Radcliffe Jr J. Total pancreatectomy for hyperinsulinism due to an islet-cell adenoma: survival and cure at sixteen months after operation: presentation of metabolic studies. Ann Surg. 1944;119:211–21.

[48] Sakorafas GH, Farnell MB, Nagorney DM, Sarr MG, Rowland CM. Pancreatoduodenectomy for chronic pancreatitis: long-term results in 105 patients. Arch Surg. 2000;135:517–24.

[49] Sakorafas GH, Sarr MG, Rowland CM, Farnell MB. Postobstructive chronic pancreatitis: results with distal resection. Arch Surg. 2001;136:643–8.

[50] Strate T, Bachmann K, Busch P, Mann O, Schneider C, Bruhn JP, et al. Resection vs drainage in treatment of chronic pancreatitis: long-term results of a randomized trial. Gastroenterology. 2008;134:1406–11.

[51] Strate T, Knoefel WT, Yekebas E, Izbicki JR. Chronic pancreatitis: etiology, pathogenesis, diagnosis, and treatment. Int J Colorectal Dis. 2003;18:97–106.

[52] Russell RC, Theis BA. Pancreatoduodenectomy in the treatment of chronic pancreatitis. World J Surg. 2003;27:1203–10.

[53] Farkas G, Leindler L, Daróczi M, Farkas Jr G. Organ-preserving pancreatic head resection in chronic pancreatitis. Br J Surg. 2003;90:29–32.

[54] Whipple AO, Parsons WB, Mullins CR. Treatment of carcinoma of the ampulla of Vater. Ann Surg. 1935;102:763–79.

[55] Farkas G, Leindler L, Daróczi M, Farkas Jr G. Prospective randomised comparison of organ-preserving pancreatic head resection with pylorus-preserving pancreaticoduodenectomy. Langenbecks Arch Surg. 2006;391:338–42.

[56] Jimenez RE, Fernandez-Del Castillo C, Rattner DW, Warshaw AL. Pylorus-preserving pancreaticoduodenectomy in the treatment of chronic pancreatitis. World J Surg. 2003;27:1211–6.

[57] Whipple AO. Radical surgery for certain cases of pancreatic fibrosis associated with calcareous deposits. Ann Surg. 1946;124:991–1006.

[58] Köninger J, Seiler CM, Sauerland S, Wente MN, Reidel MA, Müller MW, et al. Duodenum-preserving pancreatic head resection—a randomized controlled trial comparing the original Beger procedure with the Berne modification (ISRCTN No. 50638764). Surgery. 2008;143:490–8.

[59] Efron DT, Lillemoe KD, Cameron JL, Yeo CJ. Central pancreatectomy with pancreaticogastrostomy for benign pancreatic pathology. J Gastrointest Surg. 2004;8:532–8.

[60] Müller MW, Friess H, Beger HG, Kleeff J, Lauterburg B, Glasbrenner B, et al. Gastric emptying following pylorus-preserving Whipple and duodenum-preserving pancreatic head resection in patients with chronic pancreatitis. Am J Surg. 1997;173:257–63.

[61] Gloor B, Friess H, Uhl W, Büchler MW. A modified technique of the Beger and Frey procedure in patients with chronic pancreatitis. Dig Surg. 2001;18:21–5.

[62] Jimenez RE, Fernandez-del Castillo C, Rattner DW, Chang Y, Warshaw AL. Outcome of pancreaticoduodenectomy with pylorus preservation or with antrectomy in the treatment of chronic pancreatitis. Ann Surg. 2000;231:293–300.

[63] Hatori T, Imaizumi T, Harada N, Fukuda A, Suzuki M, Hanyu F, et al. Appraisal of the Imaizumi modification of the Beger procedure: the TWMU experience. J Hepatobiliary Pancreat Sci. 2010;17:752–7.

[64] Hutchins RR, Hart RS, Pacifico M, Bradley NJ, Williamson RC. Long-term results of distal pancreatectomy for chronic pancreatitis in 90 patients. Ann Surg. 2002;236:612–8.

[65] Schoenberg MH, Schlosser W, Rück W, Beger HG. Distal pancreatectomy in chronic pancreatitis. Dig Surg. 1999;16:130–6.

[66] Hartel M, Tempia-Caliera AA, Wente MN, Z'graggen K, Friess H, Büchler MW. Evidence-based surgery in chronic pancreatitis. Langenbecks Arch Surg. 2003;388:132–9.

[67] Muller MW, Friess H, Leitzbach S, Michalski CW, Berberat P, Ceyhan GO, et al. Perioperative and follow-up results after central pancreatic head resection (Berne technique) in a consecutive series of patients with chronic pancreatitis. Am J Surg. 2008;196:364–72.

[68] Bassi C. Middle segment pancreatectomy: a useful tool in the management of pancreatic neoplasms. J Gastrointest Surg. 2007;11:421–4.

[69] Jha AA, Kumar M, Galagali A. Management options in chronic pancreatitis. Med J Armed Forces India. 2012;68(3):284–7. doi:10.1016/j.mjafi.2012.04.009

[70] Roggin KK, Rudloff U, Blumgart LH, Brennan MF. Central pancreatectomy revisited. J Gastrointest Surg. 2006;10:804–12.

[71] Morrow CE, Cohen JI, Sutherland DE, Najarian JS. Chronic pancreatitis: long-term surgical results of pancreatic duct drainage, pancreatic resection, and near-total pancreatectomy and islet autotransplantation. Surgery. 1984;96:608–16.

[72] Williamson RC, Cooper MJ. Resection in chronic pancreatitis. Br J Surg. 1987;74:807–12.

[73] Müller MW, Friess H, Kleeff J, Dahmen R, Wagner M, Hinz U, et al. Is there still a role for total pancreatectomy? Ann Surg. 2007;246:966–75.

Section 3

Cystic Pancreatic Neoplasms

Chapter 4

Intraductal Papillary Mucinous Neoplasms of the Pancreas: Challenges and New Insights

Natalia Zambudio Carroll, Betsabé Reyes and
Laureano Vázquez

Additional information is available at the end of the chapter

http://dx.doi.org/10.5772/66491

Abstract

Cystic lesions of the pancreas are a common entity with almost a 25% incidence of the general population. These types of lesions are being increasingly diagnosed partly explained due to the technological advances over the past years. The management and treatment varies per cyst type. However, the most threatening cyst lesions are intraductal papillary mucinous neoplasms (IPMNs). These lesions represent nowadays a relatively new clinical entity and in many aspects remain poorly understood. The aim of this chapter is to provide a comprehensive review of the classification, diagnosis, treatment and follow-up strategy.

Keywords: IPMN, BD-IPMN, BD-IPMN, classification, malignancy risk, pathogenesis, management, surveillance

1. Introduction

In the face of this new "epidemic of pancreatic cysts," it is clear that we need to be on top of newly emerging changes in our current daily practice. Pancreatic cancer has a fateful prognosis, despite recent improvements in surgery and chemotherapy. However, most cases of intraductal papillary mucinous neoplasms (IPMNs) are considered as premalignant lesions, thus making them a target for diagnosis and prompt treatment. On the other hand, we should never forget the short- and long-term risks of surgery. This is precisely why it is so challenging to adequately manage this pathology.

Biomarkers represent an interesting opportunity, but until they can be used on a regular clinical basis, we are obliged to say knowledgeable on new insights involving radiologic characteristics and potential malignancy prior to deciding, which is the best available individualized option for each patient.

2. Classification

2.1. Anatomic classification: involvement of the pancreatic ductal system

Most IPMN arise from the pancreatic main duct or its branch ducts (**Figure 1**). Most of these tumors are unifocal, 20–30% are multifocal, and 5–10% of the IPMN diffusely affect the entire duct system of the pancreas. Depending on the involvement of the pancreatic duct, IPMNs are classified as either main duct IPMN (MD-IPMN) or branch duct IPMN (BD-IPMN). If both, main and branch ducts are involved together, then it is defined as combined-type IPMN (**Figure 2**). The clinical pathologic behavior of combined-type IPMN is similar to that of MD-IPMN. MD-IPMN is frequently more associated with this malignant transformation than is BD-IPMN, requiring surgical resection in more than a half of the patients, while most patients with BD-IPMN can be observed for a long time after the diagnosis.

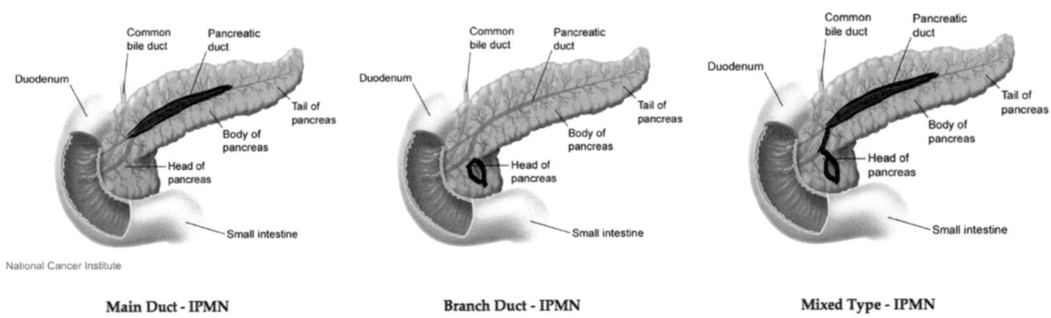

Figure 1. Types of IPMN: MD-IPMN, BD-IPMN, mixed type-IPMN. Modified from: Bliss D (Illustrator) 2001. Pancreas, Duodenum, and Small Intestine [image]. Available at: https://visualsonline.cancer.gov/details.cfm?imageid=4364.

MD - IPMN:
- Cystic tumor
- MPD: > 10mm

BD - IPMN:
- Cystic tumor in the branches
- MPD: < 6 mm

Figure 2. Differences between MD-IPMN and BD-IPMN.

2.2. Histologic classification: IPMN subtype

Immunohistochemical staining with mucin antibodies enables differentiation between tumors with different prognoses. Four subtypes of IPMNs have been characterized: gastric, intestinal, pancreatobiliary, and oncocytic. Most of BD-IPMNs are composed of gastric-type epithelium. However, intestinal type is more common in MD-IPMN. In a recent report, the four subtypes of IPMNs were associated with significant differences in survival. Patients with gastric-type IPMN had the best prognosis, whereas those with intestinal and pancreatobiliary type had a bad prognosis [1–6].

2.3. World Health Organization (WHO)

The World Health Organization (WHO) classified IPMNs into three subgroups according to degree of dysplasia: (I) IPMN with low- or intermediate-grade dysplasia; (II) IPMN with high-grade dysplasia (carcinoma in situ); and (III) IPMN with an associated invasive carcinoma. IPMN associated with PDAC (pancreatic ductal adenocarcinoma arising in association with an IPMN) was further classified into two subtypes: tubular adenocarcinoma, composed of predominantly gland-forming neoplastic cells with fibrotic stroma and absence of significant extracellular stromal mucin and colloid carcinoma (mucinous noncystic carcinoma), composed of sparsely populated strips, clusters, or individual neoplastic cells residing within extensive pools of extracellular mucin [6]. In case of IPMN with low- to intermediate-grade of dysplasia, dysplastic changes in the columnar cells are minimal or absent. The prognosis is usually favorable [7].

3. Malignancy risk

There has been an increased prevalence of pancreatic cystic neoplasms, frequently being found in elderly asymptomatic patients. This is partially caused by the greater number of cross-sectional studies being performed. Though images obtained through the use of computed tomography (CT-scan) and magnetic resonance imaging (MRI), we are able to estimate the prevalence of pancreatic cysts in 2.5% of the population. This figure increases over time; around the age of 70 years or older, 10% of the population has pancreatic cysts and 20–50% of them are IPMN [8].

The real risk of malignancy may be very low, but the diagnosis is associated with anxiety and usually leads to further medical testing in order to confirm malignancy. The most frequently used tests are likely to include: consultations con gastroenterologists and/or oncologists, endoscopic ultrasound with or without percutaneous biopsy, and occasionally surgery [6, 8, 9]. This is one of the reasons why more and more studies are focusing on evaluating the malignancy rate for pancreatic cancer distinct from IPMN and also for pancreatic cancer arising from IPMN. Figures are rather variable, but over the course of several years, we have been able to see how the rates for malignancy, especially in SB-IPMN, are found to be lower.

Not only IMPNs are associated with pancreatic malignancies but also it is known that extrapancreatic malignancies are more frequently found in these patients.

3.1. Pancreatic malignancies

3.1.1. Pancreatic cancer arising from IPMN

3.1.1.1. MD-IPMN

The malignancy risk in this type of situation is very clear which makes the decision to perform surgery also much easier. Many studies have estimated the overall risk ranges between 36 and 92% [10–13]. Overall, the prognosis after resection is generally favorable as long as its invasion remains within minimally invasive or in T1a status (depth of stromal invasion <5 mm).

3.1.1.2. BD-IPMN

In this case, there are more controversial figures. Estimated rates here can range from 6 to 47% [8, 11–13]. In 2013, Gardner et al. [8] lower the current 25% lifetime risk of malignant transformation and presented the prevalence of mucin-producing adenocarcinoma in patients diagnosed with pancreatic cysts to be 33.2 per 100,000 patients. A linear increment was detected when studying male patients between the ages of 80–84. In that group, the prevalence was 38.6 per 100,000 patients. Only one systematic review by Crippa et al. [14] is considered to be the first meta-analyses focused in the risk of developing pancreatic malignancies, including malignant BD-IPMNs and PDAC, as well as the risk of death due to pancreatic malignancy in patients undergoing nonoperative management for BD-IPMNs. The estimated overall pancreatic malignancy rate is 3.7%, an incidence of malignancy in 7 cases per 1000 per years and an annual risk on only 0.7%. This is the rate that is entirely comparable with the 90-day postoperative mortality rate following pancreatic resections found at many high-volume centers. Thus, choosing surgery in these cases does not justify for avoiding the unlikely progression from "low-risk" BD-IPMN to invasive tumors.

3.1.2. Pancreatic cancer distinct from IPMN

There appears to be a "field defect," which may give rise to both IPMN and pancreatic duct adenocarcinoma (frequently related to gastric subtype) occurring in 2–5% of patients diagnosed with IPMN [6, 10]. Also, Crippa et al. [14] lower the previous rates with an estimate of incidence of only 2 cases per 1000 per year and an annual risk of 0.2%.

3.2. Extrapancreatic malignancies

Colorectal, gastric, bile duct, renal cell, and thyroid cancers are relatively frequently associated with IPMNs [15–17].

4. Pathogenesis

IPMNs are mucinous cystic lesions of the pancreas that are characterized by neoplastic, mucin-secreting, and papillary cells projecting from the pancreatic ductal surface. They arise from the epithelial lining of the main pancreatic duct or its side branches. Intraductal proliferation of mucin-producing columnar cells is the main histologic characteristic of IPMNs, and

http://dx.doi.org/10.5772/66491

intraluminal growth causes dilatation of the involved duct and its proximal segment. They are usually found in the head of the pancreas as a solitary cystic lesion, but in 20–30% of the cases, they may be multifocal, and in 5–10% of cases, they may involve the pancreas diffusely [18–20]. In BD-IPMN, malignant tumors can be found in 6–46% and in MD-IPMN in 57–92%, making that MD-IPMN leads to worse prognosis [5].

4.1. Progression to pancreatic cancer

IPMNs are thought to follow an orderly progression from a benign neoplasm to invasive carcinoma of the pancreas, they range from premalignant lesions with low-grade dysplasia to invasive malignancy, and they have a clear tendency to become invasive carcinoma [5, 21–24]. It has been estimated a 5–6 year progression rate, depending on the subtype. They are graded according to the most atypical area in the lesion as:

- Low-grade dysplasia (adenoma).
- Moderate dysplasia (borderline).
- High-grade dysplasia (carcinoma in situ).
- Invasive carcinoma.

5. Clinical presentation

5.1. Risk factors

It has been described that previous history of diabetes, especially with insulin dependency, chronic pancreatitis, or a familial history of pancreatic ductal adenocarcinoma (PDAC), may have a higher risk for IPMN [25]. Also, several studies have noticed that the presence of auto-immune disease in general population is around 5%; however, in patients diagnosed with IPMN, the number rises up to 22%. IPMNs can be associated with systemic diseases such as: systemic lupus erythematous and rheumatoid arthritis an inflammatory bowel disease, leading to think that IMPNs may be one manifestation of a more systemic disease [26].

5.2. Symptoms

Most IPMNs are diagnosed between 60 and 70 years of age. There is a slightly higher prevalence in men than women [7]. Some patients present symptoms at the time of diagnosis (7–43%), being more frequent the presence of abdominal pain, jaundice, and previous history of pancreatitis. Other symptoms are as follows: weight loss, nausea or vomiting, and diabetes [5, 6, 27].

6. Evaluation for malignancy

Several tests can be performed when confronted with a possible IPMN. Regarding this subject, some changes have occurred recently, most of them centering on the use of EUS-FNA (endoscopic ultrasonography/fine-needle aspiration) and endoscopic retrograde cholangiopancreatography (ERCP) and analyses of the obtained fluid (**Figure 3**).

6.1. Cross-sectional imaging

Magnetic resonance cholangiopancreatography (MRCP) and computerized axial tomography scan (CAT scan) are useful as the first step, and perhaps the only one, if results are very clear (see management) (**Figure 4**). It is useful to describe:

- Anatomical characteristics: lymph node involvement and main pancreatic duct involvement.
- Mural nodules: IPMN with >3 mm nodules is highly suggestive of malignancy.

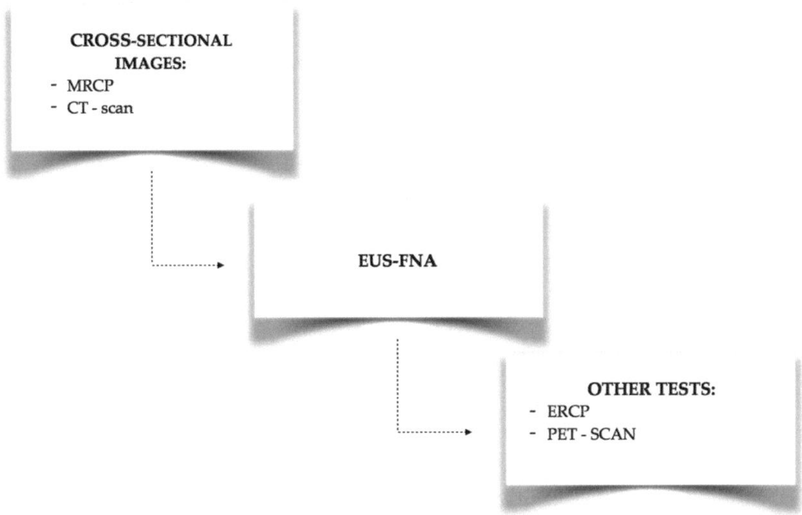

Figure 3. General sequence when diagnosing IPMNs.

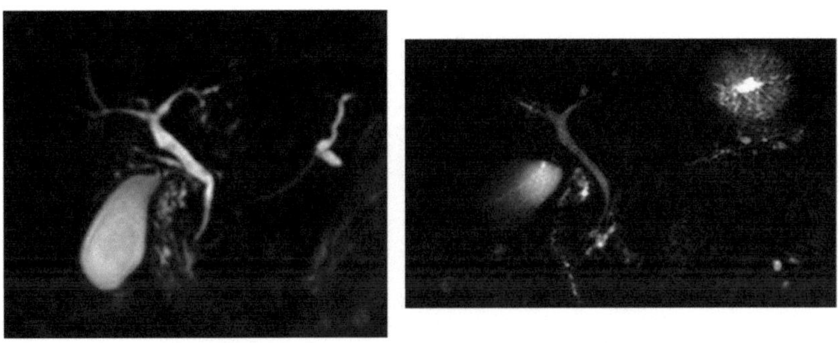

Figure 4. MRCP images of MD-IPMN (left) and BD-IPMN (right).

6.2. EUS-FNA

This technique has been evolving, and more hospitals are incorporating it into their routine diagnostic tests, helping to introduce its more general application and obtaining information by:

- Describing sonographic characteristics: mural nodes and invasion.
- Performing pancreatic and cyst fluid analysis: cellularity, CEA determination and molecular markers KRAS with or without GNAS mutation, TP53, PIK3CA, p16/CDKN21, SMAD4, or PTEN mutation (28).

On the 2012 international consensus guidelines [28], certain recommendations were made as to when to use EUS-FNA:

- Pancreatic cysts with worrisome features.
- Pancreatic small cyst with worrisome features.
- >3 cm cysts with no worrisome features, especially if elderly patients to verify the findings.
- Distinction of BD-IPMN versus serous cyst neoplasm (SCN) with CEA determination.

Nonetheless, the more recent American Gastroenterological Association (AGA) guideline on the management of pancreatic cysts [29] issues a conditional recommendation: "pancreatic cysts with at least two high-risk features, such as size ≥3 cm, a dilated main pancreatic duct, or the presence of an associated solid component, should be examined with endoscopic ultrasonography with fine-needle aspiration (EUS-FNA)" (**Figure 5**).

Macroscopically, highly viscous fluid is the first clue that the cyst is mucinous cyst. Furthermore, high concentration of CEA reflects the presence of a mucinous epithelium, and it is elevated in both IPMNs and MCNs. Thus, it is quite beneficial to distinguish mucinous cysts from non-mucinous. A cut-off CEA level of 192 ng/mL has the sensitivity of 73%, specificity of 84%. Due to connectivity to the pancreatic ductal system, amylase level may be elevated in IPMNs.

In conclusion, the most recent papers encourage the use of EUS-FNA in the initial diagnostic tests [15, 30] to identify smaller cysts with high grade or invasive pathology [30] and to detect mural nodules otherwise missed on cross-sectional imaging or malignant cytology in lesions >3 cm. The high specificity and accuracy of EUS strongly position it as the optimum tool for diagnosing malignant BD-IPMNs, particularly in patients without worrisome features and with smaller cysts [31]. It is particularly important to consider that inherent risks can be derived from this test, including complications associated with these endoscopic procedures such as difficulty in cytological interpretation of samples and relatively low sensitivity [31].

6.2.1. Biomarkers

DNA analysis of pancreatic cyst fluid demonstrated that KRAS mutation is highly specific (96%) for mucinous cysts, but the sensitivity is only 45%. KRAS is an early oncogenic mutation in the adenoma-carcinoma sequence but cannot discriminate a benign from malignant mucinous cyst. A recent study [32] demonstrated that the "GNAS mutation

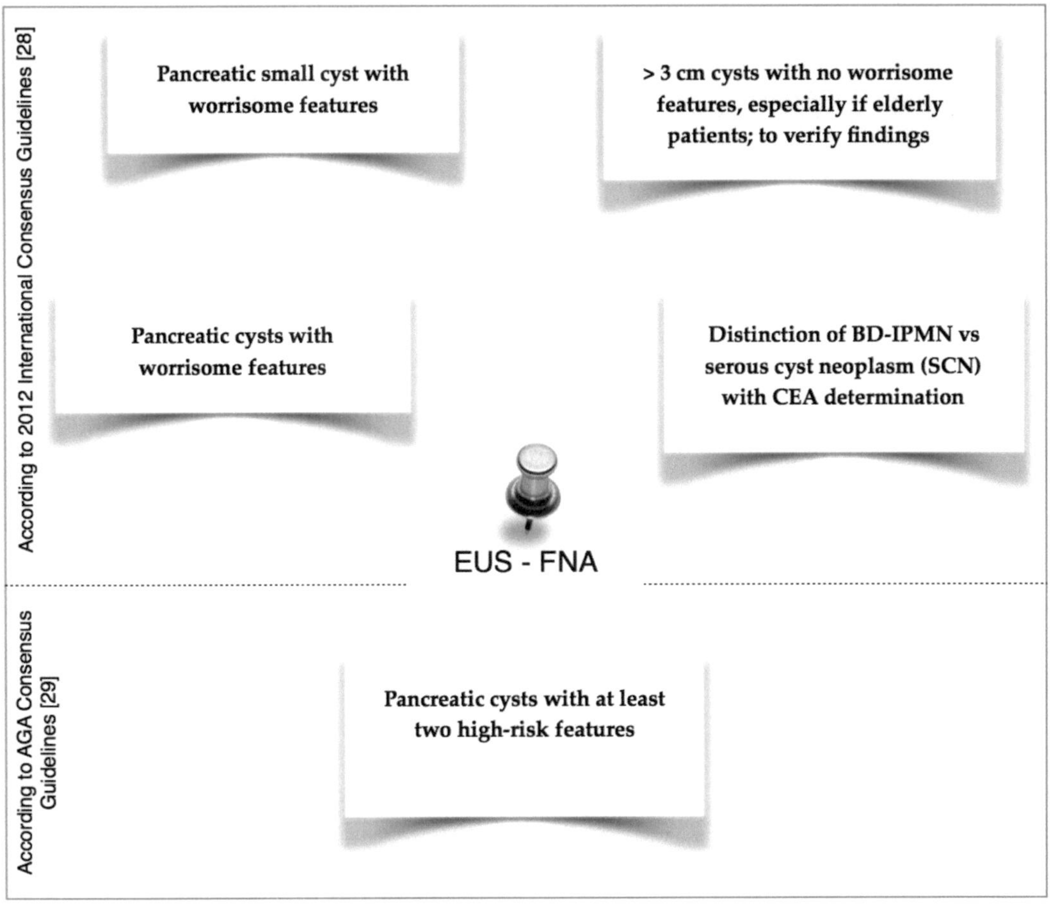

Figure 5. Use of EUS-FNA according to 2012 International Consensus Guidelines [28] and AGA Guidelines [29].

detected in cyst fluid can separate IPMN from MCN, but similar to KRAS mutations, it does not predict malignancy. The absence of a GNAS mutation also does not correlate with a diagnosis of MCN because not all IPMNs will demonstrate a GNAS mutation [33–35]. A GNAS mutation was present in 66% of IPMNs." But a recent mutations study in GNAS at codon 201 has been identified in duodenal fluid samples even before the IPMN lesion, which was identified on radiologic imaging [36]. Moreover, one study reports that 33% of incipient IPMNs analyzed have a GNAS mutation, suggesting that a large proportion of incipient IPMNs are part of the IPMN pathway, and these mutations occur early in this process [6, 37].

A recent study identified glucose and kynurenine to be differentially expressed between non-mucinous and mucinous pancreatic cysts [38]. Metabolic abundances for both were significantly lower in mucinous cysts compared with non-mucinous cysts. The clinical utility of these biomarkers will be addressed in future studies although it is clear that it will be of great utility when differentiating benign vs. malignant cysts.

6.3. Other procedures

6.3.1. ERCP

For sampling of fluid brushes in the 2012 International Consensus Guidelines for the management of IPMN, routine use of this test was not recommended and was left only for scientific purposes [28]. However, as professionals are becoming more familiarized with it and results are increasingly being more accurate, newer studies are encouraging cytology of the pancreatic juice and it is starting to be considered a reliable predictor of malignancy in IPMN [39]. Cytological examination alone is often non-diagnostic due to the low cellularity of the aspirated fluid. A positive or negative diagnosis can be obtained through a cytology analyses with a 100% specificity. Moreover, if a high-grade epithelial atypia is found in the cyst fluid, it is correlated with an 80% chance of malignancy [40].

6.3.2. PET scan

Positron emission tomography has been proposed as a useful technique for diagnosing and staging different malignancies. Several studies have investigated the outcomes in IPMN cases, concluding that dual-phase F-18 fluorodeoxyglucose positron emission tomography with computed tomography (FDG-PET/CT) has an overall specificity of 92–95% and a sensitivity of 88–94% when trying to differentiate malignant IPMNs vs. benign lesions. It has been proposed that PET scans should be performed in older patients, cases at increased surgical risk, or when the feasibility of parenchyma-sparing surgery demands a reliable preoperative exclusion of malignancy [41, 42].

7. Management

To date, three consensus guidelines have been proposed to manage pancreatic cystic lesions beginning with the original 2006 Sendai guideline, which was revised in 2012 by the International Association of Pancreatology (IAP) in Fukuoka, and the recent AGA guideline [43–45].

All guides agree that due to the higher risk of malignancy, all symptomatic cysts should be further evaluated or resected, depending on the clinical circumstances.

Invasive carcinoma in patients with asymptomatic cysts is very rare, especially in cysts <10 mm. In such cases, no further work-up will be needed; however, follow-up is still recommended [43–46]. For better characterization of the lesions, pancreatic protocol CT or gadolinium-enhanced MRI with magnetic resonance cholangiopancreatography (MRCP) is recommended for cysts >10 mm [47]. The most recent consensus among radiologists [10] suggests that MRI is preferable for evaluating cysts due to its high-contrast resolution, the identification of septum, nodules, and duct communications. Also, MRI is the preferable follow-up test because it avoids excessive exposure to radiation [47].

According to Fukuoka guidelines (1), there are:

- **"Worrisome features"**:
  - Cyst of ≤3 cm.
  - Thickened enhanced cyst walls.
  - MPD of 5–9 mm.
  - Non-enhanced mural nodules.
  - Abrupt change in the MPD caliber with distal pancreatic atrophy.
  - Lymphadenopathy.
- **"High-risk stigmata":**
  - Obstructive jaundice in a patient with a cystic lesion of the pancreatic head.
  - Enhanced solid component, MPD size of 10 mm.

All patients with cysts of 3 cm in size without "worrisome features" should undergo surveillance according the size stratification. Patients with cysts of >3 cm and no "worrisome features" can also be considered for EUS to verify the absence of thickened walls or mural nodules, particularly if the patient is elderly. All smaller cysts with "worrisome features" should be evaluated by EUS to further risk stratify the lesion [48].

7.1. Surgery

If surgery is considered for a pancreatic cyst, patients are referred to a center with demonstrated expertise in pancreatic surgery. Surgery is the only treatment option in patients with IPMN of the pancreas with high-grade dysplasia or IPMNs that have progressed to invasive carcinoma (**Figure 6**).

7.1.1. Indications

- High-grade dysplasia or Invasive carcinoma.
- High-risk stigmata + positive cytology.
- High-risk stigmata confirmed by MRI and EUS.
- Symptomatic cyst.
- Younger patients with cyst >2 cm owing to cumulative risk.

Positive cytology on EUS-guided FNA has the highest specificity for diagnosing malignancy. If there is a combination of high-risk features on imaging, then this is likely to increase the

http://dx.doi.org/10.5772/66491

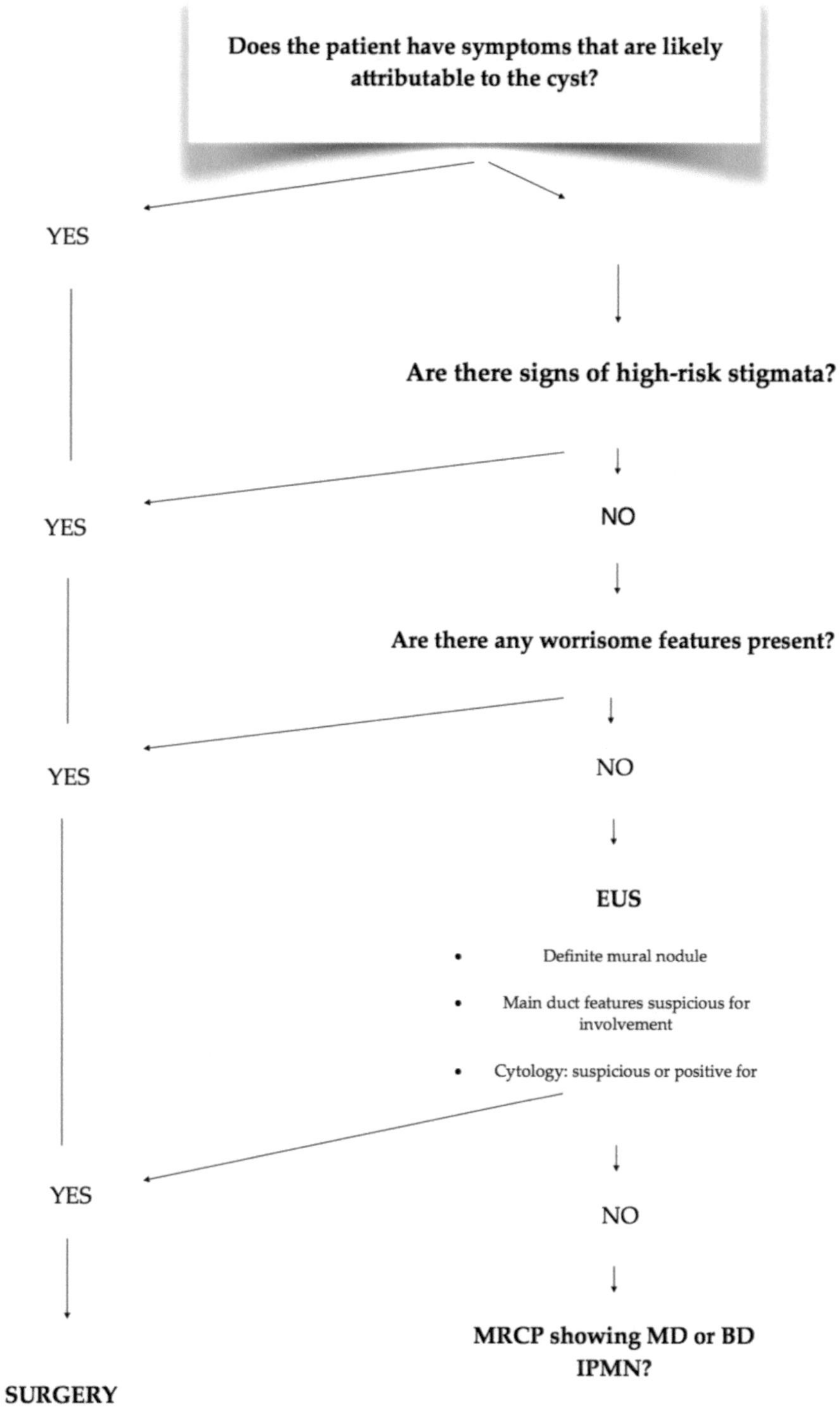

Figure 6. Proposed algorithm for surgery indications in IPMNs.

risk of malignancy. Even in the face of a negative cytology, if EUS and MRI confirm high-risk stigmata, the specificity is likely to be high. However, no currently available data can demonstrate the impact of multiple high-risk features. Molecular techniques to evaluate pancreatic cysts remain an emerging area of research [23, 49, 50], but had the benefits of surgery outweigh the risks in this selected population [51].

The most important aspect of resection is to achieve complete removal of a tumor with a negative margin. If a positive margin is found in a high-grade dysplasia, additional resection of the pancreas should be performed. However, there is no consensus regarding further resection in the case of a low- or moderate-grade dysplasia [51, 52].

Total pancreatectomy should be contemplated only in younger patients who can manage the comorbidities related to diabetes and exocrine insufficiency or in patients with a history of diabetes [53, 54]. The choice of surgery will be determined by the location of the tumor and the extent of involvement of the gland. It is not clearly established that multifocality corresponds to a higher risk of invasive cancer; in most cases with more than one lesion, the dominant or concerning lesions are resected; and the others are observed with follow-up imaging [1].

Regarding the BD-IPMN that occurs in elderly patients, the annual malignancy rate is only 2–3%. These factors support a conservative management with follow-up in patients who do not have risk factors predicting malignancy. Younger patients (<65 years) with a cyst size of >2 cm may be candidates for resection owing to the cumulative risk of malignancy [27]. BD-IPMN of >3 cm without these signs can be observed without immediate resection, particularly in elderly patients. The decision needs to be individualized and to depend not only on the risk of malignancy but also on the patient's conditions and cyst location [51].

7.2. Adjuvant therapy

It has not yet been determined whether or not to offer postresection adjuvant therapy to patients with IPMNs that have progressed to invasive carcinoma; it also undefined as to the optimal strategy for postoperative therapy (chemoradiotherapy versus chemotherapy alone) remains undefined [55]. A recent study by McMillan et al. [56] suggests that patients classified as AJCC stage II through IV, presenting with positive lymph nodes, positive resection margins or poorly differentiated tumors, may benefit from adjuvant chemoradiotherapy over chemotherapy alone in terms of overall survival, except for patients who had AJCC pathologic stage II disease.

8. Follow-up

The AGA recommends discussing the risks and benefits of a management strategy with the patient as a good clinical practice for nearly all diseases and interventions. Patients need to receive a full explanation of all therapeutical options so they can choose the best treatment in accordance with the most recent guidelines. Patients who have a limited life expectancy do not derive any benefit from surveillance, because it is inappropriate for patients who are not surgical candidates due to severe comorbidities.

http://dx.doi.org/10.5772/66491

The Fukuoka consensus has high sensitivity of the diagnosis of IPMN and prediction of malignancy [57], although the cyst size from the "high-risk stigmata" to "worrisome features" is still a matter of controversy [57–60]. A systematic review of the literature suggests that size >3 cm increased the risk of malignancy by approximately 3 times and the presence of a solid component increased the risk of malignancy approximately eight times [58].

8.1. MD-IPMN

The management depends on the degree of ductal dilation, ≥10 mm, if the duct is (**Figure 7**)

- **≥10 mm in diameter:** resection of MD-IPMN is recommended for patients who have good performance status with reasonable life expectancy. This recommendation is based on the high rate of malignancy in MD-IPMN [28].
- **5–9 mm:** we need additional evaluation with EUS and fine-needle aspiration. Surgery is then indicated if there is evidence of worrisome features. But the association of malig-

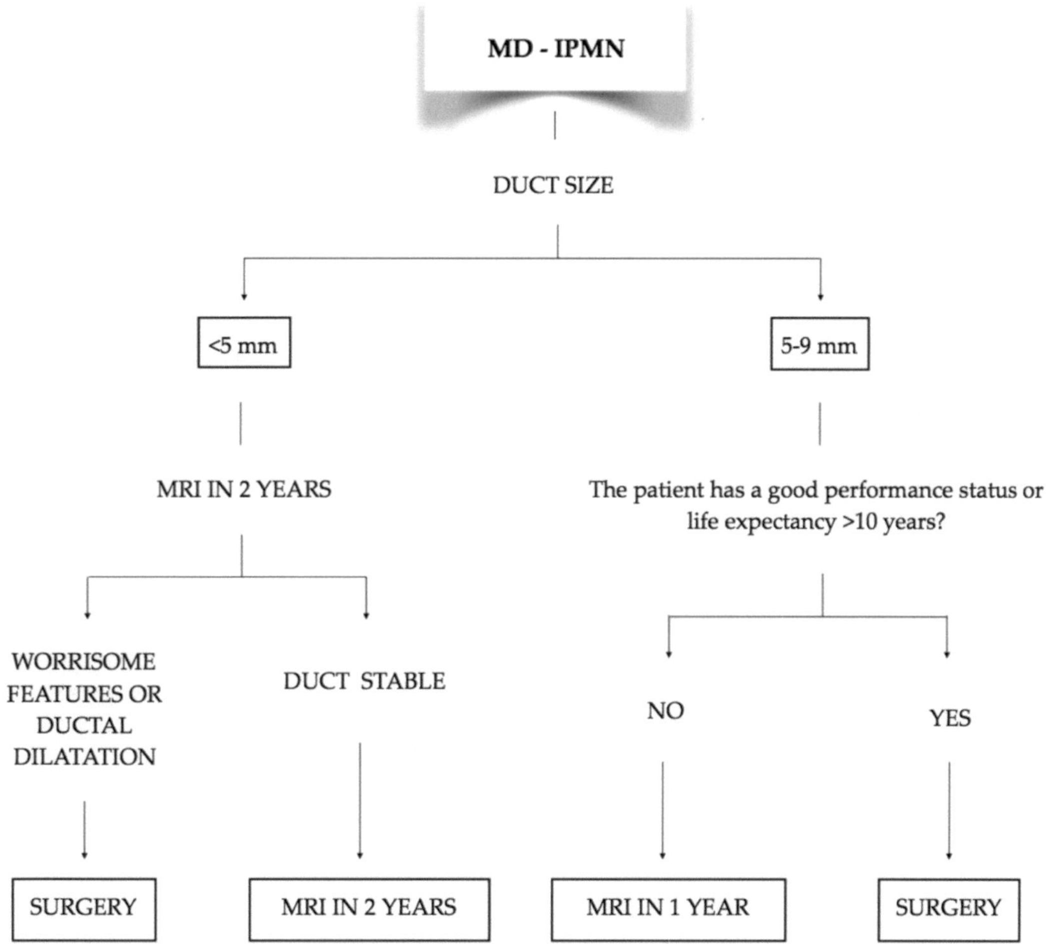

Figure 7. Follow-up for MD-IPMN <10 mm.

nancy with this degree of pancreatic duct dilation has not been well characterized. If the patient has a longer life expectancy, up to 10 years, he should be operated. For patients not undergoing surgery, we perform a magnetic retrograde cholangiopancreatography (MRCP) a year later. Surgery should be considered if the duct increases in size or if intramural nodules develop. If the duct is stable, we should repeat imaging every 2 years and continue it as long as the patient is a good surgical candidate.

- **<5 mm:** follow-up with MRCP in 2 years. As with other IPMNs, surgery is indicated if the duct increases in size or if intramural nodules develop. If the duct is stable on repeat imaging, we lengthen the surveillance interval to every 2–3 years and continue surveillance as long as the patient remains a good surgical candidate.

8.2. BD-IPMN

Resection is generally indicated if there are high-risk stigmata and if patient has symptoms attributable to the IPMN. Besides, surgery is indicated if there is evidence of worrisome features or positive cytology. We must always take into account the patient's age, life expectancy, and performance status [28] (**Figure 8**)

- **≥30 mm:** repeat MRCP in 1 year. If the IPMN is stable, continue surveillance with MRCP every 2 years.
- **10–30 mm:** repeat MRCP in 1 year. If the IPMN is stable, continue surveillance with MRCP every 2 years. After 5 years, the surveillance interval can be lengthened to every 3 years.
- **<10 mm:** repeat in 1 year. If the IPMN is stable, continue surveillance with MRCP every 2 years. After 5 years, surveillance can be discontinued.

Follow-up is made if the patient is a good surgical candidate. If, during surveillance, there are changes in the IPMN, a EUS-FNA should be performed.

MRI is the preferred surveillance imaging modality over computed tomography. The length of surveillance for IPMN is another concern for every clinician. If there is no change in size or characteristics, the AGA suggests that patients without worrisome pancreatic features undergo MRI for surveillance in 1 year and then every 2 years after, for a total of 5 years. The review of the literature suggests that the risk of malignant transformation of pancreatic cysts is approximately 0.24% per year. The risk of cancer in cysts without a significant change over a 5-year period is lower but this recommendation has very low evidence quality. Therefore, more studies are needed [45]. In addition, the Fukuoka consensus suggests for BD-IPMN follow-up: yearly follow-up if lesion is <10 mm in size, 6–12 monthly follow-up for lesions between 10 and 20 mm, and 3–6 monthly follow-up for lesions >20 mm [28]. The optimal surveillance approach, however, remains unclear.

8.3. Combined main duct and branch duct IPMN

Each lesion is managed, as it would be if it were the only lesion.

http://dx.doi.org/10.5772/66491

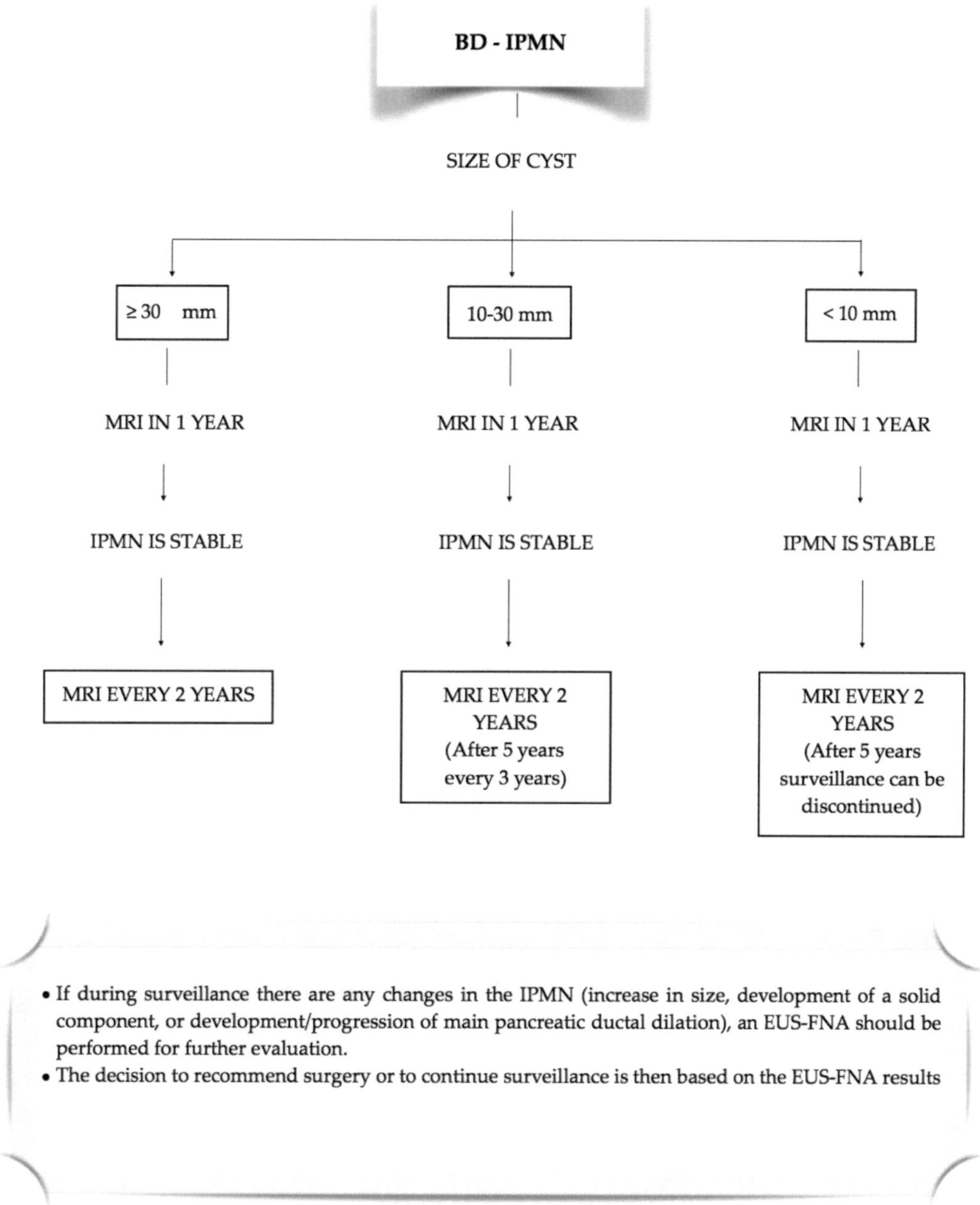

Figure 8. Follow-up algorithm for BD-IPMN.

8.3.1. Surveillance following surgery

- Noninvasive IPMN: the risk of developing a recurrence in the remaining pancreas is at least 5%. So we have to perform the follow-up with MRCP by including a lengthening in the surveillance interval if no changes are detected after several years. If there is another nonresected IPMN, follow-up should continue as stated above [23, 61].

- Invasive carcinoma: studies say that the risk of IPMN recurrence is 25–50% [62], and it recommended surveillance every 6 months [28]. If we diagnose patients, a recurrence of IPMN will need EUS for evaluation.

Acknowledgements

We would like to recognize the work of Doreen Carroll helping with the reviewing and editing of the article, and Dr. Lidia Alcalá Mata for the help obtaining MRCP images.

Author details

Natalia Zambudio Carroll[1*], Betsabé Reyes[2] and Laureano Vázquez[1]

*Address all correspondence to: nataliazambudio@gmail.com

1 Department of Surgery, Hospital San Agustín, Linares, Spain

2 Department of Surgery, Hospital Nuestra Señora de la Candelaria, Tenerife, Spain

References

[1] Tanaka M, Fernández-del Castillo C, Adsay V, Chari S, Falconi M, Jang J-Y, et al. International consensus guidelines 2012 for the management of IPMN and MCN of the pancreas. Pancreatology. 2012:12(3):183–97.

[2] Kobari M, Egawa S, Shibuya K, et al. Intraductal papillary mucinous tumors of the pancreas comprise 2 clinical subtypes: Differences in clinical characteristics and surgical management. Arch Surg. 1999 Oct 1;134(10):1131–6.

[3] Terris B, Ponsot P, Paye F, Hammel P, Sauvanet A, Molas G, et al. Intraductal papillary mucinous tumors of the pancreas confined to secondary ducts show less aggressive pathologic features as compared with those involving the main pancreatic duct. Am J Surg Pathol [Internet]. 2000;24(10):1374–1375.

[4] Furukawa T, Hatori T, Fujita I, Yamamoto M, Kobayashi M, Ohike N, et al. Prognostic relevance of morphological types of intraductal papillary mucinous neoplasms of the pancreas. Gut. 2011 Apr 1;60(4):509–16.

[5] Grützmann R, Post S, Saeger HD, Niedergethmann M. Intraductal papillary mucinous neoplasia (IPMN) of the pancreas: its diagnosis, treatment, and prognosis. Dtsch Ärztebl Int. 2011 Nov;108(46):788–94.

[6] Farrell JJ. Prevalence, diagnosis and management of pancreatic cystic neoplasms: current status and future directions. Gut Liver. 2015 Sep;9(5):571–89.

[7] Shi C, Hruban RH. Intraductal papillary mucinous neoplasm. Hum Pathol. 2012;43(1):1–16.

[8] Gardner TB, Glass LM, Smith KD, Ripple GH, Barth RJ, Klibansky DA, et al. Pancreatic cyst prevalence and the risk of mucin-producing adenocarcinoma in United States adults. Am J Gastroenterol. 2013 Oct;108(10):1546–50.

[9] Nagata N, Kawazoe A, Mishima S, Wada T, Shimbo T, Sekine K, et al. Development of pancreatic cancer, disease-specific mortality, and all-cause mortality in patients with nonresected IPMNs: a long-term cohort study. Radiology. 2015 Jul 13;278(1):125–34.

[10] Tanaka M. International consensus on the management of intraductal papillary mucinous neoplasm of the pancreas. Ann Transl Med. 2015 Nov 3(19):286.

[11] Yamada S, Fujii T, Murotani K, Kanda M, Sugimoto H, Nakayama G, et al. Comparison of the international consensus guidelines for predicting malignancy in intraductal papillary mucinous neoplasms. Surgery. 2016 Mar;159(3):878–84.

[12] Goh BKP, Lin Z, Tan DMY, Thng C-H, Khor CJL, Lim TKH, et al. Evaluation of the fukuoka consensus guidelines for intraductal papillary mucinous neoplasms of the pancreas: results from a systematic review of 1,382 surgically resected patients. Surgery. 2015 Nov;158(5):1192–202.

[13] Fritz S, Buchler M, Klauss M, Bergmann F, Strobel O. Pancreatic main-duct involvement in branch-duct IPMNs: an underestimated risk. Ann Surg. 2014 Nov;260(5):848–56.

[14] Crippa S, Capurso G, Cammà C, Fave GD, Castillo CF, Falconi M. Risk of pancreatic malignancy and mortality in branch-duct IPMNs undergoing surveillance: a systematic review and meta-analysis. Dig Liver Dis. 2016 May;48(5):473–9.

[15] Han DH, Lee H, Park JY, Kwon W, Heo JS, Choi SH, et al. Validation of international consensus guideline 2012 for intraductal papillary mucinous neoplasm of pancreas. Ann Surg Treat Res. 2016 Mar;90(3):124–30.

[16] Sugiyama M, Atomi Y. Extrapancreatic neoplasms occur with unusual frequency in patients with intraductal papillary mucinous tumors of the pancreas. Am J Gastroenterol. 1999 Feb;94(2):470–3.

[17] Choi M, Kim S, Han S, Jang J. High incidence of extrapancreatic neoplasms in patients with intraductal papillary mucinous neoplasms. Arch Surg. 2006 Jan;141(1):51–6.

[18] Brugge WR. Diagnosis and management of cystic lesions of the pancreas. J Gastrointest Oncol. 2015 Aug;6(4):375–88.

[19] Farrell JJ, Brugge WR. Intraductal papillary mucinous tumor of the pancreas. Gastrointest Endosc. 2002 May;55(6):701–14.

[20] Sahani DV, Lin DJ, Venkatesan AM, Sainani N, Mino-Kenudson M, Brugge WR, et al. Multidisciplinary approach to diagnosis and management of intraductal papillary mucinous neoplasms of the pancreas. Clin Gastroenterol Hepatol. 2009 Mar;7(3):259–69.

[21] Yoon WJ, Brugge WR. Pancreatic cystic neoplasms: diagnosis and management. Mod Manag Benign Malig Pancreat Dis. 2012 Mar;41(1):103–18.

[22] Brugge WR, Lauwers GY, Sahani D, Fernandez-del Castillo C, Warshaw AL. Cystic neoplasms of the pancreas. N Engl J Med. 2004 Sep 16;351(12):1218–26.

[23] Salvia R, Castillo CF, Bassi C, Thayer SP, Falconi M, Mantovani W, et al. Main-duct intraductal papillary mucinous neoplasms of the pancreas: clinical predictors of malignancy and long-term survival following resection. Ann Surg. 2004 May;239(5):678–87.

[24] Sohn TA, Yeo CJ, Cameron JL, Hruban RH, Fukushima N, Campbell KA, et al. Intraductal papillary mucinous neoplasms of the pancreas: an updated experience. Ann Surg. 2004 Jun;239(6):788–99.

[25] Capurso G, Boccia S, Salvia R, Del Chiaro M, Frulloni L, Arcidiacono PG, et al. Risk factors for intraductal papillary mucinous neoplasm (IPMN) of the pancreas: a multicentre case-control study. Am J Gastroenterol. 2013 Jun;108(6):1003–9.

[26] Roch AM, Rosati CM, Cioffi JL, Ceppa EP, DeWitt JM, Al-Haddad MA, et al. Intraductal papillary mucinous neoplasm of the pancreas, one manifestation of a more systemic disease? Am J Surg. 2016 Mar;211(3):512–8.

[27] Weinberg BM, Spiegel BM, Tomlinson JS, Farrell JJ. Asymptomatic pancreatic cyst neoplasms: maximizing survival and quality of life using markov-based clinical nomograms. Gastroenterology. 2010 Feb;138(2):531–40.

[28] Tanaka M, Fernández-del Castillo C, Adsay V, Chari S, Jang J-Y, Kimura W, et al. International consensus guidelines 2012 for the management of IPMN and MCN of the pancreas. Pancreatology. 2012;12:183–97.

[29] American Gastroenterological Association Institute Guideline on the Diagnosis and Management of Asymptomatic Neoplastic Pancreatic Cysts. Vege V, Ziring B, Jain R, et al. Gastroenterology 2015;148:819–822

[30] Nguyen AH, Toste PA, Farrell JJ, Clerkin BM, Williams J, Muthusamy VR, et al. Current recommendations for surveillance and surgery of intraductal papillary mucinous neoplasms may overlook some patients with cancer. J Gastrointest Surg Off J Soc Surg Aliment Tract. 2015 Feb;19(2):258–65.

[31] Ridtitid W, DeWi JM, Schmidt CM, Roch A, Stuart JS, Sherman S, et al. Management of branch-duct intraductal papillary mucinous neoplasms: a large single-center study to assess predictors of malignancy and long-term outcomes. Gastrointest Endosc. 2016 Sep;84(3):436–45

[32] Michaels PJ, Brachtel EF, Bounds BC, Brugge WR, Bishop Pitman M. Intraductal papillary mucinous neoplasm of the pancreas. Cancer Cytopathol. 2006 Jun 25;108(3):163–73.

[33] Pitman MB, Centeno BA, Daglilar ES, Brugge WR, Mino-Kenudson M. Cytological criteria of high-grade epithelial atypia in the cyst fluid of pancreatic intraductal papillary mucinous neoplasms. Cancer Cytopathol. 2014 Jan 1;122(1):40–7.

[34] Molin MD, Matthaei H, Wu J, Blackford A, Debeljak M, Rezaee N, et al. Clinicopathological correlates of activating GNAS mutations in intraductal papillary mucinous neoplasm (IPMN) of the pancreas. Ann Surg Oncol. 2013 Nov;20(12):3802–8.

[35] Sahora K, Castillo CF. Intraductal papillary mucinous neoplasms. Curr Opin Gastroenterol. 2015 Sep;31(5):424–9.

[36] Kanda M, Sadakari Y, Borges M, Topazian M, Farrell J, Syngal S, et al. Mutant TP53 in duodenal samples of pancreatic juice from patients with pancreatic cancer or high-grade dysplasia. Clin Gastroenterol Hepatol Off Clin Pract J Am Gastroenterol Assoc. 2013 Jun;11(6):719–30.e5.

[37] Matthaei H, Wu J, dal Molin M, Shi C, Perner S, Kristiansen G, et al. GNAS sequencing identifies IPMN-specific mutations in a subgroup of diminutive pancreatic cysts referred to as "incipient IPMNs." Am J Surg Pathol. 2014 Mar;38(3):360–3.

[38] Sakorafas GH, Smyrniotis V, Reid-Lombardo KM, Sarr MG. Primary pancreatic cystic neoplasms revisited. Part III. Intraductal papillary mucinous neoplasms. Surg Oncol. 2011 Jun;20(2):e109–18.

[39] Hara T, Ikebe D, Odaka A, Sudo K, Nakamura K, Yamamoto H, et al. Preoperative histological subtype classification of intraductal papillary mucinous neoplasms (IPMN) by pancreatic juice cytology with MUC stain. Ann Surg. 2013;257(6):1103–11.

[40] Kang MJ, Lee KB, Jang J-Y, Kwon W, Park JW, Chang YR, et al. Disease spectrum of intraductal papillary mucinous neoplasm with an associated invasive carcinoma: invasive IPMN versus pancreatic ductal adenocarcinoma-associated IPMN. Pancreas. 2013 Nov;42(8):1267–74.

[41] Saito M, Ishihara T, Tada M, Tsuyuguchi T, Mikata R, Sakai Y, et al. Use of F-18 fluorodeoxyglucose positron emission tomography with dual-phase imaging to identify intraductal papillary mucinous neoplasm. Clin Gastroenterol Hepatol. 2013 Feb;11(2):181–6.

[42] Sperti C, Pasquali C, Chierichetti F, Liessi G, Ferlin G, Pedrazzoli S. Value of 18-fluorodeoxyglucose positron emission tomography in the management of patients with cystic tumors of the pancreas. Ann Surg. 2001 Nov;234(5):675–80.

[43] Fernández-del Castillo C, Targarona J, Thayer SP, Rattner DW, Brugge WR, Warshaw AL. Incidental pancreatic cysts: clinicopathologic characteristics and comparison with symptomatic patients. Arch Surg. 1960. 2003 Apr;138(4):427–34.

[44] Tanaka M, Chari S, Adsay V, Carlos Castillo F-D, Falconi M, Shimizu M, et al. International consensus guidelines for management of intraductal papillary mucinous neoplasms and mucinous cystic neoplasms of the pancreas. Pancreatology. 2006;6(1–2):17–32.

[45] Vege SS, Ziring B, Jain R, Moayyedi P, Adams MA, Dorn SD, et al. American Gastroenterological Association Institute guideline on the diagnosis and management of asymptomatic neoplastic pancreatic cysts. Gastroenterology. 2015 Apr;148(4):819–22.

[46] Das A, Wells CD, Nguyen CC. Incidental cystic neoplasms of pancreas: what is the optimal interval of imaging surveillance [quest]. Am J Gastroenterol. 2008 Jul;103(7):1657–62.

[47] Berland LL, Silverman SG, Gore RM, Mayo-Smith WW, Megibow AJ, Yee J, et al. Managing incidental findings on abdominal CT: White Paper of the ACR Incidental Findings Committee. J Am Coll Radiol. 2010 Oct;7(10):754–73.

[48] Tanaka M. Controversies in the management of pancreatic IPMN. Nat Rev Gastroenterol Hepatol. 2011 Jan;8(1):56–60.

[49] Hwang DW, Jang J-Y, Lee SE, Lim C-S, Lee KU, Kim S-W. Clinicopathologic analysis of surgically proven intraductal papillary mucinous neoplasms of the pancreas in SNUH: a 15-year experience at a single academic institution. Langenbecks Arch Surg. 2012;397(1):93–102.

[50] Sugiyama M, Izumisato Y, Abe N, Masaki T, Mori T, Atomi Y. Predictive factors for malignancy in intraductal papillary-mucinous tumours of the pancreas. Br J Surg. 2003 Oct 1;90(10):1244–9.

[51] Scheiman JM, Hwang JH, Moayyedi P. American Gastroenterological Association technical review on the diagnosis and management of asymptomatic neoplastic pancreatic cysts. Gastroenterology. 148(4):824–48.e22.

[52] Jang J-Y, Kim S-W, Ahn YJ, Yoon Y-S, Choi MG, Lee KU, et al. Multicenter analysis of clinicopathologic features of intraductal papillary mucinous tumor of the pancreas: is it possible to predict the malignancy before surgery? Ann Surg Oncol. 2005;12(2):124–32.

[53] Crippa S, Tamburrino D, Partelli S, Salvia R, Germenia S, Bassi C, et al. Total pancreatectomy: indications, different timing, and perioperative and long-term outcomes. Surgery. 2011 Jan;149(1):79–86.

[54] Stauffer JA, Nguyen JH, Heckman MG, Grewal MS, Dougherty M, Gill KRS, et al. Patient outcomes after total pancreatectomy: a single centre contemporary experience. HPB. 2009 Sep;11(6):483–92.

[55] Swartz MJ, Hsu CC, Pawlik TM, Winter J, Hruban RH, Guler M, et al. Adjuvant chemoradiotherapy after pancreatic resection for invasive carcinoma associated with intraductal papillary mucinous neoplasm of the pancreas. Int J Radiat Oncol Biol Phys. 2010 Mar 1;76(3):839–44.

[56] McMillan MT, Lewis RS, Drebin JA, Teitelbaum UR, Lee MK, Roses RE, et al. The efficacy of adjuvant therapy for pancreatic invasive intraductal papillary mucinous neoplasm (IPMN). Cancer. 2016 Feb 15;122(4):521–33.

[57] Kim, Kyung Won KW. Imaging features to distinguish malignant and benign branch-duct type intraductal papillary mucinous neoplasms of the pancreas: a meta-analysis. Ann Surg. 2014 Jan;259(1):72–81.

[58] Anand N, Sampath K, Wu BU. Cyst features and risk of malignancy in intraductal papillary mucinous neoplasms of the pancreas: a meta-analysis. Clin Gastroenterol Hepatol. 2013 Aug;11(8):913–21.

[59] Wong J, Weber J, A. Centeno B, Vignesh S, Harris CL, Klapman JB, et al. High-grade dysplasia and adenocarcinoma are frequent in side-branch intraductal papillary mucinous neoplasm measuring less than 3 cm on endoscopic ultrasound. J Gastrointest Surg. 2013;17(1):78–85.

[60] Nakata K, Ohuchida K, Aishima S, Sadakari Y, Kayashima T, Miyasaka Y, et al. Invasive carcinoma derived from intestinal-type intraductal papillary mucinous neoplasm is associated with minimal invasion, colloid carcinoma, and less invasive behavior, leading to a better prognosis. Pancreas 2011;40(4):581–7.

[61] Kang MJ, Jang J-Y, Lee KB, Chang YR, Kwon W, Kim S-W. Long-term prospective cohort study of patients undergoing pancreatectomy for intraductal papillary mucinous neoplasm of the pancreas: implications for postoperative surveillance. Ann Surg. 2014;260(2):356–63.

[62] Niedergethmann M, Grützmann R, Hildenbrand R, Dittert D, Aramin N, Franz M, et al. Outcome of invasive and noninvasive intraductal papillary-mucinous neoplasms of the pancreas (IPMN): a 10-year experience. World J Surg. 2008;32(10):2253–60.

Chapter 5

Management of Pancreatic Cystic Lesions

Vincenzo Neri

Additional information is available at the end of the chapter

http://dx.doi.org/10.5772/65117

Abstract

Objectives: In the last several decades, the knowledge of the cystic neoplasms has enlarged and the management has changed. The wide adoption in the diagnostic procedures of routine and advanced imaging has become the cornerstone of the diagnosis.

Methods: Pancreatic cystic tumors comprise neoplasms with a wide range of malignant potential. The most common include serous cystic neoplasm, mucinous cystic neoplasms (MCNs), intraductal papillary mucinous neoplasms (IPMNs), solid pseudopapillary neoplasms (SPPNs), and cystic pancreatic endocrine neoplasms (CPENs). Other cystic lesions are acute postnecrotic pseudocysts and chronic pseudocysts. Finally, the indeterminate cystic lesions have been presented.

Results: The epidemiology, pathological features, imaging characteristics, clinical evolution, and therapeutic choices of the most frequent lesions as well as less frequent forms are described. This study can be completed with the presentation of some cases of cystic pancreatic neoplasms treated in our service.

Conclusion: The improvement of imaging, endoscopic modalities, and cyst fluid studies allows now accurate and reliable diagnosis of pancreatic cystic lesions. Moreover, the enlarged knowledge of valuable pathological studies established the potential for malignant transformation of these lesions identifying higher-risk neoplasms. Finally, the management options should be based on the assessment of each type of cystic neoplasms and the distinction of pancreatic cystic neoplasms (PCNs) from other cystic lesions.

Keywords: cystic pancreatic lesions, pancreas, pseudocysts, pancreatitis, indeterminate pancreatic cystic lesions

1. Introduction

Cystic lesions of the pancreas are less frequent in relation to solid neoplasies. These lesions have attracted new and great interest. In the last several decades, the knowledge of the cystic neoplasms has enlarged and the management has changed dramatically. The wide adoption in the diagnostic procedures of routine and advanced imaging such as ultrasonography (US), computed tomography (CT), magnetic resonance imaging (MRI), magnetic resonance cholangiopancreatography (MRCP), and endoscopic ultrasound (EUS) has become the cornerstone of the diagnosis.

EUS-guided fine needle aspiration (FNA) can allow the assessment of tumor markers, chemistries, cytology, and DNA analysis. Also pathological study has played a very important role.

2. Classifications and epidemiology

The recent WHO classification 2010 of all pancreatic tumors is more extensively used. This classification encompasses epithelial tumors (benign, premalignant lesions, malignant lesions, and neuroendocrine neoplasms), mesenchymal tumors, lymphomas, and secondary tumors [1].

Based on pathological, clinical and radiologic assessments, some not recent but valuable [2], several classifications of cystic pancreatic neoplasms and lesions have been proposed. We believe interesting to note the proposed classification that fully includes all cystic lesions of the pancreas [3]. This classification includes the following cystic lesions: neoplastic epithelial (benign, borderline, and malignant), non-neoplastic epithelial, neoplastic non-epithelial (very rare), and non-epithelial non-neoplastic (very rare).

The frequency of each cystic lesions is not defined with precision, may be for observers diversity (surgeons, radiologists, and pathologists) and for the assessment of different developmental stages of lesions.

Pancreatic cystic tumors comprise a variety of neoplasms with a wide range of malignant potential: benign, borderline, and malignant. The classification proposed by Kosmahl encompasses the majority of the recently now described lesions (**Table 1**).

Many cystic neoplasms listed in the classifications are infrequent or rare pathological varieties, with minimal and not evident clinical characterization [4]. The simplified classification can be proposed that comprises two groups of lesions:

- Non-mucinous cystic lesions: inflammatory pseudocysts without a true epithelial lining (in the setting of acute and chronic pancreatitis), serous cystic neoplasms (SCNs), solid pseudopapillary neoplasms (SPPNs), and cystic pancreatic endocrine neoplasms (CPENs).
- Mucinous cystic lesions (epithelial lining produces mucinous cyst fluid): intraductal papillary mucinous neoplasms (IPMNs) and mucinous cystic neoplasms (MCNs).

http://dx.doi.org/10.5772/65117

Cystic epithelial tumors	**Non-neoplastic epithelial cysts**
Benign	Congenital cyst
Intraductal papillary mucinous adenoma	Lymphoepithelial cyst
Mucinous cystic adenoma	Retention cyst
Serous microcystic adenoma	
Serous oligocystic ill-demarcated adenoma	
von Hippel–Lindau-associated cystic neoplasm	
Benign cystic neuroendocrine tumors	
Acinar cell cystadenoma	
Cystic teratoma (dermoid cyst)	
Borderline	**Non-neoplastic non-epithelial cysts**
Intraductal papillary mucinous neoplasm borderline	Pancreatitis-associated pseudocysts
	Parasitic cysts
Mucinous cystic neoplasm borderline	
Solid pseudopapillary neoplasm	
Malignant	
Intraductal papillary mucinous carcinoma	
Mucinous cystic carcinoma	
Ductal cystic adenocarcinoma	
Serous cystadenocarcinoma	
Cystic non-epithelial tumors	
Lymphangioma	
Sarcomas	

Table 1. Classification of cystic neoplasms and lesions of pancreas [3].

This classification highlights as criterion of differentiation the presence of mucinous epithelium characterized by malignant potential.

Another criterion of classification of cystic lesions of pancreas is based on the epithelium lining of the cyst (**Table 2**).

In summary, the most common neoplasms include: serous cystic neoplasms (SCNs)/serous cystadenoma, mucinous cystic neoplasms (MCNs), intraductal papillary mucinous neoplasms (IPMNs), solid pseudopapillary neoplasms (SPPNs), and cystic pancreatic endocrine neoplasms (CPENs). There are others rare or very rare tumors: acinar cells cystadenoma, cystadenocarcinoma, cystic teratoma (dermoid cyst), and cystic pancreatoblastoma. Pancreatic cystic tumors are rare and less frequent than others pancreatic tumors. Image-based studies show prevalence of pancreatic cystic lesions ranging from 1.2 to 19% [6, 7].

No lining → Pseudocysts (pancreatitis associated)	
Lining	
Mucinous epithelium	
	MCNs
	IPMNs
Serous epithelium	
	SCNs
	VHL-associated pancreatic cysts
Squamous epithelium	
	Lymphoepithelial cysts
Acinar cells	
	Acinar cell cystadenocarcinomas
Endothelial lined cysts	
	Lymphangiomas
Degenerative necrotic changes in a neoplasm	
SPPNs	
CPENs	
Cystic ductal adenocarcinomas	

Table 2. Classification of cystic lesions of the pancreas [5].

In the autopsy series, the prevalence reaches 24% [8]. All cystic tumors of the pancreas reach about 10–15% of all cystic pancreatic lesions [7]. The exact prevalence of cystic pancreatic tumors is not defined. Autopsy study shows a prevalence of 24.3%; however, imaging studies have found the prevalence of 1.2–2.4%. On the other hand, pseudocystic lesions reach 90% of all pancreatic cystic lesions but only 45% of these patients had previous pancreatitis [6]. The economic impact that is necessary to follow these patients by imaging studies should be evaluated.

The epidemiologic and demographic features are different in the several types of cystic tumors, and they will be presented in specific sections.

3. Diagnostic perspectives and management options

The current use of imaging modalities has allowed some important results in the nosographic study: certain distinction between postnecrotic acute or chronic pseudocysts and cystic tumors; among the cystic neoplasms, the identification of clinical pathological features that allow recognizing some kinds of cystic tumors with several perspective of neoplastic evolution.

Cystic and intraductal mucinous neoplasms are pancreatic tumors of ductal origin and are characterized by cysts lined by mucinous epithelium.

Cystic tumors of the pancreas have the characteristic of precursor: they may be associated with or progress to invasive carcinoma. They are the preinvasive neoplasms, as the pancreatic intraepithelial neoplasms, but these tumors form clinically detectable masses, usually before that they become invasive, as the gastrointestinal adenoma. From these data, we take the therapeutic decision. A rough and summary monitoring of this setting clearly shows that cystic lesions are becoming increasingly more common, particularly among resection specimens. The reasons for this increase in frequency are various: important improvement in imaging techniques allows increased detention of clinically silent neoplasms; the majority of the cystic tumors are surgically removable because they are non-infiltrative in their evolution, and finally great decrease in postoperative complications and mortality rate of pancreatic surgery. The increased imaging and pathological studies and confirmation of all pancreatic cystic lesions result in better knowledge of these lesions.

A rough estimate of relative frequency of the pancreatic cystic lesions from the published data in the literature has been reported [5, 9]: pseudocysts (pancreatitis associated), 30%; IPMNs, 20%; MCNs, 10%; SCNs, 20%; acinar cell cystadenocarcinomas, lymphoepithelial cysts and lymphangiomas, <5%; SPPNs, <5%; cystic ductal adenomas, <5%; CPENs and metastasis, <5%.

The more simple classification of pancreatic cystic lesions subdivides two main classes: non-neoplastic cysts with pseudocysts non-lining and simple or congenital cysts, retention cysts that reach 80% of cases; neoplastic cysts or lining lesions that set up 20% of cases and can be defined pancreatic cystic neoplasms (PCNs) [7]. The main problem in the management of these lesions is the sure distinction between non-neoplastic cysts (pseudocysts, retention, and simple cysts) and pancreatic cystic neoplasms. Moreover, in the latter group, we need to distinguish non-mucinous from mucinous cysts that are considered being premalignant lesions. The therapeutic choices can be very different from simple follow-up to surgical resection. The WHO [1, 10] histological classification of tumors of exocrine pancreas and classification of pancreatic cystic lesions, integrated and updated by Kosmahl et al. [3] should be valuable references in the development of this subject. The specific epidemiology, histological features, imaging characteristics, clinical evolution, and therapeutic choices of the most frequent lesions as well as rare forms are described in each specific section.

4. Serous cystic neoplasms (SCNs)

SCNs can be divided into serous cystadenoma and serous cystadenocarcinoma. Serous cystadenoma is a benign neoplasm consisting of uniform glycogen-rich epithelial cells that give rise innumerable small cysts containing serous fluid. These lesions arise from centroacinar cell-intercalated duct system [11, 12], producing MUC6.

Histological and immunohistochemical data characterize the morphology and pathological evolution of serous cystadenoma. The cells lining the small cysts have clear cytoplasm with well-defined border and round uniform nuclei. They are negative for mucin stains; in these, lesions are not present the molecular genetic alterations, specific of mucinous-type ductal pancreatic neoplasia such as mutation in the K-ras, SMADH4/DPC4, TP53, and p16 genes [13]. In the pathogenesis of serous cystadenomas, the alterations of von Hippel-Lindau (VHL) gene have been demonstrated in 40% of cases [3]; therefore, serous cystadenomas are associated with von Hippel-Lindau syndrome, an autosomal dominant disorder, characterized by hemangioblastoma of central nervous system and retina, renal cysts and neoplasms, and phaeochromocytomas. The pancreatic cystic lesions in VHL syndrome usually develop earlier than central nervous system lesions.

The relative frequency of serous lesions into cystic pancreatic neoplasms ranges from 20 to 30%.

The SCNs occur predominantly in female patients (female/male ratio 3:1) of sixth–seventh decade. Almost 70% of SCNs occur in the body or tail of the pancreas and 30–40% of the patients are asymptomatic, and the lesions are detected incidentally. Symptomatic patients can present some trouble caused by size of the neoplasm such as abdominal pain, discomfort, malaise, anorexia, or objective signs as palpable mass, jaundice, and weight loss.

On imaging studies (CT or MRI), SCNs may present with two main morphologies: the more frequent, classic microcystic appearance and the less common oligocystic appearance.

Microcystic-type lesions present multiple small cysts, in one-third of cases with a central fibrous scar and calcification creating a sponge-like appearance, which can be considered pathognomonic. The size of the mass, much variable, ranges from few centimeters to 20–25 cm.

There are rare cases of oligocystic-type pattern (megacystic and macrocystic). This type consists of fewer and larger loculi, with lobulated contour without wall enhancement and usually is located in the pancreatic head [14]. The epithelial lining of these cysts may become denuded and can be difficult to distinguish from mucinous neoplasms. In this case, it can be useful to identify the characteristic glycogen-rich clear cells [15].

On EUS, the SCNs show multiple, small, anechoic cysts and thin septations. There is a vascular network on cyst wall. The aspirated cyst-fluid from EUS-FNA is low in CEA concentration, and the result of cytology is poor.

For SCNs, the risk of malignancy is <1%. SCNs with certain clinical diagnosis, little in size, from 2–2.5 to 4–5 cm, asymptomatic can be observed. The criteria of the control are based on increase of the size lesion and increase of the tumor markers (CEA). Beside the benign serous cystadenomas that are the majority of cases, there are also few malignant lesions, serous cystadenocarcinomas [16]. The structural histological findings are overlappable between serous cystadenoma and cystadenocarcinoma, and often only the metastatic potential should distinguish the malignant variants.

In the SCNs, the certainty of the preoperative diagnosis is most important for the therapeutic choice between non-operative management with follow-up and surgical treatment. Three criteria should be evaluated for surgery: likelihood of malignant evolution, symptoms caused by increase of the size of the tumor, and age of the patient.

Malignant SCNs constitute <3% of all SCNs [17], but within these cases, there are also serous cystadenocarcinomas not as evolution of benign tumors. Therefore, the global risk of malignancy of SCNs is <1% [18, 19].

A lot of the patients are asymptomatic at the diagnosis (incidental diagnosis). The likelihood of symptoms increases with the size of tumor. In fact, 22% of the patients is symptomatic with tumor <4 cm in diameter, but for tumor more than 4 cm, 77% of the patients becomes symptomatic [19].

The average age at the diagnosis frequently is 65 years or more.

The choice of treatment of SCNs can be summarized. We can consider several cases:

- old patients (>65 years), asymptomatic, size tumor <4 cm with pathognomonic imaging appearance should be observed;
- young patients (<65 years), asymptomatic, size tumor <4 cm with pathognomonic imaging appearance also should be observed;
- patients asymptomatic, size tumor >4 cm with pathognomonic imaging appearance could be observed (but the surgery can be discussed);
- patients symptomatic, size tumor >4 cm with pathognomonic imaging appearance should be proposed for surgery;
- cases with not complete diagnostic appearance or uncertain diagnosis should be proposed for surgical treatment.

In summary, surgical indications for SCNs with certain diagnosis (imaging, fluid cyst evaluation, etc.) are based on serious symptoms, great size tumors, or great increase of the size tumor in patient diagnosed and followed over time and increase of tumor marker (CEA) in fluid cyst [20].

5. Mucinous cystic neoplasms (MCNs)

These are the most frequent cystic pancreatic neoplasms. They amount for 20–40% of all cystic tumors with the prevalence of 25–30% for mucinous cystadenoma and 15% for mucinous cystadenocarcinoma.

There are two types of MCNs, both not communicate with the pancreatic duct. The cysts are lined by columnar, mucin-producing ductal epithelium and sometimes papillary epithelium. In the first type, ovarian-type stroma is located under the epithelial layer; the ovarian-type stroma is positive to estrogen and progesterone receptors [6]. Ectopic ovarian stroma can be included in the pancreas during embryogenesis and this can cause, by releasing hormones, the proliferation of epithelium and then the cystic neoplasm. This hypothesis that connects the stromal component of MCNs and ovarian tissue should be supported by morphological resemblance. This type is present almost exclusively in women of fifth–sixth decade and predominantly is located in body and tail of pancreas.

There is another type of MCNs, more common, without ovarian stroma that can be located anywhere in the pancreas and occurs in both sexes. The malignant potential is very high in MCNs based on the possible evolution of mucinous transitional epithelium. Consequently, MCNs may be classified based on the degree of dysplasia: MCNs with low-intermediate grade dysplasia, with high-grade dysplasia, and finally with associated invasive carcinoma [14]. Histological heterogeneity of MCNs is in evidence with coexistence of benign appearance and malignant epithelia. Malignancy, *in situ* or invasive, is found in 35–45% of cases [21].

The macroscopic appearance of MCNs is cystic mass, unilocular or multilocular, containing thick mucine or sometimes mixed with hemorrhagic materials. The cystic wall is well defined, fibrous, and sometimes (10%) calcified.

Clinical appearance in the symptomatic patients presents abdominal pain, palpable mass, anorexia, fatigue, weight loss, and in some cases pancreatitis. The results of routine laboratory examinations are generally non-specific. One-third of patient can be asymptomatic [22]. Imaging examinations (CT and MRI) of MCNs show large cysts with septae and in some cases peripheral thin calcification of the walls. In some experiences, the presence of peripheral calcification, wall thickening, and thick septation has been highlighted as important for malignant evolution of MCNs [23]. Overlappable data can be detected by EUS: mass formed from fluid-filled cysts with thin walls, septae, and diameter 1–2 cm without duct communication. Malignancy suspicious can be based on wall thickening, irregularity, intracystic solid mass, and increased size of all lesion.

EUS-FNA can allow the evaluation of fluid content of cysts: CEA levels are high and can be useful in the diagnosis [6]. Pathological and evolutionary characteristic of MCNs affect treatment decisions. Malignant potential of these neoplasms is the cornerstone of the therapy. Relevant is the increase in the frequency of K-ras and p53 mutations as in sequence adenoma–carcinoma of colon cancer. Consequently, there is high likelihood of evolution into cancer if untreated. In fact, there is age difference of 10 years longer between patients with cystadenocarcinoma and patients with cystadenoma [24, 25]. Based on the pathological characteristics of histologic heterogeneity, extensive histologic sampling is necessary for certainty of diagnosis (from adenoma to carcinoma). The current and unanimous guidelines propose the surgical treatment for all MCNs. The contraindications for intervention are related to the patient's conditions. The pancreatic resection is connected with the location of lesion: head, body, and tail. Duodenopancreatectomy, middle pancreatectomy, and distal pancreatectomy with or without splenectomy should be performed. Less extensive resections, such as enucleations are not recommended also because usually followed by high complications rate. Laparoscopic approaches are becoming more common and fully justified.

Cure rate of surgical resection for non-invasive MCNs (carcinoma *in situ*) is 100%. The 5-year survival rate for resected patients with invasive lesions is 40–50%; whereas the 2-year survival rate is 60–70%. Surveillance after surgery in these patients is required.

6. Intraductal papillary mucinous neoplasms (IPMNs)

The incidence of IPMNs is not well defined. In the recent years, their detection is increased based on the technical improvement of imaging examinations and the better knowledge of pathological features. Some data from the literature report that incidence range from 20 to 50% of all pancreatic cystic neoplasms [6, 26, 27]. Tumor arises from epithelium of the main pancreatic duct or its side branches. The lesions are lined by the intraductal proliferations of ductal columnar mucin-secreting epithelium with papillary projections that cause obstruction and dilatation of the duct. Tumors localized in the main pancreatic duct can spread in the rest of the duct. Men and women are equally affected. The neoplasm can be located anywhere in the pancreas. The most frequent localization of lesion is in the head of the gland and in 20–30% of cases can be multifocal. In 5–10% of cases, the pancreas can be diffusely interested [26, 27]. There are two varieties of this neoplasm, following its localization: main duct type (MD-IPMNs), most frequent (57–92%), and side branches type (BD-IPMNs), localized in the side branches of ductal system, less frequent (6–46%) [28]. In the combined type of IPMNs, main and branch ducts are both involved. IPMNs encompass epithelial changes from adenoma as premalignant lesions to carcinoma *in situ*, based on the progression of dysplasia, and finally invasive carcinoma. The degree of dysplasia allows the classification of IPMNs: IPMNs with low- or intermediate-grade dysplasia, IPMNs with high grade, and IPMNs with invasive carcinoma.

The characteristic behavior of IPMNs progresses toward malignancy. There is, in the observational studies, an age difference, 6 years longer, between patients with malignant tumors and patients with mucinous adenoma [29]. The communication with pancreatic duct system is characteristic. According to histological features (architecture and cytology), four types of IPMNs, such as gastric, intestinal, pancreatobiliary, and oncocystic, have been described. Gastric-type epithelium is frequent in side branches type with better prognosis (malignant potential 28%); intestinal-type and pancreatobiliary-type epithelia are more frequent in main duct type with bad prognosis (malignant potential 60%) [30]. Several patients can be symptomatic with non-specific symptoms. Clinical appearances can be usually abdominal discomfort or pain, malaise, nausea, and vomiting. Frequently, first clinical appearance is acute pancreatitis generally with benign evolution, due to mucous obstruction of the pancreatic ducts. Acute pancreatitis can be recurrent in 20% of cases. In most cases, IPMNs are asymptomatic. IPMNs with invasive carcinoma should be associated with more evident clinical data such as weight loss, jaundice, and diabetes.

IPMNs usually are diagnosed in elderly (sixth decade). Because high likelihood of malignant evolution of these lesions, there is an age difference, 6 years longer, between patients with malignant or benign lesions [29]. The results of blood examinations, as liver function tests, lipase, amylase, serum CA 19-9, and CEA, and routine tests are non-specific for these pancreatic cystic neoplasms.

Imaging examinations are decisive for diagnosis. They can be less invasive such as US, CT, MRI, and more invasive such as EUS, endoscopic retrograde cholangiopancreatography (ERCP).

Transabdominal US has limited diagnostic role. This examination can show dilatation of the main duct with cystic images around the ducts and thick mucinous content. Sometimes, US can detect the duct communications. CT and MRI are currently employed in the diagnostic assessment of IPMNs. These examinations can detect morphological features of the lesions: size and location, calcification, pancreatic duct dilatation, appearance of the cysts with septae, and thickening of wall. These morphological appearance detected by imaging examinations can identify IPMNs excluding other cystic pancreatic lesions and can distinguish the MD-IPMNs from BD-IPMNs. MRI and CT can also demonstrate the communication between the duct and cyst.

In the past years, endoscopic retrograde cholangiopancreatography (ERCP) was crucial imaging examination in the diagnosis of IPMNs. ERCP may detect dilated main pancreatic duct with mucinous filling and/or intraductal proliferations. These features are characteristic of MD-IPMNs. Whereas in the BD-IPMNs, the examination shows cystic lesions due to dilatation of affected branch ducts that communicate with main pancreatic duct.

In some cases, the imaging studies show a dilated pancreatic duct but not the intraductal tumor. Moreover, the dilation can be proximal and distal to the tumor, because of overproduction of mucous. Classically, the endoscopic observation of open Vater's papilla and mucin extrusion has been reported.

Unfortunately, ERCP is invasive procedure and its diagnostic use has been limited. In the recent years, EUS plays an important role in the diagnostic program of pancreatic diseases. EUS should be useful in the differentiation of types of IPMNs. EUS findings in MD-IPMNs can be a characteristic of morphological changes of these lesions such as various extension and degree of duct dilatation and, in some cases, the presence of intraductal tumor. The recurrent acute pancreatitis can show several parenchymal damages such as edema and enlargement of the gland or signs of parenchymal atrophy. Characteristics of BD-IPMNs are the lesions formed by multiple little cysts (few millimeters) with internal septation, mucous, wall nodule, or thickening, intracystic papillary projections. The Wirsung's duct should be moderately dilated [31].

Based on EUS findings, some criteria of malignancy in IPMNs were defined: great dilatation (>10 mm) of the main pancreatic duct and evident, large intraductal tumor (>10 mm) in MD-IPMNs; large cystic lesions (>40 mm) with thick, irregular septation, wall thickening, mural nodule in BD-IPMNs. We can also add to these criteria of malignancy the vascular invasion and lymph node metastases. The accuracy of EUS malignancy criteria ranges from 40 to 90% [32, 33]. Fine needle aspiration biopsy (FNAB) during EUS allows taking samples for biochemical, cytological, and DNA analyses. The first macroscopic finding is the mucinous fluid characteristic of MCNs and IPMNs. High concentration of CEA should be characteristic of mucinous lesions, such as high level of amylase because duct system communication. Brugge has emphasized the cutoff CEA level for differentiating mucinous from non-mucinous pancreatic cystic lesions: the CEA level of 192 ng/ml has the sensitivity of 73% and specificity of 84% [34]. Unfortunately, this analysis not distinguish MCNs from IPMNs and benign from malignant lesions. Cytological study should be useful for the diagnosis of mucinous lesions with the presence of epithelial cells (different from glycogen-rich clear cells of serous cystadenoma). Moreover, the presence of high-grade cytological atypia relevant to malignancy can be detected [35]. DNA analysis of pancreatic cyst fluid shows K-ras mutation, characteristic for mucinous lesions, and GNAS mutation more present in IPMNs. The latter can differentiate IPMNs from MCNs [36].

The planned interventions for treatment of IPMNs are duodenopancreatectomy or distal/middle pancreatectomy based on location of lesions. We need to take into account that the tumors localized in the main pancreatic duct can spread in the rest of the duct. Consequently, the surgical planification can have changes with possible extension of pancreatic resection to allow negative or low-grade dysplasia at surgical margins. In fact, intraoperative frozen section diagnosis of the transection margin shows positive results in 20–50% of cases [28]. Surgical indications for IPMNs are based on risk of malignancy that is different for MD-IPMNs and for BD-IPMNs. The frequency of malignant potential in MD-IPMNs is 61.6% and the frequency of invasive IPMNs is 43.1% [32]. The malignant potential in BD-IPMNs reaches 28% and the frequency of the invasive lesions is 18%. Therefore, the indication for pancreatic resection is justified and recommended in the majority of the patients with MD-IPMNs by international consensus guidelines [32]. On the contrary, surgical indications in the patients with BD-IPMNs are more debatable. IPMNs, with some not negligible differences between main duct type and branch duct type, encompass epithelial changes from adenoma, carcinoma *in situ*, and invasive carcinoma. The lesions benign at the beginning progress toward malignancy. This characteristic of biological evolutivity makes difficult and complex the surgical indications or the timing of intervention after a possible observation period. Beside the positive and specific diagnosis of each type of cystic pancreatic neoplasm as IPMNs or MCNs, SCNs are crucial for the next diagnostic step, recognizing the malignancy of the neoplasm. In the difficult diagnosis of IPMN, the criteria based on CT imaging suggested by international consensus guidelines should be useful [32]. These criteria have been subdivided as "high-risk stigmata" and "worrisome features." The first are obstructive jaundice in a patient with cystic lesion of the head of the pancreas, enhancing solid component within cyst, main pancreatic duct size of 5–9 mm, or main pancreatic duct >10 mm in size. The "worrisome features" are cyst size >3 cm, thickened/enhancing cyst walls, non-enhancing mural nodule, and lymphadenopathy [32]. Ablation therapies of cystic neoplasms have been proposed: EUS-guided injection of cytotoxic agents (e.g., paclitaxel, ethanol) and radiofrequency ablation. These procedures are not widely employed and their results are not defined and can be evaluated with difficulty, also because these ablation therapies have been used for various PCNs [37–39]. The results of surgical treatment for non-invasive disease are very positive with 5-year overall survival of 100%; for invasive disease, 5-year overall survival drops to 50–60% [28]. Recurrence rate of IPMNs can be evaluated after surgical resection. The mean recurrence rate is 15% in the remnant pancreas (ranges from 7 to 30%). The recurrence of IPMNs as invasive disease ranges from 3.4 to 44% [40, 41]. The differential diagnosis between IPMNs and chronic pancreatitis can be difficult in some cases. Usually, alcohol abuse is frequent in chronic pancreatitis. Several clinical and morphological features are common to both diseases: main duct and branch duct dilatation, intracystic and intraductal calcifications, and recurrent episodes of pancreatitis. Moderate and segmental dilatation of main pancreatic duct with intraductal lithiasic obstruction, moderate dilatation of the branch ducts communicating with main duct, and finally the widespread of the pancreatic ductal system are characteristic of chronic pancreatitis. On the contrary, segmental and marked dilatations of the branch ducts with little calcifications are characteristics of IPMNs.

7. Solid pseudopapillary neoplasms (SPPNs)

SPPNs represent 9% of all cystic pancreatic tumors and have the major incidence in young female patients (second–third decade). SPPNs are a neoplasm of unknown, not well-defined origin: in fact, in the past, various descriptive names were employed. The macroscopic appearances of SPPNs are large solid masses (8–10 cm in size) and well encapsulated, and often the cut section shows areas of hemorrhage, cystic degeneration, and solid areas. The microscopic features are polygonal epithelioid cells that form solid pseudopapillary structures alternated hemorrhagic necrotic pseudocyst. There is also evident extensive vascular network, often with infiltrative growth pattern. Alterations in the antigen-presenting cell/beta-catenin pathway [42] and vimentine positive can be present. The histologic picture may resemble closely to pancreatic endocrine neoplasms (PEN) but chromogranin is negative. In some cases, histologic criteria of malignancy such as high nuclear grade, venous invasion, and atypical cells may be observed; the metastatic spread is possible (10–15% of cases). SPPNs can be located in all side of the pancreas. Clinical appearances are abdominal pain, palpable mass, nausea/vomiting, jaundice, and weight loss. The imaging examinations (CT, MRI, and EUS) show a solid and cystic masses with a well-defined and thick capsule with sometimes peripheral calcifications without septations. EUS-FNA provides little information. SPPNs can be considered lesions with low malignity and rare occurrence of metastasis, usually hepatic (10–15%). The recommended treatment is surgery and the complete resection is often possible (94%); the cure rate reaches 85–95% of patients [6, 44]. The pancreatic resection is based on the location of neoplasm in the gland [43, 44].

8. Cystic pancreatic endocrine neoplasms (CPENs)

CPENs encompass 8% of all pancreatic cystic tumors and about 15% of pancreatic neuroendocrine tumors [45, 46]. The majority of CPENs are non-functioning and asymptomatic. These neoplasms usually are diagnosed in elderly patients (sixth–seventh decades) without sex prevalence. They can be associated with multiple endocrine neoplasia types. The diagnosis, generally incidental, is based on imaging examinations (US, MRI, and CT). Cystic mass is usually with hypervascular rim, and in several cases, there is septation or a solid component [45]. The lesions are generally well circumscribed with regular wall around areas of cystic degeneration.

EUS-guided FNA can reveal low levels of CEA. Immunohistochemical staining for chromogranine and synaptophysin is present. Malignant potential of CPENs is not clearly defined because it is difficult to detect malignancy on biopsy. The lesions are considered premalignant, and surgical treatment is indicated especially for lesions plus than 2 cm in size. The resective surgery presents excellent results with very long survival (plus than 85% of patient treated) [46]. Observational strategy has been proposed [47] for CPENs based on the similar experience with non-functioning pancreatic endocrine neoplasms (PENs) [48]. The results of non-operative choice are not defined.

9. Acute postnecrotic pseudocysts

Pancreatic pseudocysts are inflammatory lesions. They are evolutions and complications of chronic and acute pancreatitis. The etiologies of pancreatitis are various: alcoholic, biliary, or traumatic. The pseudocysts represent about 80% of all cystic lesions of the pancreas. The pseudocyst wall has no epithelial lining unlike the true cysts [49]. Histologically, the pseudocyst wall consists of fibrosis and inflammatory tissue. Moderate and severe acute pancreatitis are characterized by fluid necrotic collections in or near the pancreas at the beginning without wall. With the flogistic evolution, the fluid necrotic collections are surrounded by granulation and fibrous tissue [50]. Acute postnecrotic pseudocysts are the final evolution of necrotizing pancreatic gatherings, characterized by complete separation of the tissues, with liquid content and a fibrous wall [51]. The incidence of acute pseudocysts is low, at 5–16%. Several clinical imaging and chemistries features can be useful for differential diagnosis between pseudocysts and cystic pancreatic tumors. In the history, there is usually previous pancreatitis; the cystic walls are regular and thin, without calcification: in the 65–70% of cases, there is the communication with Wirsung's duct; in the intracystic fluid, CEA, CA19-9, and mucous cells, on the contrary increased amylase and lipase, are absent. The evolution of a lesion with a fibrous wall and the formation of a pseudocyst can be completed in several weeks and in some cases in a longer period (12–16 weeks). Small cysts (<5–6 cm) can develop for many months without clinical appearance. In some cases, spontaneous improvement until the resolution of the pseudocysts can occur [52].

Diagnosis of acute postnecrotic pseudocysts is greatly facilitated by the history of previous episodes of acute pancreatitis. The imaging examinations (transabdominal US, CT, MRI, and MRCP) are crucial for positive diagnosis (sensitivity of CT is very high 90–100%) [49]. Characteristic picture on CT is roundish cyst, fluid filled, without septations, and surrounded by a thick wall around the pancreas. EUS can be used for further evaluation but usually do not add other information on CT. EUS-guided FNA and cyst fluid analysis can demonstrate high amylase concentration.

The size of pseudocysts (plus than 6–7 cm) and the clinical presentation and evolution (lesions symptomatic and/or persistent over many months) can direct the treatment [53].

The choice of therapeutic procedure should be based on the very frequent connection of the acute pseudocysts with pancreatic ducts [53]. The percutaneous US/CT-guided drainage is usually complicated by pancreatic fistula with persistent leakage from the drain, infection, and repeated changes of the drain [53, 54]. Therefore, the intervention of choice must provide persistent drainage of pancreatic secretion by a cystodigestive anastomosis or fistulas [53].

Another pathological characteristic of acute pseudocysts is the close connections with various adjacent intestinal organs (stomach, duodenum, and small intestine) according to the anatomical site where the pseudocyst develops [53].

Drainage of the pseudocysts by endoscopic technique has been proposed [55, 56]: this is performed by creating a small opening between the cyst and the stomach. The disadvantage of this techniques is incomplete drainage with recurrence of pseudocysts and infections because the communication can be small and in site not declive [53, 57]. The surgical cystodigestive anastomosis can employ the more adjacent intestinal organ (stomach or duodenum or small intestine) and can perform cystogastrostomy or cystojejunostomy or cystoduodenostomy [52, 53].

For cysts located in the body or tail of pancreas, the cystojejunostomy or cystogastrostomy is performed depending on the development of the cyst above or under the mesocolon. For pseudocysts located on the head of the pancreas, cystoduodenostomy is usually performed. The same surgical procedures can be performed with a laparoscopic approach with the advantage of the minimal invasiveness [53].

10. Chronic pseudocysts

In the chronic pancreatitis parenchymal fibrosis and ducts, dilatation can cause chronic pseudocysts [53]. Chronic pancreatitis encompasses various complications. Most frequent are pseudocyst formation, mechanical obstruction of the duodenum, or common bile duct. Pseudocysts occur in about 10% of patients with chronic pancreatitis. There are great pathological differences from acute and chronic pseudocysts. The first usually develop from peripancreatic fluid accumulations that cause the pseudocysts formation in the setting of acute pancreatitis. On the contrary, chronic pseudocysts develop as a result of ductal disruptions [53]. Pseudocysts may be single or multiple, various in size. In fact, the pancreatic pseudocysts generally are caused and long maintained by some leaks from the pancreatic ducts that give the constant filling by pancreatic secretions [50]. A long history and clinical evolution of chronic pancreatitis can give usually a clear diagnostic direction. Chronic recurrent abdominal pain characterizes the clinical appearance of the disease. The other common symptoms are nausea and vomiting, early satiety. Jaundice can occur in 10% of patients with a slow start due to bile duct compression by the pseudocyst or the pancreatic flogosis. The imaging examinations, particularly EUS, allow, beside the cystic lesion, to detect the characteristic parenchymal features of chronic pancreatitis: the damage of the pancreatic duct system, parenchymal fibrosis, and calcifications [53]. The Rosemont classification [58] of chronic pancreatitis, based on EUS findings, identifies major criteria such as main pancreatic duct calculi and lobularity and minor criteria with cysts, dilated ducts >3.5 mm, irregular pancreatic duct contour, and dilated side branches >1 mm.

The surgical treatment of chronic pancreatitis should be based on the clinical and pathological scenario: two types of surgical procedures with the aim of improving or eliminating ductal hypertension by intestinal anastomotic drainage can be performed [53]. Resectional procedures allow eliminating the areas of chronic inflammation frequently in the head of the pancreas. A late complication of chronic pancreatitis encompasses evident ductal dilatation. The incidence of these chronic pseudocysts is high: 20–40% [59]. The pseudocysts can be connected with adjacent organs such as stomach or duodenum. Consequently, endoscopic approach can be performed with mini-invasive intent, cystogastrostomy, or duodenocystostomy [60]. The morbidity of this procedure is 3–11%, without mortality. The treatment of chronic pseudocysts by drainage through the duodenal papilla and ductal system also has been proposed by endoscopy. This procedure with ERCP allows putting in place the transpapillary endoprotesis as drainage. In addition, the transluminal stones removal and/or lithotripsy can be possible, if intraductal stones are present [60–62]. The surgical management has shown good results in the treatment of chronic pseudocysts, pancreatic duct dilatation with stenosis, and stones. The Puestow procedure and its modifications of Partington and Rochelle [63, 64] are the standard surgical drainage methods in chronic pancreatitis with pseudocyst and/or dilated ducts. These interventions involve the anastomosis between dilated main duct and pseudocystic wall with a Roux-en-Y loop of jejunum. The results show low morbidity (<10%) and low mortality (<1%) with relief from abdominal pain in 85–90% of the patients [65–67]. Sometimes, with a dilated pancreatic duct, a fibrotic inflammatory mass may be present in the pancreas. In these cases, the interventions that couple drainage and resective procedures defined "hybrid" can be chosen: Beger, Frey interventions, and some variants [67–69].

11. Indeterminate pancreatic cystic lesions

Cystic lesions of the pancreas today are an important diagnostic challenge. In each case the specific diagnosis must be defined: pseudocysts, SCNs, MCNs, IPMNs, and SPPNs are the most common lesions. Perhaps more important is to establish the malignant potential and the objective data of a neoplastic degeneration. The diagnostic procedures to choose should be geared toward minimally invasiveness. Imaging examinations are at the first line: CT, MRI, MRCP, and PET are minimally invasive and have shown various degrees of sensitivity and specificity. ERCP and EUS–FNA are invasive and can give some useful information. If imaging findings allow the certain diagnosis of specific lesion of which is well known the malignant potential and the characteristic features of malignant evolution, the therapeutic choices (surgery or observation) are enough defined. Moreover, clinical symptomatic picture adds further certainty to the treatment program. There are also, among cystic pancreatic neoplasms, some well-defined diagnoses characterized by imaging and clinical data for which the management is uncertain and debatable. In summary, there are two problems in the management of cystic pancreatic lesions. Firstly, the difficulty in the diagnostic definition and/or in the detection of malignancy; moreover, also, in some cases, the positive diagnosis of the lesions is characterized by particular pathological and clinical features that cause uncertainty in the choice of treatment between surgery, observation program, and for how many times the control can be prolonged.

All clinical, pathological, and imaging findings with also analysis of cyst fluid examination by EUS-FNA have been reported above in the detailed report of each cystic lesions of the pancreas.

This knowledge crucial for the diagnosis and management should be integrated by the classification that separates pancreatic cystic lesions in two categories. There are pancreatic cysts benign, not premalignant, such as SCNs, pseudocysts, lymphoepithelial cysts, and lymphangioma, and pancreatic cysts premalignant and malignant such as MCNs, IPMNs, SPPNs, and CPENs [70]. Roughly, the first conclusion can be the indication of surgical resection for premalignant lesions and observation for benign or indolent lesions. The indeterminate cystic lesions can be located between the cysts frankly benign such as pseudocysts or serous cystadenoma or lymphangioma and, on the other hand, the cystic lesions frankly malignant or with clear findings of malignant evolution such as MD-IPMNs, IPMNs associated with invasive carcinoma, MCNs with increased size, cyst-wall irregularity, and intracystic solid regions. In the indeterminate cystic lesions, the management choices can be debatable and uncertain. In this group, small cysts with not certain diagnosis, small BD-IPMNs, or MCNs can be considered. Characteristic in this setting is the asymptomatic pancreatic cyst incidentally detected on abdominal CT. The improvement of an unclear diagnosis can be achieved with MRI and MRCP. If the data obtained with these examinations are not conclusive (e.g., main duct <1 cm; thick cyst wall size >2 cm), the diagnostic process can continue with invasive procedure such as EUS-FNA. The detection of nodule or solid mass or main duct >1 cm and cytology positive for malignancy is crucial for the surgical resection. In the patients without these diagnostic data, the conservative option marked by periodic controls with CT or MRI or EUS (repeat the control test in 6 months) can be evaluated [70]. In the patients with clear diagnosis (CT, MRI, EUS, and clinical data), serous cystadenoma asymptomatic can be followed with periodic imaging control with MRI or CT (repeat the control test in 1 year); if symptomatic, overall in young patient (<65 years), surgery should be considered. Patients with MD-IPMNs, mixed-type IPMNs, SPPNs, and MCNs should be proposed for surgical resection. BD-IPMNs characterized by main pancreatic duct >1 cm, cystic lesion in the head of pancreas, jaundice, solid component, main duct with thickened wall, and mural nodule, which are features concerning malignancy, can undergo surgical resection, if, without these findings, CT, MRI, and EUS (repeat the control test in 6 months) may be followed conservatively.

There is almost unanimously consensus [32, 71] for surgical indications in patients with MCNs, SPPNs, MD-IPMNs, and mixed-type IPMNs. Patients with serous cystadenoma should be directed to conservative management. Surgery can be proposed only in symptomatic patients or if the diagnosis is uncertain. Patients with BD-IPMN can be observed also if the size lesion is more than 3 cm unless there are features concerning for potential malignancy.

12. Clinical cases

This chapter can be completed with the presentation of some cases of cystic pancreatic neoplasms treated in our Service. These detailed examinations can contribute to clarify several clinical pathological features.

- *First case study*: female, 35 years old. Anamnestic data: non-specific vague upper abdominal pain and postprandial fullness since 4 months. The diagnosis is incidental by US and CT.

The multislice CT shows cystic mass located in the tail of the pancreas, size 8.5 cm, unilocular, fluid content, and wall well defined, with contact but not infiltration of posterior gastric wall and splenic vessels. The cystic pancreatic lesion, with this radiologic features, may be also a postnecrotic pseudocyst.

Differential diagnosis, for a cystic pancreatic lesion with these imaging features, may be discussed between MCNs and postnecrotic pseudocysts (**Figure 1**).

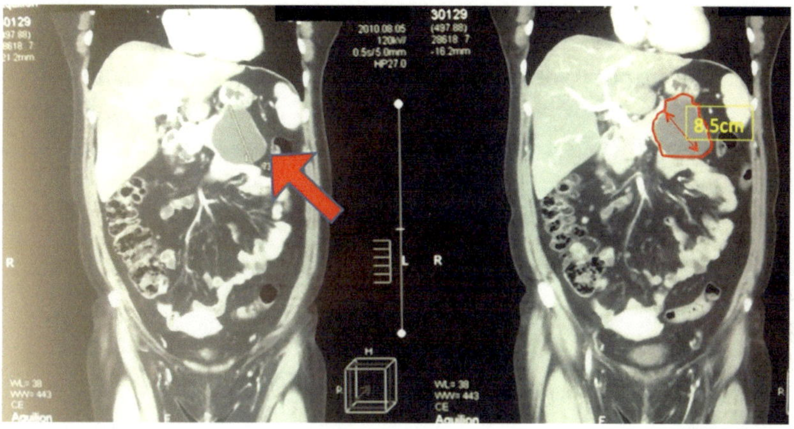

Figure 1. MCN of the tail of the pancreas (arrow).

The first question is whether other examinations for preoperative diagnosis can be useful. In these cases, the anamnestic data are most important: this patient had not in the past acute pancreatitis that can explain pseudocyst. Consequently in our opinion, other abdominal imaging cannot add other information. The preoperative diagnosis is MCN with the surgical indication: distal pancreatectomy and splenectomy.

The second question regards the method of treatment of proximal pancreatic stump. The transection (pancreatic body and splenic vein) with linear stapler and tubular drainage can be suggested. The splenic artery is treated separately.

The third question regards the incidence of pancreatic fistula in distal pancreatectomy. The most important and frequent complication of distal pancreatectomy is the pancreatic fistula. The incidence of pancreatic fistula ranges from 5 to 30% [72–75]. This variability is explained because there are no the standard definition of the fistula: there are a little gatherings or a few drainage in the postoperative period that are not diagnosed as fistula. The criteria for grading pancreatic fistula have been proposed by ISGPF [76, 77] based on drain and amylase level, persistent drainage (>3 weeks), signs of infections, sepsis, clinical conditions, and need for reoperation. The fistula can be classified, with increase of severity, as grades A, B, and C. The grade A and B usually can be treated with non-invasive approach: parenteral nutrition, somatostatine, etc. CT control can be useful. Pathological feature shows cystic lesion, size 8.5 cm, mucoid content with smooth surfaces, and thickened, glistening wall. Histological diagnosis was mucinous cystadenoma. Lymph node is negative.

The fourth question is whether surgical treatment with laparoscopic approach can be proposed. A laparoscopic approach is possible for small or medium size mucinous cystic tumors located in the body or tail of the pancreas. The laparoscopic duodenopancreatectomy is a very complex procedure not yet worldwide performed. But there are two important considerations: not to break the cyst during the intervention because the spillage of mucoid material could lead to tumor spread; moreover, the cyst should be removed intact because the pathologist can do an appropriate examination of the complete wall of the cyst.

- *Second case study*: male, 80 years old. Anamnestic data: recurrent episodes of pancreatitis with upper abdominal pain, hyperamilasemia, diabetes, mild alteration of cholestasis tests, and no alcohol consumption since 10 months. The imaging examinations (US and CT) show cystic lesions of the head of the pancreas, its size is 7 cm, mild dilation of main pancreatic duct, and choledocal duct. The MRCP confirms the same lesion and no stones or sludge in the bile duct (**Figure 2**).

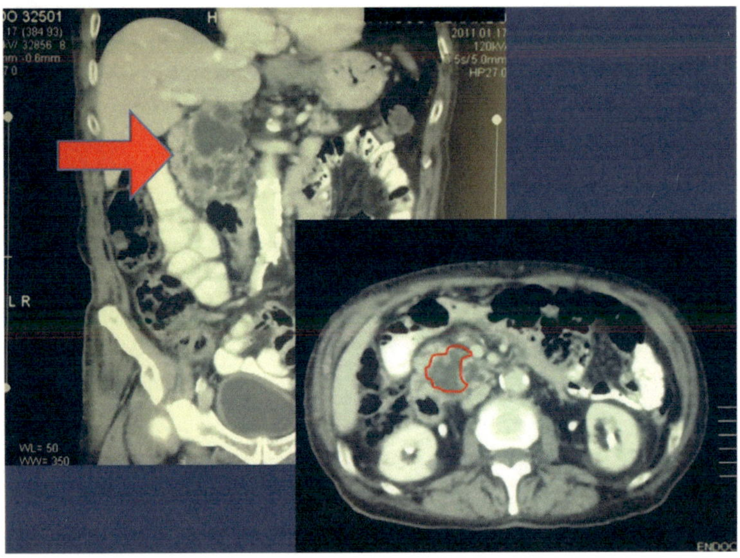

Figure 2. MD-IPMN of the head of pancreas (arrow).

Preoperative diagnosis: Because of previous episodes of acute pancreatitis and no biliary stones and alcohol consumption, the proposed diagnosis may be cystic neoplasm. In addition, in this case, we have had the pathognomonic sign: mucus extrusion through a bulging papilla at endoscopy. The diagnosis was intraductal papillary mucinous neoplasm. There are clear surgical indications: duodenpancreatectomy has been proposed.

Pathological description: head of the pancreas, increased in size (7.5 × 5.3 × 4.5 cm), and dystrophic with cystic lesions with mucus. Histology: IPMN not invasive in the pancreatic ductal ectasia with squamous metaplasia of epithelium. There is no neoplastic invasion in the lymph nodes.

In the surgical management, how to regulate the extension of pancreatic resection in IPMN is very important. First consideration: IPMNs encompass a spectrum of epithelial changes from adenoma to invasive adenocarcinoma; in addition, there is the propensity of the tumor to spread microscopically along the pancreatic ducts. Because of these histopathological features, the most simple therapeutic choice is the intraoperative control (by frozen section) to rule out the presence of the tumor in the transection margin (over the all on main duct). In this perspective, the extension of pancreatic resection is possible once or twice, but is corrected to make a total pancreatectomy? The standard choices are difficult. In the experience of Massachusetts, General Hospital has performed 63% duodenopancreatectomy, 17% distal pancreatectomy, and 19% total pancreatectomy [28]. The positive frozen-section intraoperative examination ranges from 23 to 52%. If recurrence occurs in the pancreas after first intervention, a second resection may be possible.

- *Third case study*: male, 78 years old. Anamnestic data: the patient has been operated for lung cancer 3 years ago.

In the follow-up, US of abdomen shows cystic lesion of the pancreatic head. As the most patients with serous cystadenoma, our patient was asymptomatic and the diagnosis incidental.

CT and MRI confirm cystic tumor (size 1.5 cm) in the head of pancreas, well circumscribed and multinodular. There are also mild dilation of main bile duct and Wirsung. Our conclusion was for SCN (**Figure 3**).

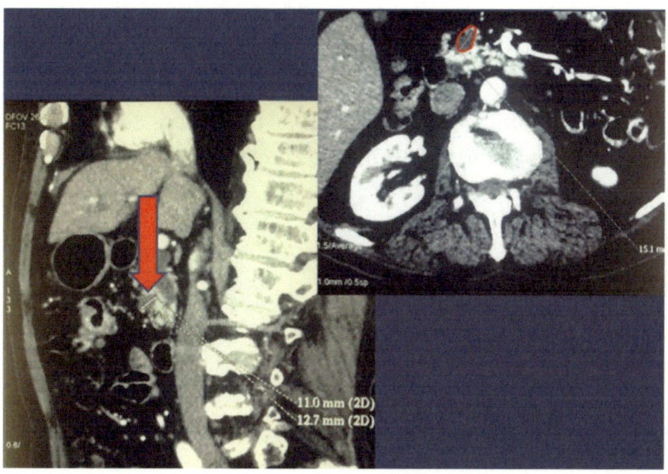

Figure 3. SCN of the head of the pancreas (arrow).

In this patient, the diagnosis may be serous cystadenoma and the therapeutic choice is the organized controls. At present, we have made three controls (by imaging) every 6 months: There is no clinical or morphological modification of the lesion.

The first question is in which patients, the prolonged observation of the cystic tumor of the pancreas may be reasonable? Serous cystadenomas are indolent, slow-growing tumors, with a very low incidence of malignancy (3%) [17]. These lesions become symptomatic with the increase in size. The reasonable therapeutic organization for serous tumors may be the following: first to take the certainty of the clinical diagnosis (serous cystic neoplasm).

Patient with little lesion (<4 cm) asymptomatic (in addition take in mind the great incidence of this tumors in sixth–seventh decade) with certain diagnosis can be undergone to non-operative treatment and followed up. Patient with the lesion bigger in size (>4 cm) symptomatic, in particular if younger, may be undergone to surgical treatment with pancreatic resection.

13. Conclusions

The improvement of imaging, endoscopic modalities, and cyst fluid studies allow now accurate and reliable diagnosis of pancreatic cystic lesions.

Moreover, the enlarged knowledge of valuable pathological studies established the potential for malignant transformation of these lesions identifying higher-risk lesions. Finally, the management options should be based on the assessment of each type of cystic neoplasms and the distinction of pancreatic cystic neoplasms from other pancreatic cystic lesions.

Acknowledgements

The author is grateful to Dr. Libero Luca Giambavicchio for his cultural support and valuable assistance in the typographical transcription of the manuscript.

Author details

Vincenzo Neri

Address all correspondence to: vincenzo.neri@unifg.it

Department of Medical and Surgical Sciences, University of Foggia, Foggia, Italy

References

[1] WHO. Classification of tumors of the Digestive System 2010, PubCam.org Pathologe 2011;32(Suppl 2):332.

[2] Warshaw AL, Compton CC, Lewandrowski K et al. Cystic tumors of the pancreas. New clinical, radiologic and pathologic observations in 67 patients. Ann Surg 1990;212:432–445.

[3] Kosmahl M, Pauser U, Peters K et al. Cystic neoplasms of the pancreas and tumor–like lesions with cystic features: a review of 418 cases and a classification proposal. Virchows Arch 2004;445:168–178.

[4] Curry CH, Eng J, Horton KM et al. CT of primary cystic pancreatic neoplasms: can CT be used for patient triage and treatment? AJR 2000;175:99–103.

[5] Adsay NV. Cystic lesions of the pancreas. Mod Pathol 2007;20:S71–S93.

[6] Yoon WJ, Brugge WR. Pancreatic cystic neoplasms: diagnosis and management. Gastroenterol Clin North Am 2012;41:103–118.

[7] Brugge WR. Diagnosis and management of cystic lesions of pancreas. J Gastrointest Oncol 2015;6(4):375–388.

[8] Kimura W, Nagai H, Kuroda H et al. Analysis of small cystic lesions of the pancreas. Int J Pancreatol 1995;18:197–206.

[9] Adsay NV, Klimstra DS, Compton CC. Cystic lesions of pancreas. Introduction. Semin Diagn Pathol 2000;17:1–6.

[10] Kloppel G, Solcia E, Longnecker DS. Histological typing of tumors of the exocrine pancreas. 2nd ed., Berlin, Springer. 1998. ISBN3-540-60280-1

[11] Compton CC. Serous cystic tumors of the pancreas. Semin Diagn Pathol 2000;17:43–56.

[12] Kosmahl M, Wagner J, Peters K et al. Serous cystic neoplasms of the pancreas: an immunohistochemical analysis revealing alpha-inhibin, neuron specific enolase, and MUC6 as new markers. Am J Surg Pathol 2004;28:339–346.

[13] Gerdes B, Wild A, Wittemberg J et al. Tumor-suppressing pathways in cystic pancreatic tumors. Pancreas 2003;26:42–48.

[14] Bai XL, Zhang Q, Masood N et al. Pancreatic cystic neoplasms: a review of preoperative diagnosis and management. J Zhejiang Univ Sci B 2013;14:185–194.

[15] Choen-Scali F, Vilgrain V, Brancatelli G et al. Discrimination of unilocular macrocystic serous cystoadenoma from pancreatic pseudocyst and mucinous cystoadenoma with CT: initial observations. Radiology 2003;228:727–733.

[16] Friebe V, Keck T, Mattern D et al. Serous cystadenocarcinoma of the pancreas: management of a rare entity. Pancreas 2005;31:182–187.

[17] Strobel O, Z'graggen K, Schmitz-Winnenthal FH et al. Risk of malignancy in serous cystic neoplasms of the pancreas. Digestion 2003;68(1):24–33.

[18] Abe H, Kubota K, Mori M et al. Serous cystadenoma of the pancreas with invasive growth: benign or malignant? Am J of Gastroenterol 1998;93:1963–1966.

[19] Tseng JF, Warshaw AL, Sahani DV. Serous cystadenoma of the pancreas: tumor growth and recommendations for treatment. Ann Surg 2005;242:413–419.

[20] Fernández-del Castillo C, Targarona J, Thayer SP et al. Incidental pancreatic cysts: clinicopathologic characteristics and comparison with symptomatic patients. Arch Surg 2003;138:427–434.

[21] Sarr MG, Carpenter HA, Prabhakar LP et al. Clinical and pathologic correlation of 84 mucinous cystic neoplasms of the pancreas: can one reliably differentiate benign from malignant (or premalignant) neoplasms? Ann Surg 2000;231:205–212.

[22] Crippa S, Salvia R, Warshaw AL et al. Mucinous cystic neoplasms of the pancreas is not an aggressive entity: lessons from 163 resected patients. Ann Surg 2008;247:571–579.

[23] Procacci C, Carbognin G, Accordini S et al. CT features of malignant mucinous cystic tumors of the pancreas. Eur Radiol 2001;11:1626–1630.

[24] Zamboni G, Scarpa A, Bogina G et al. Mucinous cystic tumors of the pancreas: clinicopathological features, prognosis, and relationship to other mucinous cystic tumors. Am J Surg Pathol 1999;23:410–422.

[25] Jimenez RE, Warshaw AL, Z'graggen K et al. Sequential accumulation of K-ras mutations and p53 overexpression in the progression of pancreatic mucinous cystic neoplasms to malignancy. Ann Surg 1999;230:501–511.

[26] Sahani DV, Lin DJ, Venkatesan AM et al. Multidisciplinary approach to diagnosis and management of intraductal papillary mucinous neoplasms of the pancreas. Clin Gastroenterol Hepatol 2009;7:259–269.

[27] Farrel JJ, Brugge WR. Intraductal papillary mucinous tumors of the pancreas. Gastrointest Endosc 2002;55:701–714.

[28] Salvia R, Fernández-del Castillo C, Bassi C et al. Main-duct intraductal papillary mucinous neoplasms of the pancreas: clinical predictors of malignancy and long-term survival following resection. Ann Surg 2004;239:678–687.

[29] Falconi M, Salvia R, Bassi C et al. Clinicopathological features and treatment of intraductal papillary mucinous tumour of the pancreas. Br J Surg 2001;88:376–381.

[30] Furukava T, Hatori T, Fujita I et al. Prognostic relevance of morphological types of intraductal papillary mucinous neoplasms. Gut 2011;60:509–516.

[31] Brugge WR. Endoscopic approach to the diagnosis and treatment of pancreatic disease. Curr Opin Gastroenterol 2013;29:559–565.

[32] Tanaka M, Fernandez de Castillo C, Adsay V et al. International consensus guidelines 2012 for the management of IPMN and MCN of the pancreas. Pancreatology 2012;12:183–197.

[33] Grutzmann R, Niedergethmann M, Pilarsky C et al. Intraductal papillary mucinous tumors of the pancreas: biology, diagnosis and treatment. Oncologist 2010;15:1294–1309.

[34] Brugge WR, Lewandrowski K, Lee-Lewandrowski E et al. Diagnosis of pancreatic cystic neoplasms: a report of the cooperative pancreatic cyst study. Gastroenterology 2004;126:1330–1336.

[35] Pitman MB, Centeno BA, Daglilar ES et al. Cytological criteria of high-grade epithelial atypia in the cyst fluid of pancreatic intraductal papillary mucinous neoplasms. Cancer Cytopathol 2014;122:40–47.

[36] Dal Molin M, Matthaei H, Wu J et al. Clinicopathological correlates of activating papillary mucinous neoplasm (IPMN) of the pancreas. Ann Surg Oncol 2013;20:3802–3808.

[37] Brugge WR. Management and outcomes of pancreatic cystic lesions. Dig Liver Dis 2008;40:854–859.

[38] Matthes K, Mino-Kenudson M, Sahami DV et al. EUS-guided injection of paclitaxel (OncoGel) provides therapeutic drug concentrations in the porcine pancreas (with video). Gastrointest Endosc 2007;65:448–453.

[39] Pai M, Seuturk H, Lakhtakia S et al. 351 endoscopic ultrasound guided radiofrequency ablation (EUS-RFA) for cystic neoplasms and neuroendocrine tumors of the pancreas. Gastrointest Endosc 2013;77:AB143–AB144.

[40] D'Angelica M et al. Intraductal papillary mucinous neoplasms of the pancreas: an analysis of clinicopathologic features and outcomes. Ann Surg 2004;239:400–408.

[41] Wada K, Kazarek RA, Traverso LW. Outcomes following resection of invasive and non invasive intraductal papillary mucinous neoplasms of the pancreas. Am J Surg 2005;189:632–636.

[42] Abraham SC, Klimstra DS, Wilentz RE et al. Solid-pseudopapillary tumors of the pancreas are genetically distinct from pancreatic ductal adenocarcinomas and almost always harbor beta-catenin mutations. Am J Pathol 2002;160:1361–1369.

[43] Papavramidis T, Papavramidis S. Solid pseudopapillary tumors of the pancreas: review of 718 patients reported in English literature. J Am Coll Surg 2005;200:965–972.

[44] Tipton SG, Smyrk TC, Sarr MG et al. Malignant potential of solid pseudo-papillary neoplasm of the pancreas. Br J Surg 2006;93:733–737.

[45] Gaujoux S, Tang L, Klimstra D et al. The outcome of resected cystic pancreatic endocrine neoplasms: a case-matched analysis. Surgery 2012;151:518–525.

[46] Bordeianou L, Vagefi PA, Sahani D et al. Cystic pancreatic endocrine neoplasms: a distinct tumor type? J Am Coll Surg 2008;206:1154–1158.

[47] Farrel JJ, Fernández-del Castillo C. Pancreatic cystic neoplasms: management and unanswered questions. Gastroenterology 2013;144:1303–1315.

[48] Lee LC, Grant CS, Salomao DR et al. Small nonfunctioning, asymptomatic pancreatic neuroendocrine tumors (PNETs) role for nonoperative management. Surgery 2012;152:965–974.

[49] Habashi S, Draganov PV. Pancreatic pseudocysts. World J Gastroenterol 2009;15:38–47.

[50] Brun A. Agarwal N, Pitchumoni CS. Fluid collections in and around the pancreas in acute pancreatitis. J Clin Gastroenterol 2011;45:614–625.

[51] Carter R. Percutaneous management of necrotizing pancreatitis. HPB 2007;9(3):235–239.

[52] Werner J, Warshaw A. Cystic disease of the pancreas pseudocysts, postinflammatory cystic fluid collections and other non-neoplastic cysts. In: Surgery of the pancreas. Trede M, Carter D (eds). 2nd ed., Churchill Livingstone, New York, NY, USA; 1997. p. 405–415.

[53] Neri V. Role of surgery in the treatment of pancreatitis and its complications. In: Acute and chronic pancreatitis. Rodrigo L (eds). Intech Open Publisher, Rijeka, Croatia; 2015. p. 121–151. doi:10.5772/58932

[54] Nealon WH, Walser E. Main pancreatic duct anatomy can direct choice of modality for treating pancreatic pseudocysts. Ann Surg 2002;235:751–758.

[55] Ferrucci JT, Muller PR. Interventional approach to pancreatic fluid collections. Radiol Clin North Am 2003;41:1217–1226.

[56] Naoum E, Zavos A, Goudis K et al. Pancreatic pseudocysts: 10 years of experience. J Hepatobil Pancreat Surg 2003;10:373–376.

[57] Giovannini M. Endoscopic ultrasonography-guided pancreatic drainage. Gastrointest Endosc Clin N Am 2012;22:221–230.

[58] Catalano MF, Sahai A, Levy M et al. EUS-based criteria for the diagnosis of chronic pancreatitis: the Rosemont classification. Gastrointest Endosc 2009;69(7):1251–1261.

[59] Mier J, Luque-de Leon E, Castillo A et al. Early versus late necrosectomy in severe pancreatitis. Am J Surg 1997;173(2):71–75.

[60] Binmoeller KF, Sochendra N. Endoscopic ultrasonography in the diagnosis and treatment of pancreatic pseudocysts. Gastrointest Endosc Clin N Am 1995;5:805–816.

[61] Elefthieriadis N, Dinu F, Delhaye M. Long-term outcome after pancreatic stenting in severe chronic pancreatitis. Endoscopy 2005;37:223–230.

[62] Vitale GC, Cothron K, Vitale EA et al. Role of pancreatic duct stenting in the treatment of chronic pancreatitis. Surg Endosc 2004;18:1431–1434.

[63] Puestow CB, Gillesby WJ. Retrograde surgical drainage of pancreas for chronic relapsing pancreatitis. AMA Arch Surg 1958;76:898–907.

[64] Partington PF, Rochelle RE. Modified Puestow procedure for retrograde drainage of the pancreas duct. Ann Surg 1960;152:1037–1043.

[65] Brandley EL III. Long term results of pancreatojejunostomy in patients with chronic pancreatitis. Am J Surg 1987;153:207–213.

[66] Mannel A, Adson MA, Mcllerath DC et al. Surgical management of chronic pancreatitis: long-term results in 141 patients. Br J Surg 1988;75:467–472.

[67] Andersen DK, Frey CF. The evolution of the surgical treatment of chronic pancreatitis. Ann Surg 2010;251:18–32.

[68] Beger HG, Schlosser W, Friess HM et al. Duodenum preserving head resection in chronic pancreatitis changes the natural course of the disease: a single center 26 year experience. Ann Surg 1999;230:512–519.

[69] Gloor B, Friess H, Uhl W et al. A modified technique of the Beger and Frey procedure in patients with chronic pancreatitis. Dig Surg 2001;18:21–25.

[70] Lee LS. Evaluation and management of pancreatic cystic lesions. J Clin Outcomes Manage 2013;20:129–142.

[71] Del Chiaro M, Verbeke C, Salvia R et al. European experts consensus statement on cystic tumors of the pancreas. Dig Liver Dis 2013;45:703–711.

[72] Sledzianowski JF, Duffas JP, Muscari F et al. Risk factors for mortality and intra-abdominal morbidity after distal pancreatectomy. Surgery 2005;137:180–185.

[73] Lillemoe KD, Kaushal S, Cameron JL et al. Distal pancreatectomy: indications and outcomes in 235 patients. Ann Surg 1999;229:693.

[74] Pannegeon V, Pessaux P, Sauvanet A et al. Pancreatic fistula after distal pancreatectomy: predictive risk factors and value of conservative treatment. Arch Surg 2006;141:1071–1076.

[75] Bilimoria MM, Cormier JN, Mun Y et al. Pancreatic leak after left pancreatectomy is reduced following main pancreatic duct ligation. Br J Surg 2003;90:190–196.

[76] Machado NO. Pancreatic fistula after pancreatectomy: definitions, risk factors, preventive measures and management—Review. Int J Surg Oncol 2012; Article ID 602478.

[77] Bassi C, Dervenis C, Butturini G et al. Postoperative pancreatic fistula: an international study group (ISGPF) definition. Surgery 2005;138:8–13.

Section 4

Pancreatic Cancer

Chapter 6

Hereditary Pancreatic Cancer

Erkut Borazanci and Susan Haag

Additional information is available at the end of the chapter

http://dx.doi.org/10.5772/65067

Abstract

Pancreatic cancer is estimated to surpass breast cancer to become the third leading cause of cancer-related death in the USA in 2016. The 5-year overall survival is 7%, and most individuals are diagnosed with advanced disease. Thus, there is a need to improve the early detection of pancreatic cancer in order to detect and improve survival in the same way that mammograms and colonoscopies have improved survival for individuals with breast and colorectal cancer. This chapter discusses the genetics of hereditary pancreatic cancer, the current available screening options, and the use of biomarkers for early detection of pancreatic cancer.

Keywords: pancreatic cancer, genetics, screening, early detection, hereditary, familial

1. Introduction

Pancreatic cancer remains a deadly disease despite decades of research and treatment advances. In 2016 in the USA, it is estimated that pancreatic cancer will become the third leading cause of cancer-related deaths with over 53,000 individuals diagnosed and over 41,000 deaths [1]. Only 9% of newly diagnosed pancreatic cancer is localized and the 5-year overall survival is 7%, which lags behind other solid tumor malignancies [1]. It is estimated that by the year 2030, pancreatic cancer will be the second leading cause of cancer death in the USA [2]. Thus, due to most pancreatic cancers presenting at a later stage with poor overall survival, early detection methods must be implemented to improve treatment outcomes. Pancreatic cancer has been shown through several studies to have a hereditary disposition with estimates ranging from 3 to 16% of newly diagnosed cases [3, 4]. There are several germline mutations that have shown to be at risk for the development of pancreatic cancer, including *BRCA1, BRCA2, ATM, PALB2, CDKN2A, STK11, PRSS1, MEN1, MSH2, VHL, TP53, PALLD, EPCAM, MLH1, MSH6, APC,* and *FANCC* [5, 6].

Currently, there are no guidelines for pancreatic cancer screening from the American Cancer Society, National Comprehensive Cancer Network, and the US Preventative Task Force. The International Cancer of the Pancreas Screening (CAPS) Consortium convened in 2011 to examine the best available evidence regarding pancreatic cancer screening to provide guidelines [7]. This book chapter focuses on what constitutes hereditary pancreatic cancer and what risk factors are associated with pancreatic cancer development. We also examine recent literature discussing further methods of early detection of pancreatic cancer.

2. Familial pancreatic cancer genetics

Estimates vary in the literature, but it is recognized that approximately 3–16% of cases of pancreatic cancer have a hereditary component [3, 4, 8, 9]. What constitutes the definition of hereditary pancreatic cancer also varies between known germline mutations with associations with pancreatic cancer to a family history of pancreatic cancer. In individuals with a family history of pancreatic cancer, the risk increases several fold with each first-degree relative (sibling, child, or parent) who is affected. In families with pancreatic cancer, one first-degree relative with pancreatic cancer increased risk by twofold. This risk was increased to nearly threefold if the individual was diagnosed before the age of 60 years [10]. A National Familial Pancreas Tumour Registry (NFPTR) study indicated that the risk of pancreatic cancer increased to 57-fold with three or more affected family members with pancreas cancer [8]. Typically, individuals with hereditary pancreatic cancer also are diagnosed at younger ages (<50 year) compared with those with sporadic pancreatic cancer, which occurs at 61 years of age and older [11]. Also of note is that tobacco use can lead to an increased risk of pancreatic cancer in those individuals at risk due to hereditary pancreatic cancer [11].

There are several genetic syndromes that are related to an increased risk of pancreatic cancer and are summarized in **Table 1**. Hereditary breast and ovarian cancer (HBOC) is associated by germline mutations of *BRCA1* and *BRCA2* [12]. These same mutations also carry a significant risk for the development of pancreatic cancer, with the relative risk varying by at lead two to threefold in those individuals with *BRCA1* and *BRCA2* mutations [13, 14]. The *BRCA1* gene encodes a nuclear phosphoprotein that plays a role in maintaining genomic stability and also acts as a tumor suppressor. The protein is associated with the BRCA1 associated genome surveillance complex (BASC) along with RNA polymerase II with the histone deacetlylase complexes. The protein plays a role in transcription along with DNA repair of double-strand breaks and recombination [15]. *BRCA2* encodes for a protein that is also associated with double-strand break repair and homologous recombination. It is also associated with multiple proteins, including RAD51 and PALB2 [16]. *PALB2* (partner and localizer of BRCA2) has also recently been recognized as a significant germline mutation associated with HBOC and involved in the development for pancreatic cancer [17]. The roles of these mutations in the pathogenesis of pancreatic cancer has not always been clear in preclinical animal models, but it is agreed that they contribute to defective DNA repair that leads to accumulation of damaged DNA and genomic instability that would lead to pancreatic cancer development [18].

Syndrome	Gene (s) involved	Clinical features
Hereditary breast and ovarian cancer (HBOC)	*BRCA1, BRCA2, PALB2*	Breast cancer, ovarian cancer, male breast cancer, uveal melanoma, stomach cancer, biliary cancer, endometrial cancer.
Ataxia-telangiectasia	*ATM*	Cerebellar ataxia, telangiectasia of the conjunctiva and skin, immunodeficiency, leukemia.
Lynch	*MLH1, MSH2, MSH6, PMS2*	Colorectal cancer, endometrial cancer, ovarian cancer, stomach cancer, small bowel cancer, transitional cell cancer, glioma, and sebaceous neoplasms.
Peut-Jeghers (PJS)	*STK11*	Mucocutaneous pigmentation, hamartomatous polyps; colorectal, stomach, small bowel, testicular, breast, cervical, and ovarian cancer
Familial adenomatous polyposis (FAP)	*APC, MUTYH*	Colorectal cancer, desmoid tumors, medulloblastomas, osteomas, fibromas, supernumerary teeth, gastric polyps
Familial atypical mole and multiple melanoma (FAMMM)	*CDNK2A*	Melanoma, CNS malignancies, Acute Lymphoblastic leukemia.
Familial pancreatitis	*PRSS1, CFTR, SPINK1, CASR, CTRC, CPA1*	Pancreatitis, cystic fibrosis, diabetes
Li-Fraumeni	*TP53*	Sarcomas, breast cancer, Gliomas, Choroid plexus carcinomas, and adrenocortical carcinomas
Fanconi's anemia	*FANCC, FANCG*	Aplastic anemia, bone marrow failure, acute myeloid leukemia, myelodysplatic syndrome

Table 1. Inherited syndromes associated with increased risk of pancreatic cancer.

Other DNA repair mechanism-based genes implicated in familial pancreatic cancer include the gene *ATM*, whose product works with several proteins involved in DNA damage and subsequently the cell cycle [19]. The gene *ATM* is more commonly known in relation to Ataxia-telangiectasia which is manifested by progressive cerebellar ataxia, oculomotor apraxia, telangiectasia of the conjunctiva and skin, immunodeficiency, sensitivity to ionizing radiation, and an increase rate of malignancies such as leukemia. In one series of 166 familial pancreatic cancer probands, 2.4% carried deleterious mutations [19]. Lynch syndrome, which is an autosomal dominant disorder caused by a germline mutation in one of either *MLH1, MSH2, MSH6*, or *PMS2*. The genes *MLH1, MSH2, MSH6*, and *PMS2* function as DNA mismatch repair genes. Lynch syndrome can also occur because of loss of expression of *MSH2* due to deletion in the *EPCAM* gene [20]. Typical affected family members of lynch have an increased risk of colon cancer but are at risk for several other malignancies, including pancreatic cancer [21]. The risk of pancreatic cancer in families with Lynch syndrome has been reported to be as high as an 8.6-fold increase with a cumulative risk of 3.7% by age of 70 years [22]. Another familial syndrome associated with colon cancer is familial adenomatous polyposis (FAP). This also follows an autosomal dominant pattern of inheritance in the *APC* gene. *APC* is a tumor suppressor gene that is involved in the Wnt signaling pathway along with pathways associated with migration and adhesion, transcription, and apoptosis. Pancreatic cancer has been reported to have a relative risk of 4.46 in families with familial adenomatous polyposis [23]. A variant of FAP, attenuated familial adenomatous polyposis (AFAP) is characterized by mutations in the *MUTYH* gene [24]. To date there is no reported linkage with this gene with pancreatic cancer development although due to its involvement in DNA damage repair an association with pancreatic cancer risk may be discovered.

Peutz-Jegher syndrome (PJS) is another autosomal dominant syndrome that leads to risks in several malignancies. It is characterized clinically by multiple hamartomatous polyps in the gastrointestinal tract and mucocutaneous pigmentation. Individuals with PJS are affected by mutations in *STK11* gene which is a serine threonine kinase tumor suppressor gene. Colon, stomach, small bowel, ovarian, breast, cervical, and testicular cancer risk is increased, as is pancreatic cancer The risk of pancreatic cancer in some studies has indicated as high as a 26% risk in those with *STK11* mutations for pancreatic cancer development by the age of 70 with a relative risk of 76 [25].

Familial atypical mole and multiple melanoma (FAMMM) syndrome is yet another autosomal dominant disorder that is characterized by family members with multiple nevi along with cutaneous and ocular melanomas. This disorder involves mutations in the *p16* gene or *CDNK2* gene which also can lead to pancreatic cancer. The risk of pancreatic cancer development by the age of 75 has been reported to be between 17 and 25% [26, 27]. In some studies, there has been reported to be a 13- to 22-fold increase of pancreatic cancer [27]. CDKN2A is a tumor suppressor involved in inducing cell cycle arrest in the G1 and G2 phase. What is interesting about the *CDKN2A* gene is that somatic mutations or other alterations occur in 90% of individuals with pancreatic cancer making it an important step in tumor promotion in pancreatic cancer [28].

Chronic or recurrent acute pancreatitis also has a hereditary component that has become associated with pancreatic cancer development [29]. In families with hereditary pancreatitis, the risk for pancreatic cancer increases substantially past the age of 50, with the risk being 10% by the age of 50, increasing to 19% by the age of 60, and then to 54% by the age of 75 years in one study [30]. In individuals who smoke with hereditary pancreatitis, the risk of pancreatic cancer increase by twofold if they are current or former smokers and pancreatic cancer in these individuals occurs 20 years earlier [31]. The genetics of hereditary pancreatitis is complex. Germline mutations in the serine protease 1 gene (*PRSS1*) follows an autosomal dominant pattern for hereditary pancreatitis. The gene function of this enzyme functions as a protectant against trypsin. Trypsin is a digestive enzyme secreted by the pancreas into the duodenum and control of its activity is through several proteins including PRSS1, serine protease inhibitor Kazal 1 (SPINK1), cystic fibrosis transmembrane conductance regulator (CFTR), chymotrypsinogen C (CTRC), and calcium-sensing receptor (CASR) [32]. The repeated exposure of trypsin and resulting pancreatitis has been shown preclinically to induce pancreatic fibrosis and inflammation [33]. Biallelic alterations in the aforementioned gene *SPINK1*, leads to an autosomal recessive pattern of chronic pancreatitis [34]. *SPINK1* encodes a pancreatic secretory trypsin inhibitor and is regulated as an acute phase reactant being expressed during the inflammatory process acting as a feedback inhibitor in trypsin [34]. *CFTR* follows an even more complex genetic pattern with regards to hereditary pancreatitis [35]. CFTR functions as an ion channel involved in the transport of chloride and thiocyanate and is associated with cystic fibrosis, a condition manifested by pancreatic insufficiency, failure to thrive, sinus disease, and respiratory disease [36]. Homozygotes mutations of the *CFTR* gene lead to severe chronic pancreatitis but compound heterozygote mutations may also lead to chronic pancreatitis [37]. Homozygous mutations carry a risk of 40–80-fold for chronic pancreatitis over the general population [37]. Individuals who carry only one allelic mutation of the *CFTR* gene still are at an increased risk of chronic pancreatitis three- to fourfold over the general population. Those individuals with heterozygous *CFTR* mutations typically have coexisting germline mutations in either *SPINK1* or *CTRC* [38]. The *CTRC* gene carries a risk for chronic pancreatitis but usually in conjunction in individuals with mutations in either *CFTR* or *SPINK1* [39]. *CTRC* encodes the enzyme Chymotrypsin C that helps degrades trypsin. Other genes associated with recurrent acute and chronic pancreatitis have also been discovered. *CLDN2* encodes a protein that function in tight junction and is involved in ion and water transportation. Mutations in this gene have been associated with chronic pancreatitis particularly in those individuals who consume alcohol. It has recently been described to be involved in pancreatic acinar cells [40]. And finally, the gene *CPA1* encodes a pancreatic digestive enzyme whose mutations have been found to be involved in early onset of chronic pancreatitis. The mutation appears to be involved in endoplasmic reticulum stress as opposed to direct trypsin activity in regards to the development of chronic pancreatitis [41].

There are other syndromes that do not have nearly as strong evidence as the aforementioned syndromes for pancreatic cancer risk, but studies have indicated there are associations. Li-Fraumeni syndrome is an autosomal dominant disorder that is a result of germline mutations in the tumor protein p53 gene (*TP53*) [42]. *TP53* is a tumor suppressor gene that has a major role in regulating the cell cycle in response to DNA damage. In its absence, cells containing damaged DNA survive and proliferate leading to malignant transformation. Typical malignancies at risk with germline mutations in *TP53* include osteosarcomas, rhabdomyosarcomas, breast cancer, gliomas, and adrenocortical carcinomas [42]. However, in a study of 24 families with confirmed *TP53* germline mutations, the risk of pancreatic cancer was 7.3-fold compared to the general population [43]. Fanconi anemia is an autosomal recessive or X-linked disorder that results in congenital malformations along with pancytopenia and macrocytic anemia and is characterized by germline mutations in the *FANC* family of genes [44]. These groups of genes are involved in DNA repair and interact with the BRCA pathway. Mutations in the *FANCC* and *FANCG* genes have been reported in families that have developed young onset (less than 55 years of age) pancreatic cancer [45, 46].

As genetic sequencing become more cost effective for the greater population there will likely be more genes discovered in relation to the risk of pancreatic cancer. Traditional sequencing of gene discovery may uncover additional germline mutations along with single nucleotide poylmorphisms (SNPs). Epigenetic sequencing analysis may also unveil methylated promoters that place an individual at risk for the development of pancreatic cancer. An example of whole genomic sequencing identifying new risks in the human genome came from a study examining over 1890 individuals with pancreatic cancer and compared with 2654 controls that showed an association between a locus on 9q34 and pancreatic cancer through the SNP rs505922 [47]. This SNP maps to the first intron of the ABO blood group gene which leads credence to prior epidemiologic evidence suggesting that individuals with blood group O may have a lower risk of pancreatic cancer than those with groups A or B [47].

3. Other risk factors for pancreatic cancer development

Other risk factors exist for the development of pancreatic cancer and may be associated with changes in the human genome based upon enhanced environmental susceptibility with specific germline alterations. What is currently known is that obesity plays a risk for the development of pancreatic cancer. Two longitudinal US cohort studies, the Health Professionals Follow-up study and the Nurses' Health Study, had decades of follow-up through questionnaires which examined the risk of Body Mass Index (BMI), height, and level of physical activity. Individuals with a BMI of at least 30 kg/m^2 had an elevated risk of pancreatic cancer compared with those with a BMI less than 23 kg/m^2 with a relative risk of 1.72. Height was also associated with an increased pancreatic cancer risk of 1.81 RR when comparing the tallest category (equal to or greater than 185.4 cm in men, greater than 167.6 cm in women) to the shortest category (less than or equal to 172.7 cm in men, less than 157.5 cm in women). In individuals with moderate physical activity defined as equal to or greater than 11.0 MET hours per week in men and equal to or greater than 10.8 MET hours per week in women, the risk of pancreatic cancer was reduced by 59% in men and 48% in women [48]. The "Western" dietary pattern of high intake of saturated fats and smoked or processed meats has also been shown to influence the risk of pancreatic cancer development. In a 7-year prospective study, those that had the highest quintile of intake of processed meat had a 68% increased risk compared with those in the lowest quintile. Higher intake pork and red meat compared with the lowest quintiles were also associated with a 50% risk of pancreatic cancer [49]. A meta-analysis of 11 prospective studies published in 2012 confirmed that processed meat consumption was associated with an increased risk of pancreatic cancer in men but not in women. The relative risk in men was 1.29 [50]. Other social risk factors that are modifiable include tobacco use and alcohol use, particularly heavy alcohol use since it contributes to the development of pancreatitis. Heavy alcohol use is defined as having at least nine drinks per day [51]. Tobacco use leads to a 2.2-fold increased risk of developing pancreatic cancer and cessation must take place for 20 years prior to returning to the risk of nonsmokers [52]. Of note is that exposure of second-hand smoke confers an odds ratio of 1.21 relative to those individuals with no exposure [53]. The risk increases in active smokers by cigarette pack-years.

Diabetes has been recognized more and more as a tremendous risk factor for pancreatic cancer development. Due to one of the functions of the pancreas in regulating glucose metabolism, diabetes is a common presenting finding for pancreatic cancer. In one dose-response meta-analysis of prospective observational studies, it was shown that every 0.56 mmol/L increase in fasting blood glucose is associated with a 14% increase in the rate of pancreatic cancer [54]. This roughly translates to around a 0.35% change in the Hemoglobin A1C (HgbA1C). In another meta-analysis examining 44 studies of diabetes and pancreatic cancer risk, the duration of diabetes was associated with increased risk. For individuals with longer duration of diabetes, the relative risk slowly decreased, with RR being 1.64 for having diabetes for at least 2 years, then RR of 1.58 for diabetes at least five years, and 1.50 RR for having diabetes for at least 10 years [55]. In a nested case-control study within the Health Improvement Network in the UK, new onset of type 2 diabetes was associated with an estimate odds ratio (OR) of 2.16 of pancreatic cancer [56].

Other environmental risk factors include Hepatitis B virus infection and *Helicobacter pylori* infection. Both have been seen in studies and likely warrant further analysis. In a meta-analysis of nine studies involving 3033 patients, the risk of *H. pylori* infection was associated with an OR of 1.47 of developing pancreatic cancer. When broken down into regions such as East Asia the OR goes up to 2.01, but in North America it is 1.17 [57]. The association of hepatitis B virus has also been seen albeit in a single institution study of 476 pancreatic cancer patients and 879 healthy controls. The adjusted odds ratio (AOR) of hepatitis B exposure and pancreatic cancer was 2.5 in anti-Hepatitis B core antigen positive (HBc) patients, 2.3 in anti-HBc positive/anti-Hepatitis B surface antigen (HBsAg) positive patients, and the AOR was 4 for anti-HBc positive/antiHBs negative patients [58]. A cohort of over 66,000 men and women were followed in the Vitamins and Lifestyle study from 2000 to 2008. During follow up, 151 individuals developed pancreatic cancer. Magnesium intake was studied, and for every 100 mg/day decrement in magnesium intake, there was a 24% increase in the incidence of pancreatic cancer through multi-variate analysis that included age, gender, body mass index, and nonsteroidal anti-inflammatory drug (NSAID) use. Thus, magnesium intake may be beneficial for primary prevention of pancreatic cancer [59]. The etiology of why magnesium would be protective for pancreatic cancer is not completely clear. There have been associations with magnesium and the improvement in insulin sensitivity. Deficiency in magnesium may also be associated with free radical formation that leads to DNA damage and cancer development [60], and magnesium may act as a scavenger of harmful chemicals [61].

The microbiome is a burgeoning field involving the study of the microbial flora in humans and its effect on health. Human flora in the mucocutaneous surfaces are composed of a variety of aerobic and anaerobic bacteria. The human microbiome is altered by several environmental factors along with host hygiene such as alcohol use, periodontitis, and the use of antibiotics. The microbiome may play a greater role in inflammation and the eventual development of several malignancies, including pancreatic cancer [62]. A study examining the microbiome by oral wash samples from 361 individuals who developed pancreatic cancer and comparing it to 371 matched controls showed the presence of two species of bacteria, *Porphyromonas gingivalis* and *Aggregatibacter actinomycetemcomitans* associated with an increased risk of pancreatic cancer [63]. The presence of *P. gingivalis* in oral wash samples was associated with a 59% increased risk for pancreatic cancer and the presence of *A. actinomycetemcomitans* was associated with a 119% increased risk. These findings do not establish a true causal link but are intriguing and warrant greater investigation as influencing the microbiome may have a dramatic in pancreatic cancer prevention.

4. Methods of early detection of pancreatic cancer

Because pancreatic cancer carries a poor prognosis, identifying those individuals at risk for developing it is vital due to a phenomenon called anticipation. Anticipation in genetics is defined as when a genetic disorder is passed on the next generation, the symptoms of the genetic disorder become apparent at an earlier age. This is true in several familial forms of cancer such as breast or colorectal and influences when an individual is recommend screening modalities such as mammogram or colonoscopy. In a large study examining 1223 individuals from 106 families with familial pancreatic cancer, anticipation was noted. For individuals affected with pancreatic cancer, the median age of death from pancreatic cancer was 70 years old in generation one, 64 years old in generation two, and 49 years old in generation three [64].

In 2010, the International Cancer of the Pancreas Screening (CAPS) consortium was formed to help organize global pancreatic screening [7]. The consortium was composed of 50 experts from 10 countries in the fields of epidemiology, genetics, gastroenterology, radiology, oncology, surgery, and pathology. This group was composed of physicians, research scientists, and genetic counselors from a wide variety of practice settings including community-based practices and academic centers. The consensus on who should be offered screening was based upon best available evidence. For individuals with three or more blood relatives with pancreatic cancer, with at least one affected first-degree relative (FDR) should be considered for screening. FDR denotes either a parent, brother, sister, or child. Those with at least two affected FDRs should be considered for screening. And finally those with two affected blood relatives with pancreatic cancer with at least one FDR should be considered. For those individuals with only a young onset pancreatic cancer relative (not an FDR), there was no consensus reached on offering screening. In regards to mutation carriers, those with Peutz-Jeghers regardless of family history should be considered for screening. For *BRCA2* mutation carriers with one or more affected FDR with pancreatic cancer and those with two or more affected family members (even without a FDR) should be considered for screening. For *PALB2* mutation carriers with one or more affected FDR should be considered for screening. For individuals with *p16* germline mutations with one or more affected FDR with pancreatic cancer should be considered for screening. For individuals with Lynch syndrome with one or more affected FDR with pancreatic cancer should be considered for screening. The age to initiate screening was not agreed upon nor the age to end screening. The consensus regarding screening modalities was utilizing endoscopic ultrasound (EUS) and magnetic resonance imaging (MRI)/magnetic resonance cholangiopancreatography (MRCP) [7]. Computed tomography (CT) of the abdomen has the disadvantage of utilizing radiation as opposed to MRI/MRCP's reliance of magnetic fields. Furthermore, in a screening program utilizing either CT, MRI, or EUS, CT scans were inferior in detecting pancreatic lesions. CT scans detected pancreatic abnormalities in 11% of the individuals compared with 33.3% for MRI and 42.6% for EUS [65]. As always, the risks of these modalities must be considered, particularly with EUS. Regarding the routine follow up per the CAPS consortium, a 12-month interval was recommended but no consensus on what tests to repeat. Surgical intervention for pancreatic lesions was also recommended to be considered after multidisciplinary assessment, preferably within research studies [7].

There are a handful of published studies on screening for pancreatic cancer. One study published in 2010 from Columbia University Medical Center/NewYork Presbyterian Hospital utilized a screening program similar to the recommendations put forth from the CAPS consortium. In this study, individuals with a family history of pancreatic cancer were allowed to enroll in a prospective screening study and were placed into three risk groups: average, moderate, or high risk. The individuals in average risk were those with one family member with pancreas cancer diagnosed over the age of 55 years old. Individuals with moderate risk were defined as those with two first-, second-, or third-degree relatives with pancreatic cancer or those with one first-degree relative with pancreatic cancer less than 55 years of age. A second-degree relative denotes an aunt, uncle, grandparent, grandchild, niece, nephew, or half-brother or half-sister. A third-degree relative denotes a great grandparent, great grandchildren, and first cousins. Individuals were defined as high risk for pancreatic cancer if there were three or more first-, second-, or third-degree relatives with pancreatic cancer; two or more first-degree relatives with pancreatic cancer; one first-degree relative and one second-degree relative if one was diagnosed at 55 years or younger, and any genetic syndrome associated with pancreatic cancer such as BRCA, Peutz-Jeghers Syndrome, Lynch, Familial Melanoma, or hereditary pancreatitis. Depending upon the individual's risk, they were offered basic blood testing (average risk) or blood testing with MRI (moderate risk) or blood testing, EUS, and MRI (high risk). In these asymptomatic individuals, pancreatic cancer was detected in two of them- one resectable and one stage IV pancreatic cancer. Four patients has intraductal mucinous neoplasms (IPMN) lesions, two individuals were diagnosed with ovarian cancer, one individual with retroperitoneal carcinoid, and one with papillary carcinoma of the thyroid [4]. All told, 18% of the 51 asymptomatic individuals in the program were found to have a preneoplastic or neoplastic lesion. In a follow-up report on their website, 7 of the 29 individuals that have continued screening have also been found to have abnormalities of the pancreas [66]. In another study enrolling 411 asymptomatic individuals performed through a multi-institutional collaboration in Europe, surveillance was offered through individuals at risk for pancreatic cancer [67]. Individuals with a confirmed *CDKN2A* mutation or with a personal history of melanoma and a known mutation in the family were eligible along with individuals from families with two or three first-degree relative with pancreatic cancer. All individuals were offered MRI/MRCP along with EUS every third year of screening. For individuals with *CDNK2A* mutations, 13 (7.3%) developed pancreatic cancer. The resection rate in those individuals was 75% and the 5-year survival was 24%. In the familial pancreatic cancer cohort, 13 individuals (6.1%) underwent a surgical resection, but only four had high-risk lesions. In a cohort of 10 individuals with *BRCA1/2* or *PALB2* mutation, one individual (3.8%) developed pancreatic cancer [67]. Various screening studies have been published throughout the past several years examining several at risk-populations. Routine screening for pancreatic cancer in all healthy individuals currently is not recommended.

Biomarkers for pancreatic cancer continue to be developed. As mentioned previously, the occurrence of diabetes typically precedes pancreatic cancer and bears monitoring in those individuals at risk for pancreatic cancer development. Carbohydrate antigen aka cancer antigen 19–9 (CA 19–9) is the most common pancreatic cancer serum biomarker. However, this biomarker's sensitivity and specificity are not high as several benign conditions involving the gastro-biliary system can cause its elevation [68]. Furthermore, in individuals with negative Lewis phenotype, the CA 19–9 is not elevated, even in the setting of widely metastatic pancreatic cancer. Therefore, the development of newer biomarkers is of interest for pancreatic cancer and those at risk for developing it. A study originating from MD Anderson and Dr. Raghu Kalluri's lab looked at exosomes, which are lipid-bilayer-enclosed extracellular vesicles that contain protein and nucleic acids. The identification of cell surface proteoglycan, glypican-1 (GPC1) is specifically enriched in cancer cells, particularly pancreatic cancer. The assay itself simply uses a small amount of peripheral blood. In comparing individuals without cancer and those with pancreatic cancer, the expression of GPC1 was always elevated in individuals with pancreatic cancer. In a study examining the GPC1 levels in response to surgical resection of pancreatic cancer, individuals who had a greater decrease of detectable GPC1 levels than those that did not correlated to an improved overall survival [69]. Thus, GPC1 may be a biomarker of interest for individuals at risk for pancreatic cancer. Another study identified elevated plasma levels of branched-chain amino acids (BCAAs) are associated with an increased risk of future pancreatic cancer diagnosis. The study examined cases of pancreatic cancer with matched controls from four prospective cohort studies with blood collected at least 2 years before cancer diagnosis with the median time between blood collection and pancreatic cancer diagnosis being 8.7 years. Several metabolites were analysed, and the BCAAs isoleucine, leucine, and valine stood out as an increased risk of greater than twofold for pancreatic cancer development [70]. Circulating BCAAs are elevated in obese individuals and those with insulin resistance [71]. These findings also suggest that muscle protein loss happens much earlier than anticipated in pancreatic cancer, thus contributing further to the debilitating nature of this cancer. Other noninvasive serum approaches include the use of circulating tumor DNA (ctDNA). In a study of patients who underwent resection of their primary pancreatic tumor, the detection of ctDNA preceded the presence of measurable recurrent pancreatic cancer on CT by 9.9 months [72]. Other clinical studies have examined the use of urinary KRAS in advanced cancers requiring very small copy numbers of the KRAS ctDNA [73]. The implications of this and other work suggests that noninvasive testing is improving for detecting pancreatic cancer and may be a consideration for clinical trial design in cohorts of those individuals at risk of the developing pancreatic cancer.

5. Future directions

Pancreatic cancer remains a difficult cancer to diagnose and treat. The identification of individuals who are at risk for pancreatic cancer is important for several reasons. The first significant benefit is for the individual to be aware of their risk and to undergo a surveillance program for the early detection of pancreatic cancer. This program should be compromised of multi-disciplinary panel composed of oncologists, gastroenterologists, radiologists, pathologists, and genetic counsellors. The benefit of early detection for an individual at high risk is for improved survival for pancreatic cancer. Through remarkable work from Johns Hopkins and Dr. Christine Iacobuzio-Donahue's lab from autopsy series, pancreatic cancer appears to take about 20 years from the first mutated cell to clinical presentation and metastasis [74]. This provides a window of opportunity in regards to early detection of the disease and a chance to change the natural course of pancreatic cancer in an individual. The other benefits lie in identifying individuals at risk for pancreatic cancer development and offering these individuals opportunities to participate in clinical trials examining biomarkers—through either serum, urine, or imaging or a combination. The improvement in the overall 5-year survival in breast cancer was not born out of improved treatment for metastatic breast cancer, but through the use of mammography, increased awareness of the cancer, and optimal management of localized disease through a multi-modality approach. In an editorial by Hait and Levine, they argued that the main focus by oncologists has been in treating tumors that are genetically complex [75]. Their argument focuses on examining premalignant lesions and the likelihood of dealing with less genetically complex lesions with treatment. One example of this approach is the use of imatinib, a Bcr-abl inhibitor that is incredibly effective against chronic myelogenous leukemia (CML). The effectiveness of this drug is measured by complete haematological response (CHR). During the chronic phase of CML where the cancer genome is relatively simple, the CHR is 95% for imatinib. As the tumor becomes more genetically complex through disease progression of accelerated phase and then myeloid blast crisis, the CHR falls to 38% and 7%, respectively [75]. This is what oncologists deal with pancreatic cancer, a cancer that has likely metastasized by the time of clinical presentation, hence the low response rates of current therapies.

The oppurtunity to detect pancreatic cancer early through better assays may also allow for intervention. For instance, an individual without confirmed histological confirmation by way of EUS with an elevated biomarker that is highly sensitive and specific to pancreatic cancer may consider watchful waiting or treatment. The treatment may include agents such as metformin, a biguanide which reduces weight and decreases fasting plasma insulin concentrations by enhancing insulin sensitivity via activation of 5'-AMP-activated protein kinase (AMPK) [76]. Metformin has also shown benefit in preclinical models in pancreatic cancer [77]. In a study of individuals who underwent resection for pancreatic cancer, metformin use was associated with an improved survival [78]. The use of immunotherapeutic agents that have so far been met with disappointment in treating advanced pancreatic cancer, may have significantly improved outcomes in premalignant or early pancreatic cancer. Another example of early intervention may be through the use of RANK ligand inhibitors that are available commercially such as Denosumab (Xgeva, Prolia). In a three-dimensional organoid breast cancer model from women that have *BRCA1* mutation and pre-neoplastic legions, the inhibition of RANKL substantially curtailed tumorogenesis [79]. The possibility of offering a drug like Denosumab which is administered subcutaneously and has relative few side effects as opposed to offering a women with *BRCA1* mutation risk reducing mastectomy or bilateral oophorectomy particularly at a young age would likely be appealing for most individuals.

Costs of screening protocols in individuals at risk for pancreatic cancer development have been examined and appears to be cost-effective [80]. Utilizing early detection programs through several institutions may define better the risk factors for pancreatic cancer along with initiating clinical trials for earlier intervention. The potential benefits of identifying and improving survival in individuals with pancreatic cancer is tremendous. By examining those at high risk for developing the disease, the possibility of developing a more widespread early detection tool for pancreatic cancer in the vein as mammograms may save countless lives in the future.

Author details

Erkut Borazanci[1,2*] and Susan Haag[1]

*Address all correspondence to: Erkut.borazanci@honorhealth.com

1 Honor Health, Scottsdale, AZ, USA

2 Translational Genomics Research Institute (TGen), Phoenix, AZ, USA

References

[1] Siegel RL, Miller KD, Jemal A. Cancer statistics. CA Cancer J Clin. 2016; 66(1):7–30.

[2] Rahib L, Smith BD, Aizenberg R, Rosenzweig AB, Fleshman JM, Matrisian LM.Projecting cancer incidence and deaths to 2030: the unexpected burden of thyroid, liver, and pancreas cancers in the United States. Cancer Res. 2014 Jun;4(11):2913–21.

[3] Klein AP, Hruban RH, Brune KA, Petersen GM, Goggins M. Familial pancreatic cancer. Cancer J. 2001 Jul-Aug;7(4):266–73.

[4] Verna EC, Hwang C, Stevens PD, Rotterdam H, Stavropoulos SN, Sy CD, Prince MA, Chung WK, Fine RL, Chabot JA, Frucht H. Pancreatic cancer screening in a prospective cohort of high-risk patients: a comprehensive strategy of imaging and genetics. Clin Cancer Res. 2010 Oct 15;16(20):5028–37.

[5] Hruban RH, Canto MI, Goggins M, Schulick R, Klein AP. Update on familial pancreatic cancer. Adv Surg. 2010;44:293–311.

[6] Lennon AM, Wolfgang CL, Canto MI, Klein AP, Herman JM, Goggins M, Fishman EK, Kamel I, Weiss MJ, Diaz LA, Papadopoulos N, Kinzler KW, Vogelstein B, Hruban RH. The early detection of pancreatic cancer: what will it take to diagnose and treat curable pancreatic neoplasia? Cancer Res. 2014 Jul 1;74(13):3381–9.

[7] Canto MI, Harinck F, Hruban RH, Offerhaus GJ, Poley JW, Kamel I, Nio Y, Schulick RS, Bassi C, Kluijt I, Levy MJ, Chak A, Fockens P, Goggins M, Bruno M; International Cancer of Pancreas Screening (CAPS) Consortium. International Cancer of the Pancreas Screening (CAPS) Consortium summit on the management of patients with increased risk for familial pancreatic cancer. Gut. 2013 Mar;62(3):339–47.

[8] Tersmette AC, Petersen GM, Offerhaus GJ, Falatko FC, Brune KA, Goggins M, Rozenblum E, Wilentz RE, Yeo CJ, Cameron JL, Kern SE, Hruban RH. Increased risk of incident

pancreatic cancer among first-degree relatives of patients with familial pancreatic cancer. Clin Cancer Res. 2001 Mar;7(3):738–44.

[9] Permuth-Wey J, Egan KM. Family history is a significant risk factor for pancreatic cancer: results from a systematic review and meta-analysis. Fam Cancer. 2009;8(2):109–17.

[10] McWilliams RR, Rabe KG, Olswold C, De Andrade M, Petersen GM. Risk of malignancy in first-degree relatives of patients with pancreatic carcinoma. Cancer. 2005 Jul 15;104(2):388–94.

[11] James TA, Sheldon DG, Rajput A, Kuvshinoff BW, Javle MM, Nava HR, Smith JL, Gibbs JF. Risk factors associated with earlier age of onset in familial pancreatic carcinoma. Cancer. 2004 Dec 15;101(12):2722–6.

[12] Malone KE, Daling JR, Doody DR, Hsu L, Bernstein L, Coates RJ, Marchbanks PA, Simon MS, McDonald JA, Norman SA, Strom BL, Burkman RT, Ursin G, Deapen D, Weiss LK, Folger S, Madeoy JJ, Friedrichsen DM, Suter NM, Humphrey MC, Spirtas R, Ostrander EA. Prevalence and predictors of BRCA1 and BRCA2 mutations in a population-based study of breast cancer in white and black American women ages 35 to 64 years. Cancer Res. 2006 Aug 15;66(16):8297–308.

[13] Goldgar DE. Analysis of familial breast cancer in genetic analysis workshop 9: summary of findings. Genet Epidemiol. 1995;12(6):833–6.

[14] Thompson D, Easton DF; Breast Cancer Linkage Consortium. Cancer Incidence in BRCA1 mutation carriers. J Natl Cancer Inst. 2002 Sep 18;94(18):1358–65.

[15] Hiraike H, Wada-Hiraike O, Nakagawa S, Koyama S, Miyamoto Y, Sone K, Tanikawa M, Tsuruga T, Nagasaka K, Matsumoto Y, Oda K, Shoji K, Fukuhara H, Saji S, Nakagawa K, Kato S, Yano T, Taketani Y. Identification of DBC1 as a transcriptional repressor for BRCA1. Br J Cancer. 2010 Mar 16;102(6):1061–7.

[16] Bhatia V, Barroso SI, García-Rubio ML, Tumini E, Herrera-Moyano E, Aguilera A. BRCA2 prevents R-loop accumulation and associates with TREX-2 mRNA export factor PCID2. Nature. 2014 Jul 17;511(7509):362–5.

[17] Slater EP, Langer P, Niemczyk E, Strauch K, Butler J, Habbe N, Neoptolemos JP, Greenhalf W, Bartsch DK. PALB2 mutations in European familial pancreatic cancer families. Clin Genet. 2010 Nov;78(5):490–4.

[18] Campbell PJ, Yachida S, Mudie LJ, Stephens PJ, Pleasance ED, Stebbings LA, Morsberger LA, Latimer C, McLaren S, Lin ML, McBride DJ, Varela I, Nik-Zainal SA, Leroy C, Jia M, Menzies A, Butler AP, Teague JW, Griffin CA, Burton J, Swerdlow H, Quail MA, Stratton MR, Iacobuzio-Donahue C, Futreal PA. The patterns and dynamics of genomic instability in metastatic pancreatic cancer. Nature. 2010 Oct 28;467(7319):1109–13.

[19] Roberts NJ, Jiao Y, Yu J, Kopelovich L, Petersen GM, Bondy ML, Gallinger S, Schwartz AG, Syngal S, Cote ML, Axilbund J, Schulick R, Ali SZ, Eshleman JR, Velculescu VE,

Goggins M, Vogelstein B, Papadopoulos N, Hruban RH, Kinzler KW, Klein AP. ATM mutations in patients with hereditary pancreatic cancer. Cancer Discov. 2012 Jan; 2(1): 41–6.

[20] Palomaki GE, McClain MR, Melillo S, Hampel HL, Thibodeau SN. EGAPP supplementary evidence review: DNA testing strategies aimed at reducing morbidity and mortality from Lynch syndrome. Genet Med. 2009 Jan;11(1):42–65.

[21] Møller P, Seppälä T, Bernstein I, Holinski-Feder E, Sala P, Evans DG, Lindblom A, Macrae F, Blanco I, Sijmons R, Jeffries J, Vasen H, Burn J, Nakken S, Hovig E, Rødland EA, Tharmaratnam K, de Vos Tot Nederveen Cappel WH, Hill J, Wijnen J, Jenkins M, Green K, Lalloo F, Sunde L, Mints M, Bertario L, Pineda M, Navarro M, Morak M, Renkonen-Sinisalo L, Frayling IM, Plazzer JP, Pylvanainen K, Genuardi M, Mecklin JP, Möslein G, Sampson JR, Capella G, Mallorca Group (http://mallorca-group.org). Incidence of and survival after subsequent cancers in carriers of pathogenic MMR variants with previous cancer: a report from the prospective Lynch syndrome database. Gut. 2016 Jun 3.

[22] Kastrinos F, Stoffel EM, Balmaña J, Steyerberg EW, Mercado R, Syngal S. Phenotype comparison of MLH1 and MSH2 mutation carriers in a cohort of 1,914 individuals undergoing clinical genetic testing in the United States. Cancer Epidemiol Biomarkers Prev. 2008 Aug; 17(8):2044–51.

[23] Giardiello FM, Offerhaus GJ, Lee DH, Krush AJ, Tersmette AC, Booker SV, Kelley NC, Hamilton SR. Increased risk of thyroid and pancreatic carcinoma in familial adenomatous polyposis. Gut. 1993 Oct; 34(10):1394–6.

[24] Grover S, Kastrinos F, Steyerberg EW, Cook EF, Dewanwala A, Burbidge LA, Wenstrup RJ, Syngal S. Prevalence and phenotypes of APC and MUTYH mutations in patients with multiple colorectal adenomas. JAMA. 2012 Aug 1; 308(5):485–92.

[25] Korsse SE, Harinck F, van Lier MG, Biermann K, Offerhaus GJ, Krak N, Looman CW, van Veelen W, Kuipers EJ, Wagner A, Dekker E, Mathus-Vliegen EM, Fockens P, van Leerdam ME, Bruno MJ. Pancreatic cancer risk in Peutz-Jeghers syndrome patients: a large cohort study and implications for surveillance. J Med Genet. 2013 Jan;50(1):59–64.

[26] Goldstein AM, Fraser MC, Struewing JP, Hussussian CJ, Ranade K, Zametkin DP, Fontaine LS, Organic SM, Dracopoli NC, Clark WH Jr, et al. Increased risk of pancreatic cancer in melanoma-prone kindreds with p16INK4 mutations. N Engl J Med. 1995 Oct 12;333(15):970–4.

[27] Lynch HT, Fusaro RM, Lynch JF, Brand R. Pancreatic cancer and the FAMMM syndrome. Fam Cancer. 2008;7(1):103–12.

[28] Iacobuzio-Donahue CA, Velculescu VE, Wolfgang CL, Hruban RH. Genetic basis of pancreas cancer development and progression: insights from whole-exome and whole-genome sequencing. Clin Cancer Res. 2012 Aug 15;18(16):4257–65.

[29] Lowenfels AB, Maisonneuve P, DiMagno EP, Elitsur Y, Gates LK Jr, Perrault J, Whitcomb DC. Hereditary pancreatitis and the risk of pancreatic cancer. International Hereditary Pancreatitis Study Group. J Natl Cancer Inst. 1997 Mar 19;89(6):442–6.

[30] Rebours V, Boutron-Ruault MC, Schnee M, Férec C, Le Maréchal C, Hentic O, Maire F, Hammel P, Ruszniewski P, Lévy P. The natural history of hereditary pancreatitis: a national series. Gut. 2009 Jan; 58(1):97–103.

[31] Lowenfels AB, Maisonneuve P, Whitcomb DC, Lerch MM, DiMagno EP. Cigarette smoking as a risk factor for pancreatic cancer in patients with hereditary pancreatitis. JAMA. 2001 Jul 11;286(2):169–70.

[32] Whitcomb DC. Genetic aspects of pancreatitis. Annu Rev Med. 2010;61:413–24.

[33] Archer H, Jura N, Keller J, Jacobson M, Bar-Sagi D. A mouse model of hereditary pancreatitis generated by transgenic expression of R122H trypsinogen. Gastroenterology. 2006 Dec;131(6):1844–55.

[34] DiMagno MJ, DiMagno EP. Chronic pancreatitis. Curr Opin Gastroenterol. 2005 Sep; 21(5):544–54.

[35] Weiss FU, Simon P, Bogdanova N, Mayerle J, Dworniczak B, Horst J, Lerch MM. Complete cystic fibrosis transmembrane conductance regulator gene sequencing in patients with idiopathic chronic pancreatitis and controls. Gut. 2005 Oct; 54(10):1456–60.

[36] Ratjen F, Döring G. Cystic fibrosis. Lancet. 2003 Feb 22;361(9358):681–9.

[37] Cohn JA, Mitchell RM, Jowell PS. The impact of cystic fibrosis and PSTI/SPINK1 gene mutations on susceptibility to chronic pancreatitis. Clin Lab Med. 2005 Mar; 25(1):79–100.

[38] Schneider A, Larusch J, Sun X, Aloe A, Lamb J, Hawes R, Cotton P, Brand RE, Anderson MA, Money ME, Banks PA, Lewis MD, Baillie J, Sherman S, Disario J, Burton FR, Gardner TB, Amann ST, Gelrud A, George R, Rockacy MJ, Kassabian S, Martinson J, Slivka A, Yadav D, Oruc N, Barmada MM, Frizzell R, Whitcomb DC. Combined bicarbonate conductance-impairing variants in CFTR and SPINK1 variants are associated with chronic pancreatitis in patients without cystic fibrosis. Gastroenterology. 2011 Jan;140(1):162–71.

[39] Rosendahl J, Landt O, Bernadova J, Kovacs P, Teich N, Bödeker H, Keim V, Ruffert C, Mössner J, Kage A, Stumvoll M, Groneberg D, Krüger R, Luck W, Treiber M, Becker M, Witt H. CFTR, SPINK1, CTRC and PRSS1 variants in chronic pancreatitis: is the role of mutated CFTR overestimated? Gut. 2013 Apr;62(4):582–92.

[40] Derikx MH, Kovacs P, Scholz M, Masson E, Chen JM, Ruffert C, Lichtner P, Te Morsche RH, Cavestro GM, Férec C, Drenth JP, Witt H, Rosendahl J; Pan EuropeanWorking group on Alcoholic Chronic Pancreatitis Members and Collaborators. Polymorphisms

at PRSS1-PRSS2 and CLDN2-MORC4 loci associate with alcoholic and non-alcoholic chronic pancreatitis in a European replication study. Gut. 2015 Sep;64(9):1426–33.

[41] Witt H, Beer S, Rosendahl J, Chen JM, Chandak GR, Masamune A, Bence M, Szmola R, Oracz G, Macek M Jr, Bhatia E, Steigenberger S, Lasher D, Bühler F, Delaporte C, Tebbing J, Ludwig M, Pilsak C, Saum K, Bugert P, Masson E, Paliwal S, Bhaskar S, Sobczynska-Tomaszewska A, Bak D, Balascak I, Choudhuri G, Nageshwar Reddy D, Rao GV, Thomas V, Kume K, Nakano E, Kakuta Y, Shimosegawa T, Durko L, Szabó A, Schnúr A, Hegyi P, Rakonczay Z Jr, Pfützer R, Schneider A, Groneberg DA, Braun M, Schmidt H, Witt U, Friess H, Algül H, Landt O, Schuelke M, Krüger R, Wiedenmann B, Schmidt F, Zimmer KP, Kovacs P, Stumvoll M, Blüher M, Müller T, Janecke A, Teich N, Grützmann R, Schulz HU, Mössner J, Keim V, Löhr M, Férec C, Sahin-Tóth M. Variants in CPA1 are strongly associated with early onset chronic pancreatitis. Nat Genet. 2013 Oct;45(10):1216–20.

[42] Malkin D. Li-fraumeni syndrome. Genes Cancer. 2011 Apr;2(4):475–84.

[43] Ruijs MW, Verhoef S, Rookus MA, Pruntel R, van der Hout AH, Hogervorst FB, Kluijt I, Sijmons RH, Aalfs CM, Wagner A, Ausems MG, Hoogerbrugge N, van Asperen CJ, Gomez Garcia EB, Meijers-Heijboer H, Ten Kate LP, Menko FH, van 't Veer LJ. TP53 germline mutation testing in 180 families suspected of Li-Fraumeni syndrome: mutation detection rate and relative frequency of cancers in different familial phenotypes. J Med Genet. 2010 Jun;47(6):421–8.

[44] Wang W. Emergence of a DNA-damage response network consisting of Fanconi anaemia and BRCA proteins. Nat Rev Genet. 2007 Oct;8(10):735–48.

[45] Couch FJ, Johnson MR, Rabe K, Boardman L, McWilliams R, de Andrade M, Petersen G. Germ line Fanconi anemia complementation group C mutations and pancreatic cancer. Cancer Res. 2005 Jan 15;65(2):383–6.

[46] Rogers CD, van der Heijden MS, Brune K, Yeo CJ, Hruban RH, Kern SE, Goggins M. The genetics of FANCC and FANCG in familial pancreatic cancer. Cancer Biol Ther. 2004 Feb;3(2):167–9.

[47] Amundadottir L, Kraft P, Stolzenberg-Solomon RZ, Fuchs CS, Petersen GM, Arslan AA, Bueno-de-Mesquita HB, Gross M, Helzlsouer K, Jacobs EJ, LaCroix A, Zheng W, Albanes D, Bamlet W, Berg CD, Berrino F, Bingham S, Buring JE, Bracci PM, Canzian F, Clavel-Chapelon F, Clipp S, Cotterchio M, de Andrade M, Duell EJ, Fox JW Jr, Gallinger S, Gaziano JM, Giovannucci EL, Goggins M, González CA, Hallmans G, Hankinson SE, Hassan M, Holly EA, Hunter DJ, Hutchinson A, Jackson R, Jacobs KB, Jenab M, Kaaks R, Klein AP, Kooperberg C, Kurtz RC, Li D, Lynch SM, Mandelson M, McWilliams RR, Mendelsohn JB, Michaud DS, Olson SH, Overvad K, Patel AV, Peeters PH, Rajkovic A, Riboli E, Risch HA, Shu XO, Thomas G, Tobias GS, Trichopoulos D, Van Den Eeden SK, Virtamo J, Wactawski-Wende J, Wolpin BM, Yu H, Yu K, Zeleniuch-Jacquotte A, Chanock SJ, Hartge P, Hoover RN. Genome-wide association study

identifies variants in the ABO locus associated with susceptibility to pancreatic cancer. Nat Genet. 2009 Sep;41(9):986–90.

[48] Michaud DS, Giovannucci E, Willett WC, Colditz GA, Stampfer MJ, Fuchs CS. Physical activity, obesity, height, and the risk of pancreatic cancer. JAMA. 2001 Aug 22–29;286(8): 921–9.

[49] Nöthlings U, Wilkens LR, Murphy SP, Hankin JH, Henderson BE, Kolonel LN. Meat and fat intake as risk factors for pancreatic cancer: the multiethnic cohort study. J Natl Cancer Inst. 2005 Oct 5;97(19):1458–65. Erratum in: J Natl Cancer Inst. 2006 Jun 7;98(11): 796.

[50] Larsson SC, Wolk A. Red and processed meat consumption and risk of pancreatic cancer: meta-analysis of prospective studies. Br J Cancer. 2012 Jan 31;106(3):603–7.

[51] Lucenteforte E, La Vecchia C, Silverman D, Petersen GM, Bracci PM, Ji BT, Bosetti C, Li D, Gallinger S, Miller AB, Bueno-de-Mesquita HB, Talamini R, Polesel J, Ghadirian P, Baghurst PA, Zatonski W, Fontham E, Bamlet WR, Holly EA, Gao YT, Negri E, Hassan M, Cotterchio M, Su J, Maisonneuve P, Boffetta P, Duell EJ. Alcohol consumption and pancreatic cancer: a pooled analysis in the International Pancreatic Cancer Case–control Consortium (PanC4). Ann Oncol. 2012 Feb; 23(2):374–82.

[52] Bosetti C, Lucenteforte E, Silverman DT, Petersen G, Bracci PM, Ji BT, Negri E, Li D, Risch HA, Olson SH, Gallinger S, Miller AB, Bueno-de-Mesquita HB, Talamini R, Polesel J, Ghadirian P, Baghurst PA, Zatonski W, Fontham E, Bamlet WR, Holly EA, Bertuccio P, Gao YT, Hassan M, Yu H, Kurtz RC, Cotterchio M, Su J, Maisonneuve P, Duell EJ, Boffetta P, La Vecchia C. Cigarette smoking and pancreatic cancer: an analysis from the International Pancreatic Cancer Case–control Consortium (Panc4). Ann Oncol. 2012 Jul;23(7):1880–8.

[53] Villeneuve PJ, Johnson KC, Mao Y, Hanley AJ; Canadian Cancer Registries Research Group. Environmental tobacco smoke and the risk of pancreatic cancer: findings from a Canadian population-based case–control study. Can J Public Health. 2004 Jan-Feb; 95(1):32–7.

[54] Liao WC, Tu YK, Wu MS, Lin JT, Wang HP, Chien KL. Blood glucose concentration and risk of pancreatic cancer: systematic review and dose–response meta-analysis. BMJ. 2015 Jan 2;349:g7371.

[55] Song S, Wang B, Zhang X, Hao L, Hu X, Li Z, Sun S. Long-term diabetes mellitus is associated with an increased risk of pancreatic cancer: a meta-analysis. PLoS One. 2015 Jul 29;10(7):e0134321.

[56] Lu Y, García Rodríguez LA, Malgerud L, González-Pérez A, Martín-Pérez M, Lagergren J, Bexelius TS. New-onset type 2 diabetes, elevated HbA1c, anti-diabetic medications, and risk of pancreatic cancer. Br J Cancer. 2015 Dec 1;113(11):1607–14.

[57] Xiao M, Wang Y, Gao Y. Association between Helicobacter pylori infection and pancreatic cancer development: a meta-analysis. PLoS One. 2013 Sep 26;8(9):e75559.

[58] Hassan MM, Li D, El-Deeb AS, Wolff RA, Bondy ML, Davila M, Abbruzzese JL. Association between hepatitis B virus and pancreatic cancer. J Clin Oncol. 2008 Oct 1;26(28):4557–62.

[59] Dibaba D, Xun P, Yokota K, White E, He K. Magnesium intake and incidence of pancreatic cancer: the VITamins and Lifestyle study. Br J Cancer. 2015 Dec 1;113(11): 1615–21.

[60] Blaszczyk U, Duda-Chodak A. Magnesium: its role in nutrition and carcinogenesis. Rocz Panstw Zakl Hig. 2013;64(3):165–71.

[61] Anastassopoulou J, Theophanides T. Magnesium-DNA interactions and the possible relation of magnesium to carcinogenesis. Irradiation and free radicals. Crit Rev Oncol Hematol. 2002 Apr;42(1):79–91.

[62] Zambirinis CP, Pushalkar S, Saxena D, Miller, G. Pancreatic cancer, inflammation, and microbiome. Cancer J. 2014 May-Jun:20(3): 195–202.

[63] Fan X, Alekseyenko AV, Wu J, Eric J. Jacobs, Gapstur SM, Purdue MP, Abnet CC, Stolzenberg-Solomon R, Miller G, Ravel J, Hayes RB, Ahn J. Human oral microbiome and prospective risk for pancreatic cancer: a population based, nested case control study. Oral presentation at: AACR Annual Meeting 2016; April 16–20, 2016; New Orleans, LA.

[64] McFaul CD, Greenhalf W, Earl J, Howes N, Neoptolemos JP, Kress R, Sina-Frey M,Rieder H, Hahn S, Bartsch DK; European Registry of Hereditary Pancreatitis and Familial Pancreatic Cancer (EUROPAC); German National Case Collection for Familial Pancreatic Cancer (FaPaCa). Anticipation in familial pancreatic cancer. Gut. 2006 Feb; 55(2):252–8.

[65] Canto MI, Hruban RH, Fishman EK, Kamel IR, Schulick R, Zhang Z, Topazian M, Takahashi N, Fletcher J, Petersen G, Klein AP, Axilbund J, Griffin C, Syngal S, Saltzman JR, Mortele KJ, Lee J, Tamm E, Vikram R, Bhosale P, Margolis D, Farrell J, Goggins M; American Cancer of the Pancreas Screening (CAPS) Consortium. Frequent detection of pancreatic lesions in asymptomatic high-risk individuals. Gastroenterology. 2012 Apr; 142(4):796–804.

[66] Columbia University Medical Center. Our Screening Program;[cited 17 Jul 16]; [1 screen]. New York (NY): Columbia University Medical Center, Department of Surgery; c1999-2015. Available from: http://columbiasurgery.org/pancreas/our-screening-program.

[67] Vasen H, Ibrahim I, Ponce CG, Slater EP, Matthäi E, Carrato A, Earl J, Robbers K, van Mil AM, Potjer T, Bonsing BA, de Vos Tot Nederveen Cappel WH, Bergman W, Wasser M, Morreau H, Klöppel G, Schicker C, Steinkamp M, Figiel J, Esposito I, Mocci E, Vazquez-Sequeiros E, Sanjuanbenito A, Muñoz-Beltran M, Montans J, Langer P,

http://dx.doi.org/10.5772/65067

Fendrich V, Bartsch DK. Benefit of surveillance for pancreatic cancer in high-risk individuals: outcome of long-term prospective follow-up studies from three European Expert Centers. J Clin Oncol. 2016 Jun 10;34(17):2010–9.

[68] Scarà S, Bottoni P, Scatena R. CA 19–9: biochemical and clinical aspects. Adv Exp Med Biol. 2015;867:247–60.

[69] Melo SA, Luecke LB, Kahlert C, Fernandez AF, Gammon ST, Kaye J, LeBleu VS, Mittendorf EA, Weitz J, Rahbari N, Reissfelder C, Pilarsky C, Fraga MF, Piwnica-Worms D, Kalluri R. Glypican-1 identifies cancer exosomes and detects early pancreatic cancer. Nature. 2015 Jul 9;523(7559):177–82.

[70] Mayers JR, Wu C, Clish CB, Kraft P, Torrence ME, Fiske BP, Yuan C, Bao Y, Townsend MK, Tworoger SS, Davidson SM, Papagiannakopoulos T, Yang A, Dayton TL, Ogino S, Stampfer MJ, Giovannucci EL, Qian ZR, Rubinson DA, Ma J, Sesso HD, Gaziano JM, Cochrane BB, Liu S, Wactawski-Wende J, Manson JE, Pollak MN, Kimmelman AC, Souza A, Pierce K, Wang TJ, Gerszten RE, Fuchs CS, Vander Heiden MG, Wolpin BM. Elevation of circulating branched-chain amino acids is an early event in human pancreatic adenocarcinoma development. Nat Med. 2014 Oct;20(10):1193–8.

[71] Newgard CB, An J, Bain JR, Muehlbauer MJ, Stevens RD, Lien LF, Haqq AM, Shah SH, Arlotto M, Slentz CA, Rochon J, Gallup D, Ilkayeva O, Wenner BR, Yancy WS Jr, Eisenson H, Musante G, Surwit RS, Millington DS, Butler MD, Svetkey LP. A branched-chain amino acid-related metabolic signature that differentiates obese and lean humans and contributes to insulin resistance. Cell Metab. 2009 Apr;9(4):311–26.

[72] Sausen M, Phallen J, Adleff V, Jones S, Leary RJ, Barrett MT, Anagnostou V, Parpart-Li S, Murphy D, Kay Li Q, Hruban CA, Scharpf R, White JR, O'Dwyer PJ, Allen PJ, Eshleman JR, Thompson CB, Klimstra DS, Linehan DC, Maitra A, Hruban RH, Diaz LA Jr, Von Hoff DD, Johansen JS, Drebin JA, Velculescu VE. Clinical implications of genomic alterations in the tumour and circulation of pancreatic cancer patients. Nat Commun. 2015 Jul 7;6:7686.

[73] Kirimli CE, Shih WH, Shih WY. Amplification-free in situ KRAS point mutation detection at 60 copies per mL in urine in a background of 1000-fold wild type. Analyst. 2016 Feb 21;141(4):1421–33.

[74] Yachida S, Jones S, Bozic I, Antal T, Leary R, Fu B, Kamiyama M, Hruban RH, Eshleman JR, Nowak MA, Velculescu VE, Kinzler KW, Vogelstein B, Iacobuzio-Donahue CA. Distant metastasis occurs late during the genetic evolution of pancreatic cancer. Nature. 2010 Oct 28;467(7319):1114–7.

[75] Hait WN, Levine AJ. Genomic complexity: a call to action. Sci Transl Med. 2014 Sep 24;6(255):255 cm 10.

[76] Li D, Abbruzzese JL. New strategies in pancreatic cancer: emerging epidemiologic and therapeutic concepts. Clin Cancer Res. 2010 Sep 1;16(17):4313–8.

[77] Chai X, Chu H, Yang X, Meng Y, Shi P, Gou S. Metformin increases sensitivity of pancreatic cancer cells to gemcitabine by reducing CD133+ cell populations and suppressing ERK/P70S6K signaling. Sci Rep. 2015 Sep 22;5:14404.

[78] Cerullo M, Gani F, Chen SY, Canner J, Pawlik TM. Metformin Use Is Associated with Improved Survival in Patients Undergoing Resection for Pancreatic Cancer. J Gastrointest Surg. 2016 Sep;20(9):1572–80.

[79] Nolan E, Vaillant F, Branstetter D, Pal B, Giner G, Whitehead L, Lok SW, Mann GB; Kathleen Cuningham Foundation Consortium for Research into Familial Breast Cancer (kConFab)., Rohrbach K, Huang LY, Soriano R, Smyth GK, Dougall WC, Visvader JE, Lindeman GJ. RANK ligand as a potential target for breast cancer prevention in BRCA1-mutation carriers. Nat Med. 2016 Aug;22(8):933–9.

[80] Bruenderman E, Martin RC 2nd. A cost analysis of a pancreatic cancer screening protocol in high-risk populations. Am J Surg. 2015 Sep;210(3):409–16.

Chapter 7

Contrast-Enhanced Ultrasound for the Assessment of Pancreatic Lesions

Roxana Şirli and Alina Popescu

Additional information is available at the end of the chapter

http://dx.doi.org/10.5772/65066

Abstract

Transabdominal ultrasound (US) is the first-line imaging method used to diagnose pancreatic lesions, but contrast techniques are needed to differentiate among inflammatory and malignant lesions, as well as between pseudocysts and cystic tumors. Contrast-enhanced (CE) ultrasonography has been proven to be a useful tool in this regard with performance similar to contrast-enhanced computer tomography/magnetic resonance imaging (CT/MRI), being also safer and nonirradiant. According to the EFSUMB guidelines on the nonhepatic use of contrast-enhanced ultrasound (CEUS), this method is useful to improve characterization of ductal adenocarcinoma; to differentiate between pseudocysts and cystic tumors; to differentiate vascular (solid) from avascular (liquid/necrotic) components of a lesion; to better define the dimensions and margins of a lesion, including its relationship with adjacent vessels; and to help the choice for a next imaging technique.

Keywords: contrast-enhanced ultrasound, pancreas, pancreatic adenocarcinoma, pancreatic cystic lesions

1. Introduction

The pancreas, a retroperitoneal organ, is more difficult to evaluate by ultrasound (US), mostly due to a poor acoustic window generated by the interposition of intestinal gas between the transducer and the pancreas. In order to be able to correctly evaluate the pancreas, an experienced operator is needed.

On the other hand, US is a useful tool to identify pancreatic lesions, but ultrasound alone is not enough for the differential diagnosis and staging of the identified lesions, especially if a malignant tumor is suspected.

Contrast-enhanced ultrasound (CEUS) is not useful for the detection of focal pancreatic lesions, either solid or liquid. It is useful for the characterization of ultrasound-detected lesions at this level [1]. The technique can be used in acute and chronic pancreatitis (CP), in the characterization of solid tumors: ductal adenocarcinoma or neuroendocrine tumors, in the characterization of pseudocysts or pancreatic cystic tumors.

When a pancreatic tumor is detected, an immediate and correct differential diagnosis is mandatory to establish the appropriate management [2]. Conventional ultrasound followed by CEUS can provide a rapid assessment of the pancreatic lesion's pattern and can characterize the vascularization, thus making possible a differential diagnosis immediately after detection.

CEUS has the advantage of being a real-time imaging method that allows continuous visualization of vascular enhancement pattern, as opposed to contrast-enhanced (CE) computer tomography (CT) or magnetic resonance imaging (MRI), which only take snapshots at preset time moments. Due to lack of side effects and irradiation, CEUS can be repeated immediately if inconclusive.

The most frequently used ultrasound contrast agent for pancreas examination is SonoVue (Bracco SpA, Milan, Italy), a second generation, strictly intravascular contrast agent, containing sulfur hexafluoride–filled microbubbles encapsulated in a phospholipid shell. US contrast agents have no influence on micro-vascularity and can be also used in patients with renal failure, and also allergic reactions are exceptionally rare [2, 3], as opposed to contrast-enhanced CT/MRI [4–7].

2. CEUS technique and CEUS aspect of the normal pancreas

For the CEUS examination of the pancreas, usually a 2.4 ml bolus of SonoVue is injected in an antecubital vein, followed by a 10 ml bolus saline solution. Contrast-specific US modes are required for the contrast study. They are available on specific ultrasound systems and are generally based on the cancellation and separation of linear US signals from the tissue and use of the nonlinear response from the contrast agent microbubbles [1].

The examination is performed with low mechanical index, using conventional image for orientation, and following in the same time the contrast study in a specific window. A "real-time" dynamic observation of the contrast-enhanced phases – arterial (early stage of enhancement, until 30 s) and late (delayed stage of enhancement, 30–45 until 120 s following contrast injection) – begins immediately after the contrast bolus [1]. The following aspects are followed up during CEUS: timing and intensity of enhancement and the distribution of the contrast agent.

Approximately 25–40 s following the contrast bolus, the pancreas shows a homogeneous intense enhancement due to its rich vascularity (**Figure 1**) [8]. Also due to the rich vascularity, the pancreas has a rapid "wash-out," and 2 min following the contrast bolus, the pancreas appears as hypoenhancing as compared to the nearby liver (**Figure 2**) [8]. Thus, CEUS is useful especially for delineation of avascular pancreatic lesions.

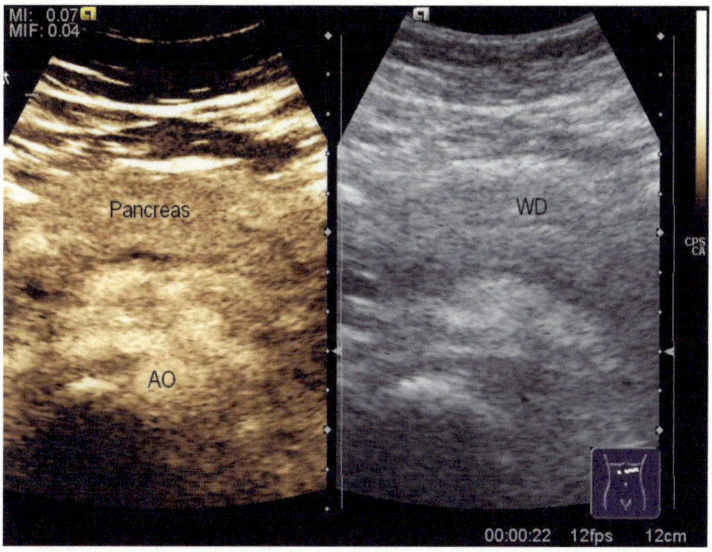

Figure 1. CEUS of the normal pancreas, arterial phase: homogeneous intense enhancement (AO—aorta).

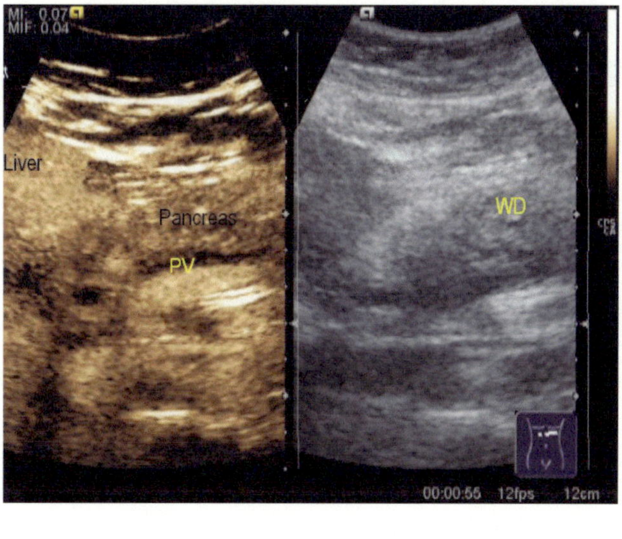

Figure 2. CEUS of the normal pancreas, late phase: the pancreas is hypoenhancing as compared to the liver (PV—portal vein; WD—Wirsung duct).

3. Acute pancreatitis (AP)

AP is a potentially severe disease with unpredictable outcome which can develop multiple complications with fast dynamics. The early differential diagnosis between a mild, edematous form and a severe, necrotic-hemorrhagic one is very important in order to be able to adapt the treatment and to be able to try to prevent the occurrence of complications. Currently, contrast-enhanced CT (CE-CT) is considered to be the reference method for the assessment and for staging AP [9]. But CE-CT is an irradiating, relatively expensive technique, and animal studies have suggested a potential risk of aggravation of AP following CE-CT due to pancreatic microcirculation impairment by the contrast agent [10–12], even if in human studies this effect has not been proven [13, 14]. Another impediment for CE-CT is the need for repetitive examinations according to the patient's evolution. This is why a safer, cheaper diagnostic tool would be useful for the diagnosis, staging, and follow-up of patients with AP.

Abdominal US is in most cases the first imaging method used to evaluate patients with AP since it is widely available, safe, rapid, and inexpensive. It is also nonirradiant, and thus, it can be repeated as often as needed to follow-up the patient's evolution. On the other hand, US has limitations due to the poor acoustic window in AP secondary to large amount of bowel gas and also due to the patient's abdominal pain which makes him unable to cooperate for an optimal evaluation.

Standard abdominal US allows only assessment of the imaging aspect of the pancreas in AP, without being able to assess vascularity. But it also reveals suggestive signs for a severe AP such as hyperechoic bursa omentalis (**Figure 3**) and presence of intra-peritoneal collections (peripancreatic, pericolic or in the Douglas space), while using Doppler US, a splenic vein thrombosis may be seen.

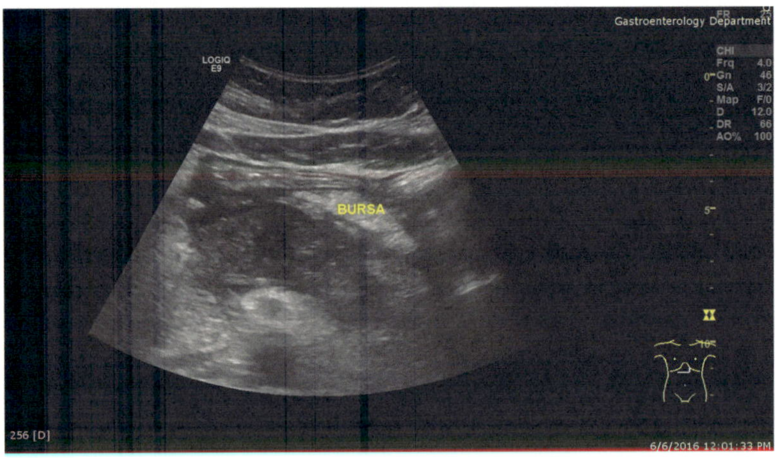

Figure 3. Acute pancreatitis, standard US: hypoechoic, inhomogeneous enlarged pancreas, hyperechoic bursa omentalis.

CEUS allows visualization of pancreatic vascularity and thus is able to reveal necrotic areas which will not enhance following the contrast bolus (**Figure 4**). But the same limitations as for standard US apply for CEUS, which is useless if the acoustic window for the pancreas is poor.

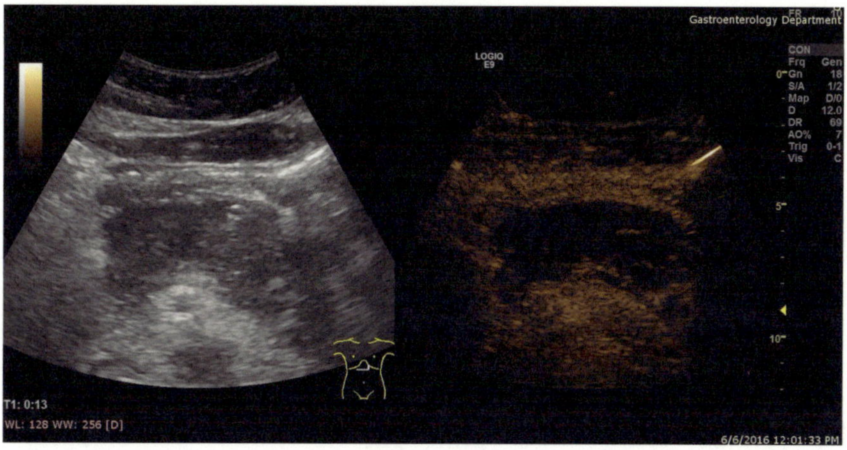

Figure 4. Severe acute pancreatitis, CEUS, arterial phase: almost the entire pancreas is unenhancing, revealing extensive necrosis.

Rickes et al. evaluated the accuracy of CEUS for the diagnosis of AP severity, considering CE-CT as the reference method, and they found out that CEUS had 82% sensitivity (Se), 89% specificity (Sp), 95% positive predictive value (PPV), and 67% negative predictive value (NPV) for diagnosing severe AP, with a much lesser cost than CE-CT [15]. Similar results were obtained by other authors, CEUS Se and Sp ranging from 86 and 97%, respectively [16], to 90.3 and 98.8%, respectively (97.4% accuracy) [17].

Thus, all these studies confirmed the value of CEUS for detecting pancreatic necrosis and for predicting the severity of AP. It showed similar results as compared with CE-CT with fewer side effects since CEUS is nonirradiant and since the US contrast agents have no influence on microvascularity and can also be used in patients with renal failure.

4. Chronic pancreatitis (CP)

During the evolution of CP, inflammatory masses can appear, a characteristic feature of pseudotumoral CP. Differential diagnosis between this entity and pancreatic cancer is often difficult not only due to the similar imaging aspect but also due to similar clinical symptoms [18]. The US aspect of pseudotumoral CP is most often of a hypoechoic, imprecisely delineated mass in the head of the pancreas. CEUS is useful to differentiate among the two entities since pancreatic adenocarcinomas are hypoenhancing following contrast (due to massive desmoplastic reaction as well as poor vascularity), while the inflammatory pseudotumor in CP will be enhancing in the arterial phase [19–21].

D'Onofrio et al. evaluated the performance of CEUS to diagnose pseudotumoral CP in a study that included 173 pancreatic masses. CEUS had 88.6% Se, 97.8% Sp, 91.2% PPV, and 96% accuracy for the diagnosis of pseudotumoral CP, while in 94% of cases the inflammatory mass showed moderate enhancement following contrast, similar to the adjacent pancreatic parenchyma [20].

A more recent study showed that the blood flow ratio between the superior mesenteric artery and the pancreatic parenchyma evaluated by CEUS correlates with the grade of chronic pancreatitis and concluded that this safe and convenient method may be useful for the early diagnose of CP [22].

A special entity is ***autoimmune pancreatitis***. It is characterized by a high level of gamma-globulins or IgG, presence of auto-antibodies, mild or absent clinical symptoms. Imaging techniques reveal an enlarged, "sausage-like" pancreas, with diffuse, irregular thinning of the Wirsung duct (WD), with possible stenosis of the retro-pancreatic main biliary duct and rarely cysts or calcifications in the pancreatic parenchyma [20]. Autoimmune pancreatitis is sometimes associated with other autoimmune diseases such as diabetes mellitus, inflammatory bowel disease, primary biliary cirrhosis, primary sclerosing cholangitis, or lupus.

On standard US, in autoimmune pancreatitis the imaging changes are most often diffuse. The pancreas is enlarged, hypoechoic and with a compressed Wirsung duct. Following contrast bolus, the pancreas is moderate or hyperenhancing in the early arterial phase, but also with inhomogeneous enhancement due to lymphocytic infiltration and fibrosis [20].

5. Solid focal pancreatic lesions

5.1. Ductal adenocarcinoma

Ductal adenocarcinomas represent 80–90% of the exocrine pancreatic tumors [23]. They have a poor prognosis, due to both their aggressiveness and the difficult diagnosis in early phases, in which effective treatment can be initiated.

On standard US, ductal adenocarcinoma most frequently appears as a hypoechoic, imprecisely delineated mass which sometimes exceeds the contour of the pancreas (which facilitates detection) (**Figure 5**), but which other times is completely embedded in the pancreatic parenchyma.

In CEUS, ductal adenocarcinoma is only slightly enhancing in the early phase, appearing as hypoenhancing as compared with the adjacent pancreatic parenchyma (**Figure 6**) probably due to the desmoplastic reaction and low mean vascular density [20, 23–25]. This pattern is present in approximately 90% of cases [2, 20, 26]. Moreover, CEUS enables a better visualization and staging of ductal adenocarcinoma by allowing a better delineation as well as assessment of vascular invasion [23, 27–29].

http://dx.doi.org/10.5772/65066

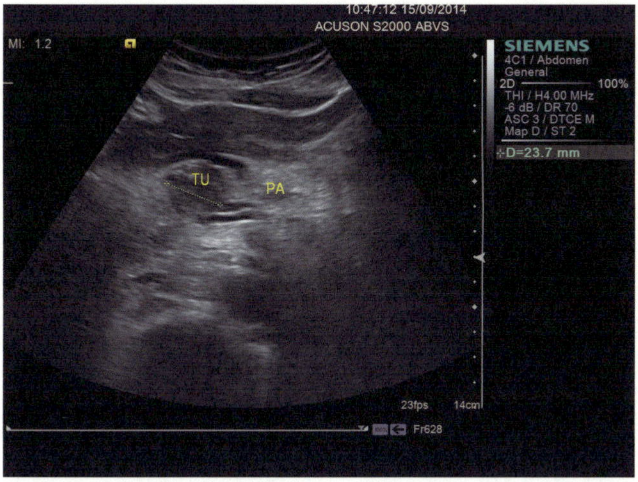

Figure 5. Ductal adenocarcinoma in the head of the pancreas, standard US: hypoechoic mass (TU arrows). PA—pancreas.

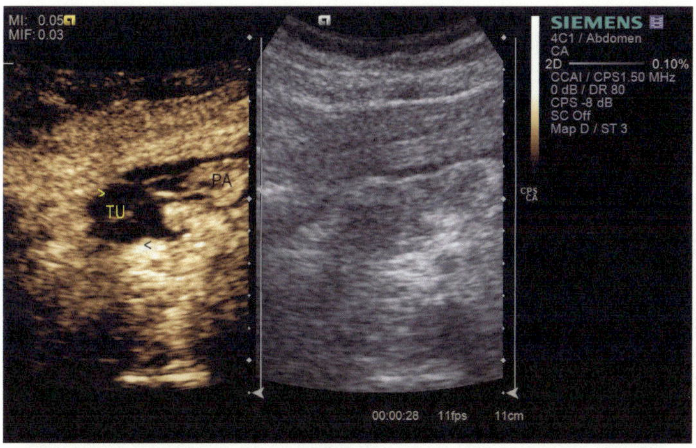

Figure 6. Ductal adenocarcinoma in the head of the pancreas, CEUS—arterial phase: hypoenhancing mass (TU—arrows) as compared to the adjacent pancreatic parenchyma (PA).

Also CEUS enables liver assessment in the late vascular phases, thus allowing visualization of eventual metastases, with a better accuracy than standard US. In the late phase (more than 120 s after the contrast bolus), liver metastases will appear as hypoenhancing focal liver lesions.

5.2. Neuroendocrine tumors

Neuroendocrine tumors may be symptomatic if they are secreting, with specific clinical signs according to the secreted hormone, or asymptomatic if they are nonfunctioning, in this case only nonspecific symptoms are present, secondary to tumoral growth.

Neuroendocrine tumors are hypervascular lesions [30]. On standard US, they have a similar aspect to ductal adenocarcinoma, as hypoechoic masses (**Figure 7**). The differential diagnosis among the two entities is extremely important, for prognosis, as well as for therapeutic strategy, and this is where CEUS can make a difference.

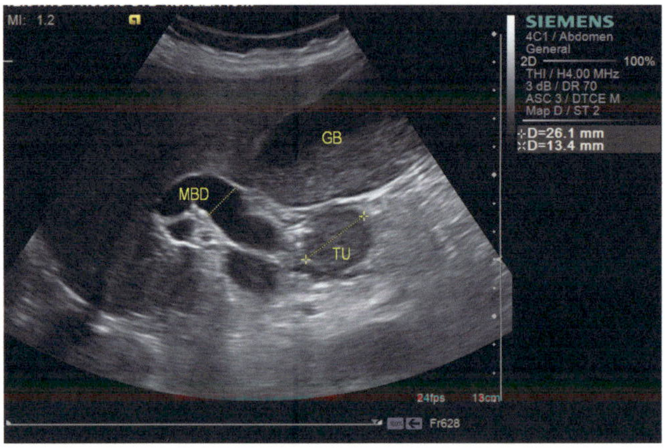

Figure 7. Neuroendocrine tumor in the pancreatic head, standard US: hypoechoic mass (TU). Dilated main biliary duct (MBD). GB—gallbladder.

On CEUS, there are different enhancing patterns according to the size and tumor vascularity [23]. Thus, large tumors show an intense enhancement in the early phase, excepting the necrotic areas that are unenhancing, while medium-sized lesions will also by enhancing in the arterial phase (**Figure 8**) [31]. Both types of lesions are hypoenhancing in the late phase (**Figure 9**). On the other hand, nonfunctioning neuroendocrine tumors can be hypovascular due to their dense hyaline stroma (they also appear as hypointense on CE-CT) [31, 32].

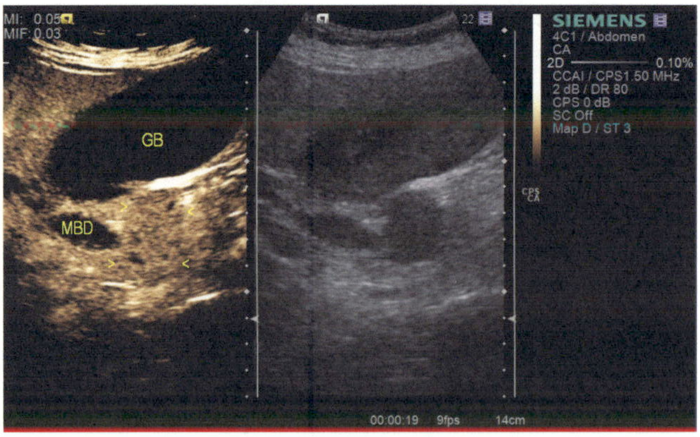

Figure 8. Neuroendocrine tumor in the pancreatic head, CEUS—arterial phase: hyperenhancing mass (arrows). Dilated main biliary duct (MBD). GB—gallbladder.

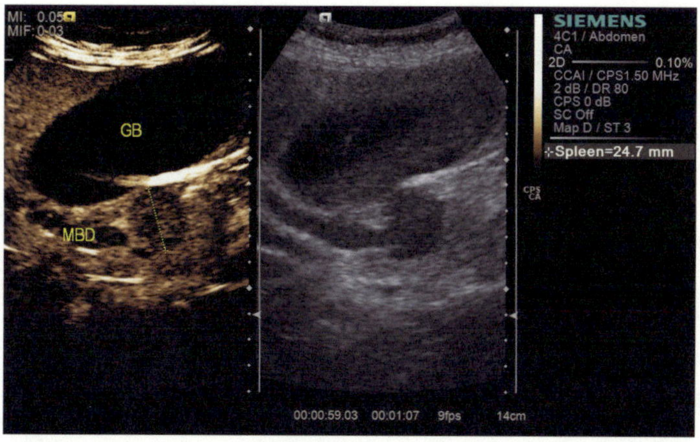

Figure 9. Neuroendocrine tumor in the pancreatic head, CEUS—late phase: hypoenhancing mass (arrows). Dilated main biliary duct (MBD). GB—gallbladder.

6. Cystic focal pancreatic lesions

6.1. Pseudocysts

Pseudocysts are the most frequent cystic pancreatic lesions and are characterized by a fibrous wall with no epithelium [33]. On standard US, they usually appear as anechoic lesions in the pancreatic area. Sometimes echoic material can be seen inside the lesions, usually in the lower areas (**Figure 10**). Association with an episode of acute pancreatitis in the recent history of the patient can be useful for a positive diagnosis.

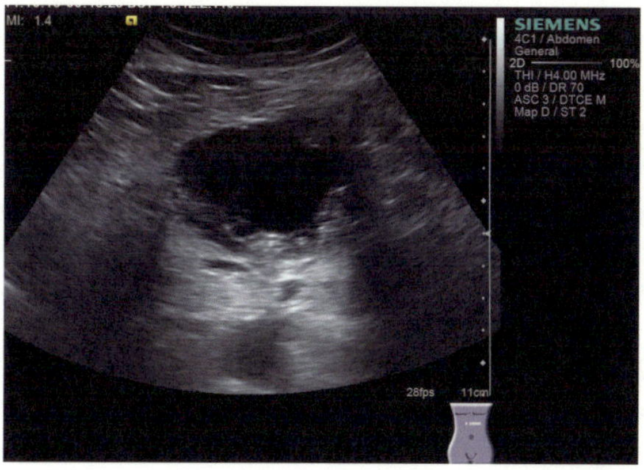

Figure 10. Pancreatic cystic lesion, standard US. Anechoic well-defined lesion, with thick, irregular walls that also have echoic protrusions.

In CEUS, pseudocysts appear as completely unenhancing due to the fact that they are avascular structures, even if in standard US they may have an echoic content (**Figure 11**). This feature is very important for the differential diagnosis with cystic pancreatic tumors [2, 23, 34]. The method has up to 100% sensitivity and specificity in characterizing these lesions [34].

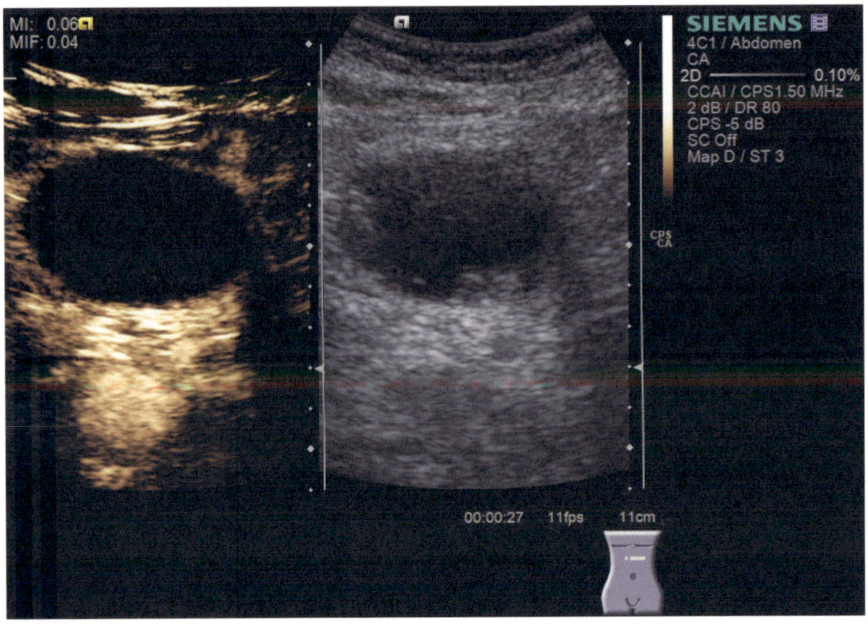

Figure 11. Pancreatic cystic lesion the same as in **Figure 10**, CEUS—arterial phase. Anechoic content with unenhancing walls and protrusions. Definitive diagnosis: pancreatic pseudocyst.

6.2. Mucinous cystadenomas and cystadenocarcinomas

Mucinous cystadenomas of the pancreas are rather rare and considered to be premalignant lesions. If found they should be resected to avoid malignant transformation. Differentiation between pancreatic serous cystadenoma and mucinous cystadenoma is difficult and is based on fine needle aspiration (FNA) that will reveal in the later high levels of carcinoembryonic antigen (CEA) in the aspirated fluid as well as a low level of pancreatic enzymes [35, 36]. They are cystic pancreatic masses, usually multilocular, rarely unilocular when they must be differentiated from pancreatic pseudocysts and from serous cystadenomas [37–41].

On standard US, mucinous cystic tumors appear as cystic masses with thick wall and septa, with echoic protrusions from the wall and with the content (mucin) not always anechoic, sometimes with peripheric calcifications (**Figure 12**). On CEUS, the cystic wall as well as the septa will enhance following the contrast bolus, being easy to differentiate from the unenhancing content (**Figure 13**). The presence of enhancing walls, protrusions, and septa is the differential element from pancreatic pseudocysts [23, 41–43].

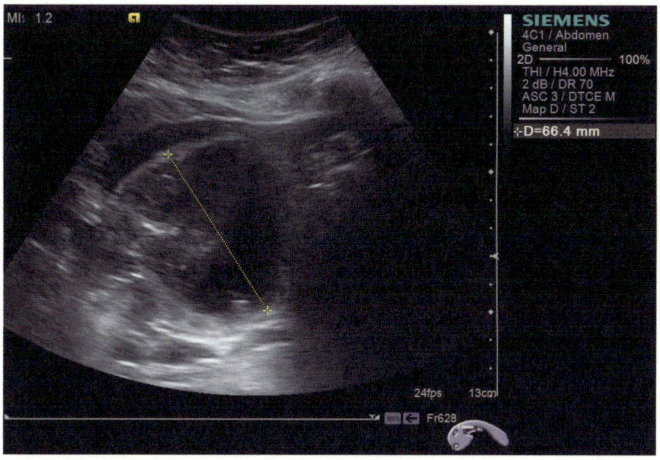

Figure 12. Large lesion in the body of the pancreas, standard US: lesion with thick walls and mixed content: anechoic component as well as echoic protrusion.

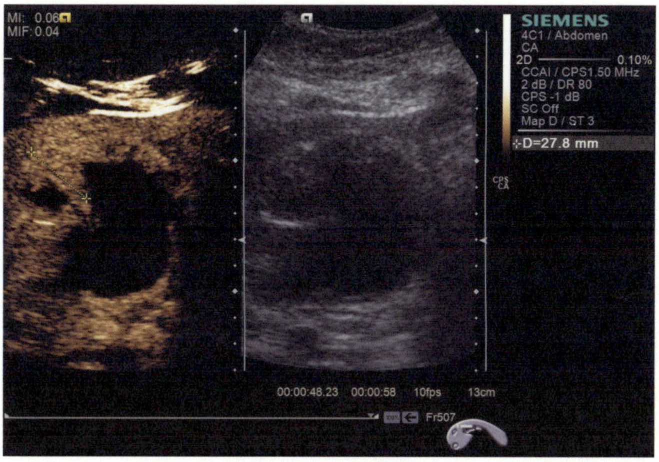

Figure 13. Large lesion in the pancreatic body: CEUS—arterial phase: the walls and the protrusion are enhancing. Conclusive for cystic tumor of the pancreatic body.

The diagnosis of intra-ductal papillary mucinous neoplasms (IPMN), main-duct or side branch-duct types, is based on MRI and endoscopic ultrasound. CEUS can be also helpful for differentiating between perfused (tumoral) and nonperfused (clot) regions [44].

6.3. Serous cystadenomas

Serous cystadenomas are benign cystic lesions, with a lobulated microcystic structure with thin and centrally oriented septa, which are vascularized on CEUS [43]. It may mimic a solid lesion, both on conventional US and on CEUS, but they are hyperenhanced on CEUS [44].

The criteria used for the differential diagnosis of pancreatic masses (standard US, Doppler US and CEUS) are presented in **Table 1**.

Lesion	Standard US	Power Doppler US	CEUS
Ductal adenocarcinoma	Hypoechoic Imprecisely delineated Dilated Wirsung duct Vascular invasion Metastases	Undetectable tumoral vessels	Poorly vascularized tumor (hypoenhancing) Marginal tumoral vessels
Acute pancreatitis	Hypoechoic Imprecisely delineated Necrotic areas Thrombosis	Rarely detectable vessels	Enhancement according to necrosis and inflammation: hyperenhancement in edematous AP with unenhancement of the necrotic areas
Chronic pancreatitis	Dilated Wirsung duct Calcifications	Rarely detectable vessels	Enhancement according to necrosis and inflammation: Hypoenhancement in CP
Neuroendocrine tumors	Hypoechoic Well delineated Undilated Wirsung duct Rare vascular invasion Metastases	Rarely detectable tumor vessels	Hyperenhancing tumors
Cystadenomas	Small cysts (<3 cm) Small size calcifications Fibrous septa Undilated Wirsung duct	Undetectable tumor vessels	Hyperenhancing tumors Arteries accompanying the fibrous septa
Cystadenocarcinomas	Large size cysts (>5 cm) Echoic areas inside the cyst and septaUndilated Wirsung duct Metastases	Rarely detectable chaotic tumor vessels	Enhancing echoic areas inside the cyst
Pseudocysts	Anechoic, well delineated lesion Signs of acute/chronic pancreatitis Signs of bleeding/calcifications Accompanying changes of the adjacent bowel	Rarely detectable tumor vessels in young lesions	Unenhancing walls

Table 1. Differential diagnosis of pancreatic masses [1, 9, 45, 46].

Several studies proved the utility of CEUS for the characterization of pancreatic tumors [2, 9, 17, 47–49]. The accuracy for the diagnosis of solid pancreatic lesions varies from 91.7% [2] to 92.9% [17] or 93.8% in other series [48].

http://dx.doi.org/10.5772/65066

In a recent meta-analysis that included 23 CEUS studies, the pooled estimate of CEUS sensitivity for the diagnosis of ductal adenocarcinoma was 0.89 (95% CI, 0.85–0.92), while the average specificity was 0.84 (95% CI, 0.77–0.89). For the differentiation of neoplastic and nonneoplastic lesions, the reported pooled sensitivity and specificity were 0.95 (95% CI, 0.93–0.96) and 0.72 (95% CI, 0.58–0.83) [50].

7. Contrast-enhanced endoscopic ultrasound (CE-EUS)

CE-EUS combines the benefits of high-resolution US to those of a contrast-enhanced imaging method. It has two subtypes with similar performance: contrast-enhanced endoscopic Doppler ultrasound (which uses a high mechanical index for examination and no special software) and contrast-enhanced low mechanical index endoscopic ultrasound (in which the examination is made in contrast mode) [51]. CE-EUS in Doppler mode is useful to differentiate between ductal adenocarcinomas (in which only arterioles are seen] and pseudotumoral chronic pancreatitis (in which both arterioles and venules can be identified by CE-EUS Doppler) [52, 53].

CE-EUS with low mechanical index has been used similarly to transabdominal CEUS to differentiate between pseudotumoral CP and ductal adenocarcinoma, but also to guide FNA in order to avoid avascular areas, improving the diagnostic accuracy of FNA [54]. Quantitative postprocedural assessment of uptake of the contrast agent has been proven useful to improve the accuracy of CE-EUS with low mechanical index for differentiating between the two entities [55, 56].

As a conclusion, we must cite the EFSUMB guidelines on the nonhepatic use of CEUS, which state that CEUS is useful to improve characterization of ductal adenocarcinoma (A;1b); to differentiate between pseudocysts and cystic tumors (A;1b); to differentiate vascular (solid) from avascular (liquid/necrotic) components of a lesion (A;1b); to better define the dimensions and margins of a lesion, including its relationship with adjacent vessels (B;2b); to help the choice for a next imaging technique (C;5) [1].

Author details

Roxana Șirli* and Alina Popescu

*Address all correspondence to: roxanasirli@gmail.com

Department of Gastroenterology and Hepatology, "Victor Babeș" University of Medicine and Pharmacy Timișoara, Romania

References

[1] Piscaglia F, Nolsoe C, Dietrich CF, Cosgrove DO, Gilja OH, Bachmann Nielsen M, et al. The EFSUMB guidelines and recommendations on the clinical practice of contrast enhanced ultrasound (CEUS): update 2011 on non-hepatic applications. Ultraschall Med 2012; 33: 33–59. doi:10.1055/s-0031-1281676

[2] D'Onofrio M, Barbi E, Dietrich CF, Kitano M, Numata K, Sofuni A, et al. Pancreatic multicenter ultrasound study (PAMUS). Eur J Radiol 2012; 81: 630–638. doi:10.1016/j.ejrad.2011.01.053

[3] Jakobsen JA, Oyen R, Thomsen HS, Morkos SK, Members of Contrast Media Safety Committee of European Society of Urogenital Radiology (ESUR). Safety of ultrasound contrast agents. Eur Radiol 2005; 15: 941–945. doi:10.1007/s00330-004-2601-0

[4] Piscaglia F, Bolondi L, Italian Society of Ultrasound in Medicine and Biology (SIUMB) Study Group on Ultrasound Contrast Agents. The safety of Sonovue in abdominal applications: retrospective analysis of 23188 investigations. Ultrasound Med Biol 2006; 32: 1369–1375. doi:10.1016/j.ultrasmedbio.2006.05.031

[5] Dillman JR, Ellis JH, Cohan RH, Strouse PJ, Jan SC. Frequency and severity of acute allergic-like reactions to gadolinium-containing i.v. contrast media in children and adults. AJR Am J Roentgenol 2007; 189: 1533–1538.

[6] Dean KE, Starikov A, Giambrone A, Hentel K, Min R, Loftus M. Adverse reactions to intravenous contrast media: an unexpected discrepancy between inpatient and outpatient cohorts. Clin Imaging Sep–Oct 2015; 39(5): 863–5. doi:10.1016/j.clinimag.2015.04.014

[7] Caschera L, Lazzara A, Piergallini L, Ricci D, Tuscano B, Vanzulli A. Contrast agents in diagnostic imaging: present and future. Pharmacol Res Aug 2016; 110: 65–75. doi:10.1016/j.phrs.2016.04.023

[8] Thorelius L. Usefulness of contrast-enhanced ultrasound in the characterization of pancreatic and renal masses. In: Albrecht T, Thorelius L, Solbiati L, Cova L, Frauscher F, ed. Contrast-enhanced Ultrasound in Clinical Practice. Springer, 2005, p. 25–35. DOI: 10.1007/88-470-0357-1_2

[9] Rickes S, Mönkemüller K, Malfertheiner P. Acute severe pancreatitis: contrast-enhanced sonography. Abdom Imaging 2007; 32: 362–364. doi:10.1007/s00261-007-9250-0

[10] Foitzik T, Bassi DG, Schmidt J, Lewandrowski KB, Fernandez-del Castillo C, Rattner DW, et al. Intravenous contrast medium accentuates the severity of acute necrotizing pancreatitis in the rat. Gastroenterology 1994; 106: 207–214. doi:10.1016/S0016-5085(94)95457-7

[11] Foitzik T, Bassi DG, Fernandez-del Castillo C, Warshaw AL, Rattner DW. Intravenous contrast medium impairs oxygenation of the pancreas in acute necrotizing pancreatitis in the rat. Arch Surg 1994; 129: 706–711. doi:10.1001/archsurg.1994.01420310038006

[12] Schmidt J, Hotz HJ, Foitzik T, Ryschich E, Buhr HJ, Warshaw A, et al. Intravenous contrast medium aggravates the impairment of pancreatic microcirculation in necrotizing pancreatitis in the rat. Ann Surg 1995; 221: 257–264. doi:10.1097/00000658-199503000-00007

[13] Carmona-Sanchez R, Uscanga L, Bezaury-Rivas P, Robles-Díaz G, Suazo-Barahona J, Vargas-Vorácková F. Potential harmful effect of iodinated intravenous contrast medium on the clinical course of mild acute pancreatitis. Arch Surg 2000; 135: 1280–1284. doi: 10.1001/archsurg.135.11.1280

[14] Uhl W, Roggo A, Kirschstein T, Anghelacopoulos SE, Gloor B, Müller CA, et al. Influence of contrast-enhanced computed tomography on course and outcome in patients with acute pancreatitis. Pancreas 2002; 24: 191–197. doi:10.1097/00006676-200203000-00011

[15] Rickes S, Uhle C, Kahl S, Kolfenbach S, Monkemuller K, Effenberger O, et al. Echo enhanced ultrasound: a new valid initial imaging approach for severe acute pancreatitis. Gut 2006; 55: 74–78. doi:10.1136/gut.2005.070276

[16] Ripolles T, Martinez MJ, Lopez E, Castello I, Delgado F. Contrast-enhanced ultrasound in the staging of acute pancreatitis. Eur Radiol 2010; 20: 2518–2523. doi:10.1007/s00330-010-1824-5

[17] Ardelean M, Sirli R, Sporea I, Bota S, Martie A, Popescu A, et al. Contrast enhanced ultrasound in the pathology of the pancreas - a monocentric experience. Med Ultrason 2014; 16(4): 325–331. doi:10.11152/mu.201.3.2066.164.mars12

[18] van Gulik TM, Reeders JW, Bosma A, Moojen TM, Smits NJ, Allema JH, et al. Incidence and clinical findings of benign, inflammatory disease in patients resected for presumed pancreatic head cancer. Gastrointest Endosc 1997; 46: 417–423. doi:10.1016/S0016-5107(97)70034-8

[19] Koito K, Namieno T, Nagakawa T, Morita K. Inflammatory pancreatic masses: differentiation from ductal carcinomas with contrast-enhanced sonography using carbon dioxide microbubbles. AJR Am J Roentgenol 1997; 169: 1263–1267. doi:10.2214/ajr.169.5.9353439

[20] D'Onofrio M, Zamboni G, Tognolini A, Malago R, Faccioli N, Frulloni L, et al. Mass-forming pancreatitis: value of contrast-enhanced ultrasonography. World J Gastroenterol 2006; 12: 4181–4184. doi:10.3748/wjg.v12.i26.4181

[21] D'Onofrio M, Malagò R, Martone E, et al. Pancreatic pathology. In: Quaia E, ed. Contrast Media in Ultrasonography. Berlin, Heidelberg: Springer-Verlag, 2005; 335–347.

[22] Azemoto N, Kumagi T, Yokota T, Hirooka M, Kuroda T, Koizumi M, et al. Utility of contrast-enhanced transabdominal ultrasonography to diagnose early chronic pancreatitis. Biomed Res Int 2015; 2015: 393124. doi:10.1155/2015/393124

[23] D'Onofrio M, Martone E, Malagò R, Faccioli N, Zamboni G, Comai A, et al. Contrast-enhanced ultrasonography of the pancreas. JOP. J Pancreas (Online) 2007; 8: 71–76.

[24] Kersting S, Konopke R, Kersting F, Volk A, Distler M, Bergert H, et al. Quantitative perfusion analysis of transabdominal contrast-enhanced ultrasonography of pancreatic masses and carcinomas. Gastroenterology 2009; 137: 1903–1911. doi:10.1053/j.gastro.2009.08.049

[25] Numata K, Ozawa Y, Kobayashi N, Kubota T, Shimada H, Nozawa A, et al. Contrast-enhanced sonography of pancreatic carcinoma: correlations with pathological findings. J Gastroenterol 2005; 40: 631–640. doi:10.1007/s00535-005-1598-8

[26] Kitano M, Kudo M, Maekawa K, Suetomi Y, Sakamoto H, Fukuta N, et al. Dynamic imaging of pancreatic diseases by contrast enhanced coded phase inversion harmonic ultrasonography. Gut 2004; 53: 854–859. doi:10.1136/gut.2003.029934

[27] Klöppel G. Pathology of the pancreas. In: Baert AL, Van Hoe DG, ed. Radiology of the Pancreas. 2nd ed. Berlin, Heidelberg: Springer-Verlag, 1999: 69–100.

[28] Faccioli N, D'Onofrio M, Malago R, Zamboni G, Falconi M, Capelli P, et al. Resectable pancreatic adenocarcinoma: depiction of tumoral margins at contrast-enhanced ultrasonography. Pancreas 2008; 37: 265–268. doi:10.1097/MPA.0b013e31816c908b

[29] Grossjohann HS, Rappeport ED, Jensen C, Svendsen LB, Hillingsø JG, Hansen CP, et al. Usefulness of contrastenhanced transabdominal ultrasound for tumor classification and tumor staging in the pancreatic head. Scand J Gastroenterol 2010; 45: 917–924. doi:10.3109/00365521003702718

[30] Procacci C, Carbognin G, Accordini S, Biasiutti C, Bicego E, Romano L, et al. Nonfunctioning endocrine tumors of the pancreas: possibilities of spiral CT characterization. Eur Radiol 2001; 11: 1175–1183. doi:10.1007/s003300000714

[31] D'Onofrio M, Mansueto G, Falconi M, Procacci C. Neuroendocrine pancreatic tumor: value of contrast enhanced ultrasonography. Abdom Imaging 2004; 29: 246–258. doi:10.1007/s00261-003-0097-8

[32] Malago R, D'Onofrio M, Zamboni GA, Faccioli N, Falconi M, Boninsegna L, et al. Contrast-enhanced sonography of nonfunctioning pancreatic neuroendocrine tumors. Am J Roentgenol 2009; 192: 424–430. doi:10.2214/AJR.07.4043

[33] Hammond N, Miller FH, Sica GT, Gore RM. Imaging of cystic disease of the pancreas. Radiol Clin North Am 2002; 40: 1243–1262. doi:10.1016/S0033-8389(02)00054-4

[34] Rickes S, Wermke W. Differentiation of cystic pancreatic neoplasms and pseudocysts by conventional and echo-enhanced ultrasound. J Gastroenterol Hepatol 2004; 19: 761–766. doi:10.1111/j.1440-1746.2004.03406.x

[35] Lewandrowski K, Lee J, Southern J, Centeno B, Warshaw A. Cyst fluid analysis in the differential diagnosis of pancreatic cysts: a new approach to the preoperative assessment of pancreatic cystic lesions. AJR Am J Roentgenol Apr 1995; 164(4): 815–819. doi: 10.2214/ajr.164.4.7537015

[36] Le Borgne J, de Calan L, Partensky C, the French Surgical Association. Cystadenomas and cystadenocarcinomas of the pancreas: a multiinstitutional retrospective study of 398 cases. Ann Surg 1999; 230(2): 152. doi:10.1097/00000658-199908000-00004

[37] Fugazzola C, Procacci C, Bergamo Andreis IA, Iacono C, Portuese A, Dompieri P, et al. Cystic tumors of the pancreas: evaluation by ultrasonography and computed tomography. Gastrointest Radiol 1991; 16: 53–61. doi:10.1007/BF01887305

[38] Sperti C, Cappellazzo F, Pasquali C, Militello C, Catalini S, Bonadimani B, et al. Cystic neoplasms of the pancreas: problems in differential diagnosis. Am Surg 1993; 59: 740–745.

[39] Demos TC, Posniak HV, Harmath C, Olson MC, Aranha G. Cystic lesions of the pancreas. AJR Am J Roentgenol 2002; 179: 1375–1388. doi:10.2214/ajr.179.6.1791375

[40] Scott J, Martin I, Redhead D, Hammond P, Garden OJ. Mucinous cystic neoplasm of the pancreas: imaging features and diagnostic difficulties. Clin Radiol 2000; 55: 187–192. doi:10.1053/crad.1999.0341

[41] D'Onofrio M, Caffarri S, Zamboni G, Falconi M, Mansueto G. Contrast-enhanced ultrasonography in the characterization of pancreatic mucinous cystadenoma. J Ultrasound Med 2004; 23: 1125–1129.

[42] D'Onofrio M, Megibow AJ, Faccioli N, Malagò R, Capelli P, Falconi M, et al. Comparison of contrast-enhanced sonography and MRI in displaying anatomic features of cystic pancreatic masses. Am J Roentgenol 2007; 189: 1435–1442. doi:10.2214/AJR.07.2032

[43] Itoh T, Hirooka Y, Itoh A, Hashimoto S, Kawashima H, Hara K, et al. Usefulness of contrast-enhanced transabdominal ultrasonography in the diagnosis of intraductal papillary mucinous tumors of the pancreas. Am J Gastroenterol 2005; 100: 144–152. doi: 10.1111/j.1572-0241.2005.40726.x

[44] D'Onofrio M, Gallotti A, Pozzi Mucelli R. Imaging techniques in pancreatic tumors. Expert Rev Med Devices 2010; 7: 257–273. doi:10.1586/erd.09.67

[45] Rickes S, Unkrodt K, Ocran K, Neye H, Lochs H, Wermke W. Evaluation of Doppler ultrasonography criteria for the differential diagnosis of pancreatic tumors. Ultraschall Med 2000; 20: 253–258. doi:10.1055/s-2000-9124

[46] Rickes S, Flath B, Unkrodt K, Ocran K, Neye H, Lochs H. Pancreatic metastases of renal cell carcinomas – evaluation of the contrast behaviour at echo-enhanced power Doppler

sonography in comparison to primary pancreatic tumors. Z Gastroenterol 2001; 39: 571–578. doi:10.1055/s-2001-16690

[47] D'Onofrio M, Gallotti A, Principe F, Mucelli RP. Contrastenhanced ultrasound of the pancreas. World J Radiol 2010; 2: 97–102. doi:10.4329/wjr.v2.i3.97

[48] Dietrich CF, Braden B, Hocke M, Ott M, Ignee A. Improved characterization of solitary solid pancreatic tumours using contrast enhanced transabdominal ultrasound. J Cancer Res Clin Oncol 2008; 134: 635–643. doi:10.1007/s00432-007-0326-6

[49] Ardelean M, Sirli R, Sporea I, Bota S, Danila M, Popescu A, et al. The value of contrast-enhanced ultrasound in the characterization of vascular pattern of solid pancreatic lesions. Med Ultrason 2015; 17(1): 16–21. doi:10.11152/mu.2013.2066.171.mars

[50] D'Onofrio M, Biagioli E, Gerardi C, Canestrini S, Rulli E, Crosara S, et al. Diagnostic performance of contrast-enhanced ultrasound (CEUS) and contrast-enhanced endoscopic ultrasound (ECEUS) for the differentiation of pancreatic lesions: a systematic review and meta-analysis. Ultraschall Med 2014; 35(6): 515–21. doi:10.1055/s-0034-1385068

[51] Dietrich CF, Sharma M, Hocke M. Contrast-enhanced endoscopic ultrasound. Endosc Ultrasound 2012; 1(3): 130–6. doi:10.7178/eus.03.003

[52] Hocke M, Schulze E, Gottschalk P, Topalidis T, Dietrich CF. Contrast-enhanced endoscopic ultrasound in discrimination between focal pancreatitis and pancreatic cancer. World J Gastroenterol 2006; 12(2): 246–50. doi:10.3748/wjg.v12.i2.246

[53] Săftoiu A, Iordache SA, Gheonea DI, Popescu C, Malos A, Gorunescu F, et al. Combined contrast-enhanced power Doppler and real-time sonoelastography performed during EUS, used in the differential diagnosis of focal pancreatic masses (with videos). Gastrointest Endosc 2010; 72(4): 739–47. doi:10.1016/j.gie.2010.02.056

[54] Seicean A, Badea R, Moldovan-Pop A, Vultur S, Botan EC, Zaharie T, et al. Harmonic contrast-enhanced endoscopic ultrasonography for the guidance of fine-needle aspiration in solid pancreatic masses. Ultraschall Med 2015. [Epub ahead of print]. doi: 10.1055/s-0035-1553496

[55] Seicean A, Badea R, Stan-Iuga R, Mocan T, Gulei I, Pascu O. Quantitative contrast-enhanced harmonic endoscopic ultrasonography for the discrimination of solid pancreatic masses. Ultraschall Med 2010; 31(6): 571–6. doi:10.1055/s-0029-1245833

[56] Săftoiu A, Vilmann P, Dietrich CF, Iglesias-Garcia J, Hocke M, Seicean A, et al. Quantitative contrast-enhanced harmonic EUS in differential diagnosis of focal pancreatic masses (with videos). Gastrointest Endosc 2015; 82(1): 59–69. doi:10.1016/j.gie.2014.11.040

Chapter 8

The Improvement of Care in Patients with Pancreatic Cancer

Christopher Riley, Nicole Villafane and
George Van Buren

Additional information is available at the end of the chapter

http://dx.doi.org/10.5772/66078

Abstract

Introduction: Pancreas adenocarcinoma (PDAC) remains a lethal malignancy with a high-mortality rate and poor long-term survival. The management of PDAC has evolved over the years to incorporate multidisciplinary care and numerous treatment modalities.

Body: We discuss the current standard of care for the management and treatment of PDAC. We also discuss the value of managing PDAC patients with multidisciplinary care, at high volume pancreas centers, with multimodality therapy, and with innovative surgical techniques.

Conclusion: PDAC is an aggressive malignancy. Nuances in the management of the disease can help to improve outcomes.

Keywords: pancreas adenocarcinoma, pancreas cancer, borderline resectable, neoadjuvant therapy, whipple, distal pancreatectomy, robotic surgery

1. Introduction

Pancreatic ductal adenocarcinoma (PDAC) is currently the 10th most commonly diagnosed cancer in the United States and the third leading cause of cancer-related mortality. It is expected to become the second leading cause of cancer-related death by 2030 [1, 2]. While most of the other more common (lung, breast/prostate, and colon) causes of cancer-related mortalities have shown signs of down-trending throughout the years, PDAC has shown an unfortunate upward trend [3]. The increasing incidence and mortality is likely multifactorial, with increasing environmental exposures, increase in survival age, or any other of the many stratifying risk factors. Regardless of the factors influencing the increasing risk of acquiring PDAC, the aggressiveness of the disease itself should be a continued target in the attempt to control or decrease the disease morbidity and mortality [3–5]. PDAC has an aggressive tumor biology with a propensity for early metastasis. Less than 20% of patients with PDAC will present with disease amenable to surgical and potentially curative therapy [1, 3].

The reason for the poor survival in PDAC patients is multifactorial. Tumor biology, lack of screening and early diagnostic test, historically morbid surgical interventions, and systemic therapies with limited efficacy are factors that have been shown to significantly affect the outcomes of patients with PDAC. The combination of the aforementioned factors has led to pessimism within the medical community about the efficacy of pancreatic disease management [6]. However, several advances have been made over the years; and with such a highly lethal disease, any margin of progress can be a large gain. Some of these advances are related to the improvement in coordination of care to overcome systemic barriers that limit the overall efficacy in caring for the disease; other advances have been technical in nature; and finally, several advances have been made in the approach of systemic therapies.

2. Multidisciplinary management team

One of the primary challenges of the modern healthcare system is the fractured nature in which care is provided [7]. Patients with PDAC may be seen by a primary care doctor or gastroenterologist but may never be seen by a medical or surgical oncologist, depending on disease recognition and provider referral. In order to accomplish a more desirable outcome, a balance must be reached between access to care and the quality of care provided. In a disease presenting with many obstacles, providers having experience in managing PDAC and patients having access to the most advanced therapies, including clinical trials, can make a significant difference in outcomes. Research into these systemic healthcare factors has spurred the production of various causal effect models; one model, in particular, demonstrates the effect of the type of provider in charge of disease management and its impact on the patient receiving expected treatment [7, 8].

Historically, the pessimistic outlook for patients with PDAC has generated skepticism regarding the efficacy of therapy and resection. These attitudes adversely affect proven beneficial disease management involving the utilization of surgical and medical interventions, particularly evident in cases of early stage pancreatic cancer [7, 9, 10]. Bilimoria et al. were able to demonstrate that despite modern improvements in survival after pancreatectomy, 51.7% of Stage I patients did not undergo surgery for potentially resectable pancreatic cancer even after accounting for patients who did not undergo surgery due to severe comorbidities, advanced age, or patient refusal. Patients were less likely to undergo surgery if they were older, were black, had lower annual incomes, had less education, or were on Medicare or Medicaid [6]. This difference in management exhibits a significant correlation with the racial and socioeconomic discrepancy. Similar discrepancies in care due to race and socioeconomic status have been reported by several studies [11, 12]. Patients were more likely to receive surgery at academic institutions, high-volume hospitals, and National Comprehensive Cancer Network or National Cancer Institute (NCCN/NCI) centers. This was the first study to describe and characterize such striking underuse of pancreatectomy while identifying factors predicting underutilization [6, 7, 11].

While the initial referral is critically important, once a patient has been referred to a surgeon or an oncologist, the provider's level of experience in managing PDAC is of equal, if not more, significance. The early involvement of a pancreatic cancer specialist has been proven to exhibit a most marked effect on early-staged disease patients [7–9]. Physicians who care for PDAC patients on a regular basis have several advantages over those who rarely treat the disease. These advantages are evident when comparing perioperative and intraoperative statistics, such as estimated blood loss, case duration, length of postoperative hospital stay, perioperative death, and need for reoperations [13]. Evidence shows us that increased surgical or disease management experience decreases disease morbidity [7, 13]. Improving morbidity, in an already highly morbid disease, will help alter the pessimism surrounding PDAC through recognition of some impactful management options.

It is known that surgery is the only curative therapy for PDAC [6]. It is also known that either adjuvant or neoadjuvant therapy is the patient's best shot for a prolonged survival [7, 14, 15]. Recent evidence regarding oncological diseases has shown that the multidisciplinary approach will have beneficial effects on disease management [7–10]. As such, the development of multidisciplinary treatment teams and multimodal therapeutic interventions has become the benchmarks of PDAC patient management. Most patients, regardless of stage, require multiple subspecialty services including surgery, gastroenterology, medical and radiation oncology, nutrition, and palliative care [7]. These teams allow for the development and collaboration of specialty expertise, bringing a variety of perspectives to each PDAC case.

Although specific team composition may vary throughout center sites, studies continue to illustrate the overall correlation of this model with improved quality of care. Studies assessing the efficacy of this model have demonstrated decreased diagnosis-to-treatment time, increased probability of receiving treatment, prolonged survival, increased involvement of multimodality therapy, and increased enrollment and participation in clinical trials. One significantly impactful factor in this model is the decreased diagnosis-to-treatment time. Evidence shows that approximately 80% of early Stage I/II diagnosed PDAC patients, not seen in specialized, multidisciplinary centers, fail to receive a potentially curative surgery or life-prolonging treatment [8, 9]. Of early-stage (Stage I/II) disease patients who did not receive surgical resection, only 28% had a surgical referral. Of early-stage patients who had received surgical intervention, it was noted that referral to a pancreatic disease specialized center or surgeon significantly impacted whether surgery was performed; 80% of early-stage patients seen in a specialized pancreatic disease clinic received surgery, whereas only 20% of comparable patients *not* seen in a specialized clinic received surgery [7, 16].

Another factor to consider multidisciplinary approach to caring for pancreatic cancer patients is the greater accessibility and probability of the use of multimodal therapy. While studies continue to show variance in the statistical significance of multimodal therapies, they remain an important element in the development of more effective interventional therapies for such an aggressive cancer. Correspondingly, the inclusion of patients in clinical trials is another benefit of multidisciplinary team centers. Studies have shown up to a two times higher likelihood of patients participating in a clinical trial when seeing a multidisciplinary team. This plays an important role in acquiring a greater understanding of the disease and the development of more effective therapies [7, 16].

Ultimately, the historical lack of multidisciplinary care is only one of multiple factors attributed to the poor survivability curve seen in PDAC patients. However, in recent years, changes in the management of PDAC have started to shift the curve toward showing improvement in the acute care of patients as well as increasing the number of long-term outcomes [17].

3. Defining the disease

The diagnosis of PDAC often remains a challenge. The utilization of various imaging modalities in the diagnosis and staging of PDAC continue to be utilized. Computed tomography (CT), ultrasonography (US), magnetic resonance imaging (MRI), and endoscopic ultrasonography (EUS) are the routinely used modalities that are relatively accessible in hospitals and specialized cancer centers. As the management of PDAC has advanced and become more aggressive analogous to the nature of the disease, imaging modalities play an important role, not only as a noninvasive option in the diagnostic phase of the disease but also in the determination of disease burden, resectability, and the monitoring of treatment efficacy [18].

CT scanning is the accepted first line investigative modality in PDAC suspected patients. This modality is usually preferred because it provides high-resolution/quality images and relatively wide availability, and its complete studies are relatively quicker than other high-resolution counterparts. CT scans are reported to provide 100% sensitivity and 72% specificity in predicting the resectability of PDAC [19]. This modality also allows for the ability to use a specific image-attaining protocol for more thorough evaluation of the pancreas. This pancreas protocol utilizes thin-sectioned slices and captures images during certain postcontrast injection time frames. Because PDAC is a hypovascular tumor, it is best detected in the late arterial phase at 35–40 s postcontrast injection, when the normal pancreatic parenchymal tissue is most optimally enhanced while the hypovascular tumor is not. At 70-s postcontrast injection, the portal venous system is optimally enhanced, which can prove helpful in assessing any extent of venous involvement and identifying possible liver metastases. These two phases are typically obtained during a pancreatic protocol CT. Of note, when there is a concern for pancreatic islet cell (endocrine) tumor exists, an earlier (20–25-s postcontrast injection), arterial phase scan is usually most beneficial, since these tumors are often hypervascular. Some of these endocrine tumors can be visualized in the portal venous phase as well, and thus dual phases of arterial and portal venous scanning are usually done for suspected pancreatic endocrine tumors. The pancreatic protocol CT scan produces images with PDAC classically appearing as a hypodense lesion relative to the pancreatic parenchyma [19, 20]. On an approximate, 10% of cases where PDAC lesions are isodense on imaging, distinguishing the tumor can be more difficult. Other signs can be present on CT imaging that increase detection of a pancreatic mass.

Lesions present in the pancreatic head can produce a secondary finding of "double duct" sign, which is the presence of simultaneous dilation of the common bile and main pancreatic ducts. This is due to the tumor in the head portion of the pancreas compressing the ducts causing obstruction and fluid build-up that result in dilation of both ducts. Tumor in the body or tail of the pancreas can result in stenosis and obstruction of the main pancreatic duct, resulting in an upstream dilation of the main pancreatic duct. These signs can be beneficial in distinguishing a more isodense lesion or in the confirmation of a smaller, hypodense PDAC lesion. However, this modality can be limited in its ability to differentiate an isodense lesion and to show possible metastatic disease when denoted by small lesions in certain areas such as the peritoneum or liver [18, 20, 21].

One of the most sensitive and high-quality image producing modalities to date is the MRI. The MRI modality in comparison to CT scans provides greater soft tissue quality. This allows for superiority in imaging of smaller tumors and fatty infiltration of the pancreatic parenchyma, and in distinguishing lesions that would show as isodense lesion on CT scan. The most effective MRI-weighted imaging sequence for assessing the pancreas is the T1-weighted, fat suppressed sequence. In this sequence, PDAC usually appears hypointense [18]. Other sequences (T2-weighted, DWI, and GRE) have been shown to be relatively inconsistent in the PDAC intensity seen on imaging; however, they are still useful in assisting thorough evaluation of the pancreatic tissue. Another advantage of the MRI is the ability to perform a more in-depth examination of the pancreatic ducts utilizing magnetic resonance cholangiopancreatography (MRCP). This technique allows for inspection of the ductal systems and ability to discern small ductal narrowing secondary to a small lesion or to detect confounding etiologies to ductal dilation such as a stone obstructing either the common bile or main pancreatic duct. MRCP, in conjunction with the MRI, can result in more efficacious detection in early stage pancreatic disease by allowing more detailed study of the pancreatic parenchyma and ductal system. Limitations of this modality in the diagnosis and interventional benefits in PDAC disease include significant time for study completion, fairly high cost, easy susceptibility to artifact and difficult accessibility in areas with limited resources [18, 21].

Ultrasonography (US) is a most likely and readily available modality than all other applicable modalities in visualizing the pancreas. US can also be done very quickly with low cost and increased portability. However, US scan of the pancreas is fairly low in quality, requires specific preimaging preparation for the patient, and requires trained and experienced people for the operation to be most effectively utilized. A minimum 6-h fast is required to better visualize the pancreas; this fast preparation improves visualization by limiting bowel gas and ensuring an empty stomach. The scan protocol evaluates different sectional cuts (transverse, oblique, and sagittal) along the pancreatic duct in the search for signs of obstruction or stenosis. This can often visualize the pathognomonic observation of double duct sign in PDAC of the pancreatic head. The PDAC lesion is often evident as a hypoechoic lesion on imaging. However, diagnostic utility of US is highly dependent upon the operator's training and experience, the burden or progression of disease, and the habitus of a patient [18, 21].

Endoscopic ultrasound (EUS) has been considered as a modality producing highly accurate detection of small (greater than 3 cm) lesions. This modality provides visualization of the pancreatic tissue and parenchyma from the stomach or duodenum. It allows for higher quality images to be obtained in comparison to standard US. EUS also has the benefit of being able to obtain specimens via fine needle aspiration. On its own, EUS is not highly effective in differentiating a chronic pancreatic disease such as chronic pancreatitis and pancreatic cancer, with evidence showing the accuracy at 76% for detecting cancer and 46% for detecting a local inflammation, whereas the combination of EUS and fine needle aspiration has shown to increase the detection percentage of pancreatic cancer to 90% and above [18]. Limitations of this modality include the necessity of conjoined procedures, including a more invasive, albeit minimally, technique. Fine need aspiration is also not a widely and readily available resource amongst all hospital and care centers.

One of the most important components of a multidisciplinary team is that the presenting state of the disease is agreed upon, and a treatment plan is constructed in accordance with national guidelines for care while also taking into account distinctive patient factors. The expertise of the multidisciplinary team and standardized national definitions regarding disease staging are associating factors best utilized concurrently in determining disease burden and the initial steps in optimizing patient management. Although pathologic staging criteria for PDAC have long been established through the American Joint Commission on Cancer (AJCC), clinical staging criteria has not been as well defined. For an extensive period of time, common language was lacking for defining the degree of tumor involvement with surrounding vasculature and the subsequent classification of whether or not it is safely resectable. From a surgical perspective, the determination for surgical intervention is based on the tumor's determined resectability. By classifying patient tumors as resectable, borderline resectable, locally advanced, and metastatic, the care team is better able to standardize treatment regimens for patients. Furthermore, more defined classifications allow for greater adherence to national guidelines [20, 22].

Although several definitions of resectability have emerged over the years, the most widely accepted classification, which has also subsequently been incorporated in the National Comprehensive Cancer Network (NCCN) criteria, was defined by Callery et al. [22]. They constructed a consensus criterion based on radiographic CT findings in the preoperative staging phase. Resectable tumors are those that (1) had demonstrated no distant metastases; (2) had shown no radiographic evidence of superior mesenteric vein (SMV) and portal vein abutment, distortion, tumor thrombus, or venous encasement; and (3) had shown clear fat planes around the celiac axis, hepatic artery, and superior mesenteric artery. Borderline resectable tumors are defined as those that (1) had shown no distant metastases; (2) demonstrated either some venous involvement of SMV/portal vein (a) with tumor abutment with or without (i) impingement and narrowing of the lumen, (ii) encasement of the SMV/portal vein without encasement of the nearby arteries, or (iii) short segment venous occlusion resulting from either tumor thrombus or encasement, (b) but with suitable vessel proximal and distal to the area of vessel involvement, which allows for safe resection and reconstruction; (3) demonstrated some gastroduodenal artery encasement up to the hepatic artery with either short segment encasement or direct abutment of the hepatic artery, without extension to the celiac axis; and (4) demonstrated tumor abutment of the SMA not to exceed more than 180° of the circumference of the vessel wall. Locally advanced tumors were defined as those that fell outside the definition of borderline resectable. Metastatic tumors were defined as those with any evidence of metastatic disease [22].

Despite the relatively high accuracy in predicting unresectable disease, current imaging modalities still lack indisputable certainty in predicting the degree of resectable disease. A complimentary tool for increasing sensitivity in assessing a tumor's resectability and stage is diagnostic laparoscopy. Per guidelines, for apparent resectable disease, utilization of laparoscopy should be used with clinical predictors that optimize yield including pancreatic head tumors greater than 3 cm, tumors of the pancreas body and tail, ambiguous findings on CT scan, or high CA 19-9 levels (>100 U/mL). In addition, locally advanced and unresectable pancreatic cancer, without radiographic evidence of distant metastasis, should also be further evaluated with laparoscopy in order to rule out subclinical metastatic disease so that the care team's therapeutic management can be optimized [20, 22].

4. High-volume centers

The outside referral to pancreatic cancer specialist, hospital, and institutional volume of patients treated for pancreas cancer matters as well. The volume of patients treated and cases seen directly correlate with the experience gained by the providers in the management care team [13, 23]. The pancreaticoduodenectomy (PD) was classically a very morbid operation with mortality after PD nearing 25% in the 1960s [6, 17]. The morbidity associated with the operation was multifactorial. However, the factor most attributable to the morbidity is the risk of pancreatic fistula development. Often unrecognized, and thus untreated, a pancreatic fistula is the development of an abnormal communication between the pancreas and other organs secondary to the leakage of pancreatic secretions from damaged pancreatic ducts. This communication can prove highly detrimental to the involved organs. A pancreatic fistula substantially contributes to the most morbid complications seen with the operation such as erosion of retroperitoneal vessels and hemorrhage, intra-abdominal abscess, sepsis, multisystem organ failure, and death [24]. Over the years, PD morbidity and mortality have improved significantly, with mortality dropping to less than 3% in some high-volume centers. The involvement of high-volume pancreatic surgical centers has greatly contributed to this decline. Multiple studies have demonstrated a relationship between hospital surgical volume and outcomes for pancreatectomy [24, 25]. Specifically illustrating that as hospital volume for pancreatic surgery increases, perioperative mortality, postoperative complications, length of stay, and overall cost decreases, and long-term survival improves [6]. In 2011, a 10-year observational study (1999–2008) examined the relationship between cancer center volume and particular cancer operations. PD was compared to several other cancer and high-risk operations including esophagectomy, lung resection, cystectomy, AAA repair, and carotid endarterectomy, among others. The study found an increase in the median number of cancer and high-risk operations performed at hospitals. Pancreatic cancer surgery exhibited the greatest observed median increase, with an approximate 200% national increase in the median number of patients receiving pancreatic cancer surgery at each hospital, an increase of 5 patients per center to 16 per center. This figure is most notably influenced by the 56% national increase in patients seen for pancreatic disease, and the 25% national decrease in the number of hospitals performing the PD procedure, which does not detract from the fact that more pancreatic cancer patients are being seen and more PD procedures are being done. The most encouraging finding is that with this increase in PDAC patients seen and PD cases performed, there has been an almost 20% decrease in the postpancreatectomy mortality (death prior to hospital discharge or within 30 days after surgery). These findings denote a strong correlation observed between the operative risk incurred and the hospital's relevant surgical case volume [25–27]. While some high-risk operations examined in the study showed minimal volume-outcome relationship, there was substantial evidence that the volume-outcome relationship for PD is particularly strong. It has also been suggested that differences in surgical technique, such as margin involvement with resection, might be influential on the volume-based differences seen in PD mortality and morbidity. Resected margins showing cancerous involvement (margin-positive) are a poor prognostic factor after PD. The study found that patients undergoing PD at low-volume pancreatic cancer centers are more likely to have margin-positive resections, either macroscopic (R2), microscopic (R1), or both [26, 27]. These findings support the concept of improved morbidity and mortality of PD at high-volume centers and emphasize the importance of PDAC patient referral to specialized, high-volume centers.

5. Improvement in surgical care of the patient

Over the last 20 years, significant advances in preoperative evaluation, surgical techniques, and postoperative care have reduced the perioperative morbidity and mortality associated with pancreatic surgery. Mortality after pancreaticoduodenectomy has dropped from 25% in the 1960s to less than 3% in some high-volume centers, with recent studies suggesting postresection long-term survival rates approaching 30%.While numerous studies and guidelines establish pancreatectomy as the primary intervention for localized PDAC, pessimism concerning pancreatic cancer disease is the likely cause of continued skepticism in the efficacy of resection. In opposition to this belief, surgeon cumulative and yearly volume in the treatment of pancreatic diseases has emerged as a surrogate marker for quality outcomes. Surgical volume produces surgical experience, and, as Birk et al. illustrated, higher volume pancreatic centers result in lower operative mortality [25]. While the number of pancreatic cancer centers is declining, the increase in case number correlating with the decrease in morbidity and mortality suggests that the market concentration of cases is providing the opportunity to obtain more experience for the surgeons performing them [25]. There has been documentation illustrating that personal surgical volume can affect patient outcome [23, 24]. This concept illustrates the importance of surgical proficiency as a contributing factor on operative morbidity and mortality, despite the complexity or high-risk nature of the operation. High-volume centers offer the opportunity for pancreatic specialized surgeons to become more experienced with the cancer operations as well as more accustomed to varying surgical expectations and complications, thus resulting in reduced operative mortality and improved outcomes. Evidence has emphasized the correlation of operative experience and case load, surgical benchmarks and the pancreatic surgical learning curve [23–25]. One study looking at approximately 2200 pancreatic surgeries performed during 1984–1991 showed a significant correlation between a surgeon's number of cases done and the mortality rate. Low-volume surgeons (<10 resections) exhibited a 16% mortality rate in comparison to higher volume surgeons (>40 resections), who exhibited a 5% mortality rate (Fisher, list paper). Fisher et al. also showed this concept to be true. The author looked at the first 11-year period of a particular surgeon's pancreatic practice, examining 162 Whipple procedures performed, divided into two categories of low-volume era (0–11 cases/year) and high-volume era (>22 cases/year). Patients in the low-volume era had a higher likelihood of exhibiting one or more complications when compared to patients in the high-volume era (58% low volume vs 46% high volume) (Fisher). Training environment, in addition to case volume, is important in acquiring and strengthening the proficiency desired for preferred pancreatic surgical outcomes [16, 23, 25]. Surgeons at academic or more specialized centers appeared to significantly progress at a greater rate, likely due to the substantial experience of the providers available to initially assist in training or mentoring more inexperienced surgeons.

6. Improvements in perioperative care

The perioperative phases of the surgically treated pancreatic cancer patient have substantially improved due to the establishment of multidisciplinary care teams, the advancement of diagnostic and interventional techniques, and the continued progression of surgical experience and proficiency. While much of this can be attributed to the development of extensive technical modalities and abilities, proper and successful recovery is also an essential factor in improving postsurgical patient outcomes. The enhanced recovery after surgery (ERAS) program is a multimodal strategy that attempts to mitigate functional loss and morbidity, while improving recovery and progression of functional capabilities in the perioperative setting. The pathways included in the ERAS strategy include various preoperative and postoperative recommendations that have significant effect on a patient's morbidity development and hospital course [28].

Significant preoperative strategies include preoperative counseling, preoperative smoking and alcohol cessation, decision to use oral bowel preparation, and anticoagulation and antimicrobial prophylaxis [28–32]. Preoperative counseling, including procedural expectations and postoperative objectives, allows for the subduing of surgical anxiety and fear. This in turn results in improved postsurgical course [28]. Preoperative smoking and alcohol cessation can substantially improve a patient's outcome. At least 1 month of abstainence from smoking and alcohol reduces the otherwise two- to threefold postoperative morbidity increase seen in these patients. Also, this concept results in a considerable reduction in the pulmonary and wound complications often present in this group [28, 29]. Oral bowel preparation is thought to reduce complications of the surgery. However, evidence has shown that there is no clinical benefit to performing mechanical bowel preparation. Data actually show that there is more of an increased risk of dehydration or electrolyte imbalance, particularly in elderly patients [28]. Thus, it is strongly recommended that mechanical bowel preparation not be used as a preoperative strategy. The malignancy of pancreatic disease in conjunction with the major surgical procedure of PD puts the patient at a substantially higher risk of acquiring a venous thromboembolic event (VTE). The evidence strongly supports the beneficial use of a heparin, preferably low-molecular-weight heparin due to its 1× daily administration, in preventing or significantly reducing the risk of VTE. Standard prophylaxis involves administration 2–12 h prior to surgery and continuation until patient has fully mobilized, with some evidence suggesting benefit of continuation until 4 weeks after discharge. Mechanical preventative measures should also be utilized in even higher risk patients. Preoperative antibiotics are another highly recommended strategy for improving postoperative course and outcome of patients. Usual antibiotic prophylaxis recommended for pancreatic surgery include either 2 g (30 mg/kg peds) of Ancef (cefazolin, first-line), clindamycin(900 mg, 10 mg/kg peds)/vancomycin (15 mg/kg adult/ped) plus gentamicin (5 mg/kg, 2.5 mg/kg peds), or the addition of 400 mg (6 mg/kg peds) Diflucan (fluconazole) for patients at high risk of acquiring fungal infection such as in cases where there is enteric drainage of the pancreas [30]. Evidence indicates that antibiotic prophylaxis should be initiated 30–60 min prior to skin incision for optimal efficacy with repeated doses intraoperatively, depending on half-life of the utilized drug.

It is noteworthy that postoperative strategies are somewhat more extensive; however, strongly recommended strategies include adequate pain control, glycemic control, early diet advancement, early mobilization, and early removal of anastomotic drains (after 72 h). Pain control in the postoperative period is often highly important in patient cooperation with postoperative, recovery goals. While specific evidence for superiority between epidural, patient controlled analgesia, and other intravenous medications is less, proper pain control evidently results in earlier progression through postoperative objectives such as early mobilization. Postoperative morbidity and mortality are greatly influenced and increased by hyperglycemia and insulin resistance. Intensive care unit postoperative patients have been documented to exhibit a lower complication risk with a reduced hyperglycemic rate. Because abdominal surgery is associated with increased levels of insulin resistance, a significant increase in baseline postoperative morbidity risk occurs since the risk of hyperglycemia increases. Insulin administration is important in keeping glucose under control; however, caution must be taken for the prevention of hypoglycemia. While evidence indicating best glucose levels is controversial, basic hyperglycemic prevention will is needed to improve outcomes despite the baseline level [28, 31]. Furthermore, optimizing nutrition, with early diet advancement, in the postoperative period remains a strongly recommended strategy as well. The majority of patients will be able to tolerate oral intake shortly after elective PD. Evidence has shown that early oral intake is safe. Recent evidence has shown that early initiation of regular diet is reasonable and safe, and that enteral tube feeds illustrate no additional or greater benefit. There is also no evidence of improved benefit or safety of provider-controlled diet advancement (e.g., sips of liquids compared to regular diet), and a patient-controlled advancement as tolerated [28]. Another often recommended postoperative strategy is early and/or scheduled patient ambulation or mobilization. Patients should begin mobilizing or trying to ambulate in the morning of postoperative day 1. This strategy significantly reduces standard postoperative complications resulting from patient inactivity such as atelectasis and VTE risk. This can be encouraged through removal of barriers to ambulating or mobilizing such as a foley, and setting incremental patient activity goals on a daily basis, such as laps around the hospital floor, moving to a chair for a set period of time, among others. This has shown to reduce the rate of postoperative complications as well as reduce hospital length of stay and improve recovery time [28, 32].

While the aforementioned concepts and strategies prove significant for the management of acute surgical patients, the overall management strategy for a pancreatic cancer patient has substantially changed. Historically, nasogastric decompression postpancreatectomy, particularly PD, was deemed necessary, not only to avoid tension on the gastrojejunostomy but also due to the concern of delayed gastric emptying, which was the most common complication after the procedure. However, it has been shown that foregoing nasogastric decompression after pancreatectomy (both PD and DP) is safe and does not result in increased frequency or severity of postoperative complications, including placement or replacement of a nasogastric tube after surgery. It also has no effect on length of stay or advancement to regular or post-gastrectomy diet [33].This evidence aligns with ERAS program recommendations for pancreatectomy patients. Nasogastric decompression should thus be reserved exclusively for selected patients, particularly approximately 10–25% [34] of patients who develop delayed gastric emptying (DGE) after PD.

Another topic of broad and current interest has been the use of intraperitoneal drains after pancreatectomy. Multiple high-volume single-institution studies have shown either no difference or a decreased overall complication rate with elimination of routine drainage. This is likely the result of the elimination of a portal of entry for bacteria and a potential source of strain on the anastomosis, the latter particularly with the use of closed suction drains. However, when routine elimination of drains was evaluated in a multicenter randomized controlled trial, there was an increase in the number of patients that had at least one? Grade 2 complication (drain 52% vs no drain 68%; $p = 0.047$) and a higher complication severity ($p = 0.027$). Not only was there an increase in morbidity, but also there was a fourfold increase in mortality from 3 to 12% in patients undergoing PD without intraperitoneal drain placement. It is important to emphasize that these results apply only to PD patients, but based on the evidence, abandonment of routine intraperitoneal drainage in this group of patients is not safe. More studies are needed to address the safety of early removal of drains in PD in compliance with ERAS protocols. As for DP, the safety of routine elimination of drains is currently being evaluated in a multicenter randomized controlled trial (NCT01441492, clinicaltrials.gov).

Finally, there is a strong recommendation for early removal of perianastomotic drains, usually within 72 h. The anastomotic drains are believed to reduce the consequential effects seen with minor pancreatic leaks. Evidence showed that early removal of a drain in low-risk pancreatic fistula patients (drain fluid amylase <5000 U/L) was associated with a significantly reduced rate of pancreatic fistula formation, abdominal complications and pulmonary complications. There has also been increased scrutiny surrounding whether drain placement is even necessary to begin with. While there is data supporting this strategy, there is also data showing otherwise [32]. Van Buren et al. studied this concept by looking at 137 PD patients in a randomized prospective multicenter trial, 68 with drain placement and 69 without. From the Level 1 data provided, it was shown that elimination of the intraperitoneal drain in PD cases resulted in a significant increase in severity and frequency of postoperative complications. Furthermore, the study also illustrated a fourfold increase in mortality (3–12%) [35]. This raises skepticism toward findings in the previous literature and supports advocating caution against eliminating the use of drains altogether. However, per ERAS recommendations, early removal of the drain is associated with fewer and reduced rate of complications [28, 35].

These strategies provide a unified protocol for perioperative management of the PD procedure that could likely prove beneficial to centers through reducing postoperative complication rates, time of recovery and hospital length of stay [28, 32]. Ultimately, it is the summation of these factors that contribute to the improvement in the postoperative outcomes of pancreatic cancer patients. While the aforementioned concepts and strategies prove significant for the management of the acute surgical patient, the overall management strategy for a pancreatic cancer patient has substantially changed [23, 25, 28, 32].

7. Technical advances

Many of the advances that are discussed above are system-based and involve the perioperative period of patient care. These have had a tremendous impact on patient outcomes in the treatment of PDAC. But of all the modalities involved, surgery remains the only treatment with the potential for cure in patients with localized pancreatic cancer. Significant improvements in preoperative evaluation and postoperative care have reduced the perioperative morbidity and mortality associated with pancreatectomy. As previously discussed, mortality after PD has dropped significantly and there have also been improvements in long-term survival rates. In addition to these changes, surgical technique itself is progressing and evolving.

In an evidence-based systematic review, Wright and Zureikat identified four key elements that have allowed minimally invasive pancreatic surgery to gain momentum: safety, oncologic efficacy, cost, and reproducibility. Even though the evidence available is not the result of randomized controlled trials but instead on case series matched with cohorts undergoing open procedures, morbidity and mortality have been shown to be comparable between minimally invasive (MI) and open techniques. This applies for both PD and DP and encompasses all modalities of MI techniques: laparoscopy, robotic-assisted surgery, and their institutional variations.

The main concern with the adoption of MI techniques for the treatment of PDAC is undoubtedly oncologic efficacy. A study by Kendrick et al. favored MI technique by demonstrating fewer delays to initiation of adjuvant chemotherapy after laparoscopic PD with similar oncologic survival when compared to that in open procedure. Another study using the National Cancer Data Base demonstrated no difference in oncologic outcomes between laparoscopic and open PD [36]. In the setting of DP cases, Lee and colleagues (reference below) showed similar oncologic outcomes and high rates of R0 resection between open and laparoscopic DP. The mean number of lymph nodes evaluated in the aforementioned series was higher with open DP (15.4) when compared with the minimally invasive techniques (10.4 with laparoscopy and 12 with robotic approach). However, there was no statistically significant difference in the number of positive lymph nodes evaluated. Although the retrospective design of these studies introduces the possibility of selection bias in terms of patient selection, surgeon preference/experience, and preoperative patient and oncologic characteristics, the available evidence so far demonstrates that laparoscopic and robotic approaches to pancreatectomy do not adversely affect oncologic outcomes and add benefits such as decreased EBL and LOS [37–39]. However, it is important to note that the sources of most of the available literature are high-volume centers, which introduces a potential source of bias and reinforces the importance of patient evaluation and treatment at high-volume centers with multidisciplinary teams.

Cost is one of the limitations of MI pancreatectomy, particularly the robotic technique. However, some authors have shown the robotic technique to be cost effective when the reduction in length of stay is taken into consideration [40, 41]. Additionally, the robotic technical skills are potentially easier to acquire when compared to laparoscopic technique. This is secondary to the advantages provided by stereotactic vision, robotic simulators, and training consoles. The learning curve defined as 80 cases for a reduction in operative time may shorten with time since the operative steps and training techniques have recently become better defined [42].

Another noteworthy technical advancement is the incorporation of vascular resection (VR) with PD. Tseng et al. described five types of venous resection and reconstruction involving the superior mesenteric vein (SMV), portal vein (PV), or superior mesenteric-portal venous (SMPV) confluence. These are tangential resection with saphenous vein patch (V1), segmental resection with splenic vein ligation and primary anastomosis (V2) or with interposition graft (V3), segmental resection without splenic vein ligation and primary anastomosis (V4) or with interposition graft (V5). In their single institution series, Tseng and colleagues demonstrated that properly selected patients with PDAC of the head of the pancreas undergoing VR had a median survival of approximately two years. There was no statistical difference between survival of patients undergoing standard PD and those undergoing PD and VR ($p = 0.177$) [43].

Adequate patient selection for PD with VR has been possible by technological advances in computer tomography and by a multidisciplinary approach involving surgeons and radiologists. While several single center studies [44–46] have demonstrated PD with VR to be safe, a retrospective cohort analysis of the National Surgical Quality Improvement Program database demonstrated increased postoperative morbidity and mortality with the inclusion of venous resection [47]. This difference can be attributed to publication bias since most of the previously published single center studies have been from high-volume centers. Based on this, PD with VR in carefully selected patients at high-volume institutions opens up the possibility of survival comparable to that of patients undergoing standard PD, even in the setting of an increased frequency of R1 resections in patients that require VR [43].

Not only has surgical technique evolved but also, operative standards of care have been improved. It is known that lymph node metastasis is a poor prognostic factor for PDAC of the pancreatic head. The retrieval of an adequate number of lymph nodes or total lymph nodes examined (TNLE) is a measure of quality of care. Not only does it lead to optimal locoregional control but also, it is of upmost importance for pathological staging. Current NCCN guidelines recommend that at least 11 lymph nodes are retrieved and examined. Gleisner and colleagues showed an association between TNLE and overall survival, but the association was not uniform through time at their institution. Standards of care improved. We have found that less than 12 lymph nodes are inadequate lymphadenectomy [48].

8. Therapeutics

The standard chemotherapy regimen for advanced pancreatic cancer has historically been monotherapy with gemcitabine [49]. In patients with metastatic PDAC, gemcitabine with nab-paclitaxel improved median overall survival (8.5 vs 6.7 months, HR = 0.72, $p < 0.001$), one-year survival (35 vs 22%), two-year survival (9 vs 4%), and improved objective response rate (23 vs 7%) when compared with gemcitabine alone [50]. The most common Grade 3 or higher toxicity events were neutropenia, fatigue, and neuropathy.

Given that the majority of patients who undergo resection with curative intent relapse within 2 years [51], the CONKO-001 trial set to evaluate the efficacy of gemcitabine as adjuvant therapy administered as a dose of 1 g/m^2 on day 1, 8, and 15 every 4 weeks for 6 months. After a median follow-up of 136 months, patients treated with gemcitabine had an increased median disease-free survival (13.4 vs 6.7 months, HR, 0.55 [95% CI, 0.44–0.69]; $p < 0.001$) and prolonged overall survival (HR, 0.76 [95% CI, 0.61–0.95]; $p = 0.01$) versus those patients who were only observed after resection. In 2010, a randomized controlled trial compared the use of fluorouracil plus folinic acid versus gemcitabine as adjuvant chemotherapy. There was no difference in survival between the two treatments [52]. Although alternative chemotherapy regimens have since emerged, utilizing other agents as either monotherapy or in combination with gemcitabine, few studies have demonstrated significantly improved results [24].

There has been increased interest in the use of neoadjuvant therapy for the treatment of pancreatic adenocarcinoma given the potential for better treatment tolerance, improved delivery to an undisturbed tumor bed, avoidance of delay in therapy, treatment of occult micrometastatic disease, and the potential of down staging borderline/unresectable tumors. In a meta-analysis evaluating 14 Phase II trials involving gemcitabine and 5-FU chemotherapy regimens (either as monotherapy or combination therapy), there was no difference in local recurrence between patients who were initially considered resectable prior to systemic therapy and those who were not. Only 1.8% of patients had a complete tumor response, while 18.8% of all patients had partial tumor response based on RECIST criteria or criteria defined by the authors of each respective study. Pathologic response was not reported. While there was no difference in survival between the groups of patients deemed resectable pretreatment and those determined to be unresectable, approximately one-third of tumors initially classified as borderline/unresectable were suitable for resection after neoadjuvant therapy [53].

Despite the lack of Phase III trials addressing neoadjuvant therapy, it is important to emphasize its role in selecting patients who will be good surgical candidates once restaged after completion of treatment. It not only allows for better patient selection based on tumor biology, but also increases the possibility of R0 resection and patient completion of multimodal therapy. In contrast to the findings described previously, a neoadjuvant approach using gemcitabine-based chemo radiation resulted in a median survival of 34 months for the patients who were candidates for PD versus 7 months for those who did no undergo surgical resection. Additionally, this study revealed that a gemcitabine-based approach to neoadjuvant therapy is superior to 5-FU and paclitaxel-based preoperative regimens in terms of better survival of patients after PD [54].

The FOLFIRINOX regimen, combining 5-flurouracil, leucovorin, irinotecan, and oxaliplatin, was first implemented in the ACCORD-11 trial conducted by the PRODIGE group. Among 342 patients with previously untreated metastatic PDA, this regimen resulted in an increase in median overall survival from 6.8 months in the gemcitabine group to 11.1 months in the FOLFIRINOX group (HR = 0.57, $p < 0.001$). However, the regimen resulted in increased Grade 3 or 4 adverse effects secondary to treatment, such as neutropenia, febrile neutropenia, thrombocytopenia, diarrhea, and sensory neuropathy. The toxicity of the regimen thus raises concern for its use in patients with more advanced age, poor ECOG status, or greater comorbidities. For this group of patients, gemcitabine with nab-paclitaxel may be a better option due to its safer toxicity profile, although response to treatment is not as impressive as that observed with FOLFIRINOX. The efficacy of FOLFIRINOX as first-line therapy in the metastatic setting has prompted the evaluation of its potential in the neoadjuvant setting for patients with borderline or locally advanced disease. FOLFIRINOX followed by chemoradiation as neoadjuvant therapy has been shown to be safe in selected patients and has been shown to result in R0 resections [55]. As FOLFIRINOX continues to become increasingly incorporated into clinical practice, further study of patients who tolerate the regimen will help determine predictive factors associated with improved response to this therapy [56–68].

9. Conclusion

Pancreas adenocarcinoma is an aggressive malignancy. Progression to a multidisciplinary approach to diagnosis, treatment, and perioperative patient management can improve patient outcomes. This can be achieved through the implementation of state-of-the-art diagnostic modalities, including imaging and endoscopic procedures, as well as the application of enhanced recovery pathways that address every aspect of the treatment process from preoperative patient optimization to postoperative rehabilitation. Advances in surgical technique, particularly the use of laparoscopy and robotic-assisted surgery, also provide benefits to patients without compromising oncologic outcomes. Lastly, advancements in systemic chemotherapy, although slower in progression, have shown some improvement in survival when combined with surgical resection and offer a treatment alternative to patients with advanced disease who are not surgical candidates.

Author details

Christopher Riley, Nicole Villafane and George Van Buren*

*Address all correspondence to: george.vanburen@bcm.edu

Division of Surgical Oncology, Elkins Pancreas Center, Michael E. DeBakey Department of Surgery, Baylor College of Medicine , Houston, USA

References

[1] Rahib, L., B. D. Smith, R. Aizenberg, A. B. Rosenzweig, J. M. Fleshman, and L. M. Matrisian. "Projecting Cancer Incidence and Deaths to 2030: The Unexpected Burden of Thyroid, Liver, and Pancreas Cancers in the United States." Cancer Research 74.11 (2014): 2913–921.

[2] Ma, J., R. Siegel, and A. Jemal. "Pancreatic Cancer Death Rates by Race Among US Men and Women, 1970-2009." JNCI Journal of the National Cancer Institute 105.22 (2013): 1694–700.

[3] Winter, J. M., M. F. Brennan, L. H. Tang, M. I. D'Angelica, R. P. Dematteo, Y. Fong, D. S. Klimstra, W. R. Jarnagin, and P. J. Allen. "Survival after Resection of Pancreatic Adenocarcinoma: Results from a Single Institution over Three Decades." Annals of Surgical Oncology Ann Surg Oncol 19.1 (2011): 169–75.

[4] Thorson, Alan G. "Progress in Cancer Care: A Rational Call To Do Better." CA: A Cancer Journal for Clinicians 60.1 (2010): 7–11.

[5] Riall, T., W. Nealon, J. Goodwin, D. Zhang, Y. Kuo, C. Townsendjr, and J. Freeman. "Pancreatic Cancer in the General Population: Improvements in Survival Over the Last Decade." Journal of Gastrointestinal Surgery 10.9 (2006): 1212–224.

[6] Bilimoria, K. Y., D. J. Bentrem, C. Y. Ko, A. K. Stewart, D. P. Winchester, and M. S. Talamonti. "National Failure to Operate on Early Stage Pancreatic Cancer." Annals of Surgery 246.2 (2007): 173–180.

[7] Schiffman, S. C., S. Abberbock, S. Winters, C. Valko, J. Steve, A. H. Zureikat, H. J. Zeh, and M. E. Hogg. "A Pancreatic Cancer Multidisciplinary Clinic: Insights and Outcomes." Journal of Surgical Research 202.2 (2016): 246–52.

[8] Pawlik, T. M., D. Laheru, R. H. Hruban, J. Coleman, C. L. Wolfgang, K. Campbell, S. Ali, E. K. Fishman, R. D. Schulick, and J. M. Herman. "Evaluating the Impact of a Single-Day Multidisciplinary Clinic on the Management of Pancreatic Cancer." Annals of Surgical Oncology 15.8 (2008): 2081–088.

[9] Gardner, T. B., R. J. Barth, B. I. Zaki, B. R. Boulay, M. M. Mcgowan, J. E. Sutton, G. H. Ripple, T. A. Colacchio, K. D. Smith, I. R. Byock, M. Call, A. A. Suriawinata, M. J.

Tsapakos, J. B. Mills, A. Srivastava, M. Stannard, M. Lisovsky, S. R. Gordon, and J. M. Pipas. "Effect of Initiating a Multidisciplinary Care Clinic on Access and Time to Treatment in Patients with Pancreatic Adenocarcinoma." Journal of Oncology Practice 6.6 (2010): 288–92.

[10] Katz, M. H. G., H. Wang, J. B. Fleming, C. C. Sun, R. F. Hwang, R. A. Wolff, G. Varadhachary, J. L. Abbruzzese, C. H. Crane, S. Krishnan, J.-N. Vauthey, E. K. Abdalla, J. E. Lee, P. W. T. Pisters, and D. B. Evans. "Long-Term Survival After Multidisciplinary Management of Resected Pancreatic Adenocarcinoma." Annals of Surgical Oncology 16.4 (2009): 836–47.

[11] Wray, C. J., E. Castro-Echeverry, E. J. Silberfein, T. C. Ko, and L. S. Kao. "A Multi-institutional Study of Pancreatic Cancer in Harris County, Texas: Race Predicts Treatment and Survival." Annals of Surgical Oncology 19.9 (2012): 2776–781.

[12] Khawja, S. N., S. Mohammed, E. J. Silberfein, B. L. Musher, W. E. Fisher, and G. Van Buren. "Pancreatic Cancer Disparities in African Americans." Pancreas 44.4 (2015): 522–27.

[13] Fisher, W. E., S. E. Hodges, M.-F. Wu, S. G. Hilsenbeck, and F. C. Brunicardi. "Assessment of the Learning Curve for Pancreaticoduodenectomy." The American Journal of Surgery 203.6 (2012): 684–90.

[14] Evans, D. B., G. R. Varadhachary, C. H. Crane, C. C. Sun, J. E. Lee, P. W. T. Pisters, J.-N. Vauthey, H. Wang, K. R. Cleary, G. A. Staerkel, C. Charnsangavej, E. A. Lano, L. Ho, R. Lenzi, J. L. Abbruzzese, and R. A. Wolff. "Preoperative Gemcitabine-Based Chemoradiation for Patients with Resectable Adenocarcinoma of the Pancreatic Head." Journal of Clinical Oncology 26.21 (2008): 3496–502.

[15] Oettle, H., P. Neuhaus, A. Hochhaus, J. T. Hartmann, K. Gellert, K. Ridwelski, M. Niedergethmann, C. Zülke, J. Fahlke, M. B. Arning, M. Sinn, A. Hinke, and H. Riess. "Adjuvant Chemotherapy with Gemcitabine and Long-term Outcomes Among Patients With Resected Pancreatic Cancer." JAMA 310.14 (2013): 1473.

[16] King, J. C., M. Zenati, J. Steve, S. B. Winters, D. L. Bartlett, A. H. Zureikat, H. J. Zeh, and M. E. Hogg. "Deviations from Expected Treatment of Pancreatic Cancer in Octogenarians: Analysis of Patient and Surgeon Factors." Annals of Surgical Oncology (2016).

[17] "Further Evidence of Effective Adjuvant Combined Radiation and Chemotherapy following Curative Resection of Pancreatic Cancer." Cancer 59.12 (1987): 2006–010.

[18] Lee, E. S. "Imaging Diagnosis of Pancreatic Cancer: A State-of-the-Art Review." World Journal of Gastroenterology 20.24 (2014): 7864.

[19] Gurusamy, K. S., and B. R. Davidson. "Diagnostic Accuracy of Different Imaging Modalities following Computed Tomography (CT) Scanning for Assessing the Resectability with Curative Intent in Pancreatic and Periampullary Cancer." Protocols Cochrane Database of Systematic Reviews (2015).

[20] Karmazanovsky, G., V. Fedorov, V. Kubyshkin, and A. Kotchatkov. "Pancreatic Head Cancer: Accuracy of CT in Determination of Resectability." Abdominal Imaging 30.4 (2005): 488–500.

[21] Shrikhande, S. V., S. G. Barreto, M. Goel, and S. Arya. "Multimodality Imaging of Pancreatic Ductal Adenocarcinoma: A Review of the Literature." HPB 14.10 (2012): 658–68.

[22] Callery, M. P., K. J. Chang, E. K. Fishman, M. S. Talamonti, L. W. Traverso, and D. C. Linehan. "Pretreatment Assessment of Resectable and Borderline Resectable Pancreatic Cancer: Expert Consensus Statement." Annals of Surgical Oncology 16.7 (2009): 1727–733.

[23] Mohammed, S., and W. E. Fisher. "Quality Metrics in Pancreatic Surgery." Surgical Clinics of North America 93.3 (2013): 693–709.

[24] Mohammed, S., G. Van Buren, II, and W. E. Fisher. "Pancreatic Cancer: Advances in Treatment." World Journal of Gastroenterology 20.28 (2014): 9354–360 (in print).

[25] Finks, J. F., N. H. Osborne, and J. D. Birkmeyer. "Trends in Hospital Volume and Operative Mortality for High-Risk Surgery." New England Journal of Medicine 364.22 (2011): 2128–137.

[26] Tseng, J., C. Raut, J. Lee, P. Pisters, J. Vauthey, E. Abdalla, H. Gomez, C. Sun, C. Crane, and R. Wolff. "Pancreaticoduodenectomy with Vascular Resection: Margin Status and Survival Duration." Journal of Gastrointestinal Surgery 8.8 (2004): 935–50.

[27] Katz, M. H. G., P. W. T. Pisters, D. B. Evans, C. C. Sun, J. E. Lee, J. B. Fleming, J. N. Vauthey, E. K. Abdalla, C. H. Crane, R. A. Wolff, G. R. Varadhachary, and R. F. Hwang. "Borderline Resectable Pancreatic Cancer: The Importance of This Emerging Stage of Disease." Journal of the American College of Surgeons 206.5 (2008): 833–46.

[28] Lassen, K., M. M. E. Coolsen, K. Slim, F. Carli, J. E. De Aguilar-Nascimento, M. Schäfer, R. W. Parks, K. C. H. Fearon, D. N. Lobo, N. Demartines, M. Braga, O. Ljungqvist, and C. H. C. Dejong. "Guidelines for Perioperative Care for Pancreaticoduodenectomy: Enhanced Recovery After Surgery (ERAS®) Society Recommendations." World Journal of Surgery 37.2 (2012): 240–58.

[29] Halaszynski, T. M., R. Juda, and D. G. Silverman. "Optimizing Postoperative Outcomes with Efficient Preoperative Assessment and Management." Critical Care Medicine 32.Supplement (2004).

[30] Bratzler, D. W., E. P. Dellinger, K. M. Olsen, T. M. Perl, P. G. Auwaerter, M. K. Bolon, D. N. Fish, L. M. Napolitano, R. G. Sawyer, D. Slain, J. P. Steinberg, and R. A. Weinstein. "Clinical Practice Guidelines for Antimicrobial Prophylaxis in Surgery." American Journal of Health-System Pharmacy 70.3 (2013): 195–283.

[31] Eshuis, W. J., J. Hermanides, J. W. Van Dalen, G. Van Samkar, O. R.C. Busch, T. M. Van Gulik, J. H. Devries, J. B.l. Hoekstra, and D. J. Gouma. "Early Postoperative Hypergly-

cemia Is Associated With Postoperative Complications After Pancreatoduodenectomy." Annals of Surgery 253.4 (2011): 739–44.

[32] Kehlet, H., and D. W. Wilmore. "Multimodal Strategies to Improve Surgical Outcome." The American Journal of Surgery 183.6 (2002): 630–41.

[33] Fisher, W.E., S. Hodges, G. Cruz, et al. "Routine Nasogastric Suction May Be Unnecessary After a Pancreatic Resection." HPB 13 (2011): 792–796.

[34] Balzano, G., A. Zerbi, M. Braga, et al. "Fast-track Recovery Programme after Pancreaticoduodenectomy Reduces Delayed Gastric Emptying." British Journal of Surgery 95 (2008): 1387–93.

[35] Buren, G. Van, M. Bloomston, S. J. Hughes, J. Winter, S. W. Behrman, N. J. Zyromski, C. Vollmer, V. Velanovich, T. Riall, P. Muscarella, J. Trevino, A. Nakeeb, C. M. Schmidt, K. Behrns, E. C. Ellison, O. Barakat, K. A. Perry, J. Drebin, M. House, S. Abdel-Misih, E. J. Silberfein, S. Goldin, K. Brown, S. Mohammed, S. E. Hodges, A. Mcelhany, M. Issazadeh, E. Jo, Q. Mo, and W. E. Fisher. "A Randomized Prospective Multicenter Trial of Pancreaticoduodenectomy With and Without Routine Intraperitoneal Drainage." Annals of Surgery 259.4 (2014): 605–12.

[36] Sharpe, S.M., M.S. Talamonti, C.E. Wang, et al. "Early National Experience with Laparoscopic Pancreaticoduodenectomy for Ductal Adenocarcinoma: A Comparison of Laparoscopic Pancreaticoduodenectomy and Open Pancreaticoduodenectomy from the National Cancer Data Base." Journal of the American College Surgery 221 (2015): 175–184.

[37] Lee, S., P. Allen, E. Sadot, et al. "Distal Pancreatectomy: A Single Institution's Experience in Open, Laparoscopic, and Robotic Approaches." Journal of the American College of Surgery 220.1 (2014): 18–27.

[38] Kooby, D., T. Gillespie, D. Bentrem et al. "Left-sided Pancreatectomy: A Multicenter Comparison of Laparoscopic and Open Approaches." Annals of Surgery; 248.3 (2008).

[39] Zureikat, A., L. Postlewait, Y. Liu, et al. (2016). "A Multi-instititional Comparison of Perioperative Outcomes of Robotic and Open Pancreaticoduodenectomy." Annals of Surgery. (In print).

[40] Waters, J.A., D.F. Canal, E.A. Wiebke, et al. (2010). "Robotic Distal Pancreatectomy: Cost Effective?" Surgery 148 (2010): 814–823.

[41] Geller, E.J., and C.A. Matthews,. "Impact of Robotic Operative Efficiency on Profitability." American Journal of Obstetrics Gynecology 211.5 (2013): 546.

[42] Wright, G.P., A. Zureikat,. "Development of Minimally Invasive Pancreatic Surgery: An Evidence-Based Systematic Review of Laparoscopic Versus Robotic Approaches." Journal of Gastrointestinal Surgery 20.9 (2016): 1658–65.

[43] Tseng, J., C. Raut, andJ. Lee,. "Pancreaticoduodenectomy with Vascular Resection: Margin Status and Survival Duration." Journal of Gastrointestinal Surgery 8.8 (2004): 935–950.

[44] Christians, K., and D.B. Evans,. "Pancreaticoduodenectomy and Vascular Resection: Persistent Controversy and Current Recommendations." Annals of Surgical Oncology 16 (2009): 789–91.

[45] Ramacciato, G., P. Mercantini, N. Petrucciani, et al. "Does Portal-superior Mesenteric Vein Invasion still Indicate Irresectability for Pancreatic Carcinoma?" Annals of Surgical Oncology; 16 (2009): 817–825.

[46] Fuhrman, G.M., S.D. Leach, C.A. Staley, et al. "Rationale for en bloc Vein Resection in the Treatment of Pancreatic Adenocarcinoma Adherent to the Superior Mesenteric-Portal Vein Confluence." Pancreatic Tumor Study Group. Annals of Surgery; 223 (1996): 154–162.

[47] Castleberry, A., R. White, S. De La Fuente, et al. "The Impact Vascular Resection on Early Postoperative Outcomes after Pancreaticoduodenectomy: An Analysis of the American College of Surgeons National Surgical Quality Improvement Program Database." Annals of Surgical Oncology; 19 (2012): 4068–4077.

[48] Gleisner, A., G. Spolverato, A. Ejaz, and T. Pawlik. "Time-related Changes in the Prognostic Significance of the Total Number of Examined Lymph Nodes in Node-negative Pancreatic Head Cancer." Journal of Surgical Oncology; 110.7 (2014): 858–63.

[49] Burris, H,, M. Moore, and J. Andersen. "Improvements in Survival and Clinical Benefit with Gemcitabine as First-Line Therapy for Patients with Advanced Pancreas Cancer: A Randomized Trial." Journal of Clinical Oncology; 15.6 (1997): 2403–2413.

[50] Von Hoff, D., T. Ervin, F. Arena, et al.. "Increased Survival in Pancreatic Cancer with Nab-placlitaxel Plus Gemcitabine." NEJM; 369.18 (2013): 1691–1703.

[51] Sener, S.F., A. Fremgen, H.R. Menck, and D.P. Winchester, "Pancreatic Cancer: A Report of Treatment and Survival Trends for 100,313 Patients Diagnosed from 1985–1995, using the National Cancer Database." *J Am Coll Surg*.189.1 (1999): 1–7.

[52] Neoptolemos, J., D. Stocken, C. Bassi, et al. "Adjuvant Chemotherapy with Fluorouracil plus Folinic Acid vs Gemcitabine Following Pancreatic Cancer Resection: A Randomized Controlled Trial." JAMA; 304.10 (2010): 1073–1081.

[53] Assifi, M,, X. Lu, G. Eibl, et al. "Neoadjuvant Therapy in Pancreatic Adenocarcinoma: A Meta-analysis of Phase II Trials." Surgery 150.3 (2011): 466–473.

[54] Evans, D., G. Varadhchary, C. Crane, et al. "Preoperative Gemcitabine-based Chemoradiation for Patients with Resectable Adenocarcinoma of the Pancreatic Head." Journal of Clinical Oncology; 26.21 (2008): 3496–3502.

[55] Christians, K,, S. Tsai, A. Mahmoud, et al. "Neoadjuvant FOLFIRINOX for Borderline Resectable Pancreas Cancer: A New Treatment Paradigm?" The Oncologist 19 (2014).: 266–274.

[56] Xiong, J., P. Szatmary, B. Chir, et al. "Enhanced Recovery after Surgery Program in Patients undergoing Pancreaticoduodenectomy: A PRISMA-Compliant Systematic Review and Meta-analysis." Medicine 95.18 (2016): 1–10.

[57] Adham, M., X. Chopin-Laly, and V. Lepilliez, et al. "Pancreatic Resection: Drain or No Drain?" Surgery 154.5 (2013): 1069–77.

[58] Conlon, K., D. Labow, D. Leung, et al. "Prospective Randomized Clinical Trial of the Value of Intraperitoneal Drainage after Pancreatic Resection." Annals of Surgery 234 (2001): 487–494.

[59] Correa-Gallego, C., M. Brennan, M. D'Angelica, et al. "Operative Drainage Following Pancreatic Resection: Analysis of 1122 Patients Resected over 5 years at a Single Institution." Annals of Surgery 258 (2013): 1051–1058.

[60] Fisher, W.E., S. Hodges, E. Silberfein, et al. "Pancreatic Resection without Routine Intraperitoneal Drainage." HPB 13 (2011): 503–510.

[61] Heslin, M., L. Harrison, A. Brooks, et al. "Is Intra-abdominal Drainage Necessary after Pancreaticoduodenectomy?" Journal of Gastrointestinal Surgery 2 (1998): 373–378.

[62] Bilimoria, K., J. Bentrem, and C. Ko, et al. "National Failure to Operate on Early Stage Pancreatic Cancer." Annals of Surgery 246.2 (2007): 173–180.

[63] Reber, H.A.. "Lymph Node Involvement as a Prognostic Factor in Pancreatic Cancer." International Journal of Pancreatology 7 (1990):125–127.

[64] Huebner, M., M. Kendrick, K.M. Reid-Lombardo, et al. "Number of Lymph Nodes Evaluated: Prognostic Value in Pancreatic Adenocarcinoma." Journal of Gastrointestinal Surgery 16 (2012): 920–926.

[65] Oettle, H., S. Post, P. Neuhaus, et al. Adjuvant chemotherapy with gemcitabine vs observation in patients undergoing curative-intent resection of pancreatic cancer: a randomized controlled trial. JAMA. 297.3 (2007): 267–277.

[66] Oettle, H., P. Neuhaus, and A. Hochhaus, "Adjuvant Chemotherapy with Gemcitabine and Long-term Outcomes among Patients with Resected Pancreatic Cancer: The CONKO-001 Randomized Trial." JAMA 310.14 (2013): 1473–1481.

[67] Therasse, P., S.G. Arbuck, E.A. Eisenhauer, J. Wander, Kaplan, et al. "New Guidelines to Evaluate the Response to Treatment in Solid Tumors." Journal of National Cancer Institute 92 (2000): 205–16.

[68] Evans, D.B., T.A. Rich, D.R. Byrd, et al. "Preoperative Chemoradiation and PD for Adenocarcinoma of the Pancreas." Archives of Surgery 127 (1992): 1335–1339.

Chapter 9

New Surgical Procedure for Pancreas Head

Yoshinobu Sato, Yoshiaki Hara, Naruhiko Sawada, Shoji Shimada, Kenta Nakahara, Daisuke Takayanagi, Fumio Ishida, Shin-EI Kudo and Junichi Tanaka

Additional information is available at the end of the chapter

http://dx.doi.org/10.5772/66493

Abstract

In this study, we demonstrate two new methods for pancreaticoduodenectomy (PD). One method is the mini-laparotomic PD by Shuriken-shaped umbilicoplasty with the real-time moving window's method. The other method is the new pancreaticojejunostomy (PJ) by punctured stent slide guiding method (PSSGM). This procedure could be performed by complete mini-laparotomy under direct vision, and the final major wound is only 2 cm of round navel. PSSGM prevents the difference of caliber between pancreatic anastomosis and the inside out of jejunal mucosa in theory. Ten cases of mini-lap PD were successfully performed under new PJ anastomosis. The pancreatic leakage (PL) was only one case of ISGPF grade A, and its frequency was 9% (1/11). Our mini-lap PD by Shuriken-shaped umbilicoplasty might be a useful way for overcoming the obstacles about safety, complication risk, cosmetic demand, and medical cost compared to laparoscopic PD. Also, our new device of PJ reconstruction by PSSGM might be an easy and useful device for the prevention of PL.

Keywords: laparoscopic pancreaticoduodenectomy, pancreaticojejunostomy, navel surgery, Shuriken-shaped umbilicoplasty, minimal invasive surgery

1. Introduction

Recently, laparoscopic surgery has been used for pancreas surgery. Laparoscopic pancreatic surgery has gradually expanded to include pancreaticoduodenectomy (PD) [1–3]. However, as the outcomes of feasibility and safety have become better yearly in the laparoscopic pancreaticoduodenectomy (LPD), a superior operative skill must be required. Therefore, LPD remains technically a difficult surgery with high rates of mortality and morbidity for usual HPB surgeons. LPD is a challenging operation for multiple reasons, including but not limited to the following: difficult access and exposure of the pancreas, which is situated in the retroperitoneum; hemorrhage control from major vasculature, a technically demanding reconstruction of the biliary and pancreatic remnants; maintaining oncologic surgical principles; and surgeon fatigue from a long operation requiring intense concentration. Limitations of the laparoscopic approach include the inability to palpate the lesion or surrounding vascular structures. Owing to the limitations of LPD, we reported a new surgical device of hybrid laparoscopic complete uncinatectomy of the pancreas by Shuriken-shaped umbilicoplasty with the sliding window's method [4] in pursuit of both safety and cosmetic advantages. In this chapter, we would like to demonstrate our modified novel technique of Shuriken-shaped umbilicoplasty with the real-time moving sliding window's method in pancreas for PD by mini-laparotomy. Our technique might be used for PD from complete mini-laparotomy to hybrid laparoscopic operation and be a useful procedure with the advantages of cosmetic, safety, and learning tools to the complete LPD.

The pancreatic fistula is a major obstacle as a complication after pancreatojejunostomy (PJ) in PD would result in intra-abdominal abscess or bleeding from arterial aneurism. A reconstruction of PJ has been reported; however, the pancreatic leakage (PL) has not disappeared. The cause for PL might be divided into two factors. First is the host's factors and second is the surgeon's factors (**Table 1**). The host's factors are their nutrition status, diabetes mellitus, pancreatitis, aging, liver cirrhosis, and so on. Those conditions might influence wound healing, immunocompetence, and susceptibility to infection. The surgeon's factors are technical problems including their surgical skill, surgical instruments, and reconstruction's method. In this study, we will also demonstrate the new PJ technique by pancreatic stent slide guiding method (PSSGM).

Case	Sex	Age	Disease	Real time sliding window's method	Operative time	Blood loss	Hospital stay	PL	BL	Other postoperative complications	Preoperative complications
1	M	66	PvC	HALS	980	2256	23	–	–	–	–
2	F	69	BDC	+ Mini-Lap	492	257	37	–	–	–	–
3	F	77	PK	+ Mini-Lap	445	389	17	–	–	–	–
4	M	78	PK	+ Mini-Lap	659	1026	18	–	–	–	DM
5	F	75	PK	+ Mini-Lap	517	673	31	–	–	–	–
6	M	77	BDC	+ Mini-Lap	485	914	17	–	–	–	–
7	M	68	PvC	+ Mini-Lap	482	344	36	Grade A	–	Bleeding of gastric anastomosis	–
8	F	70	BDC	+ Mini-Lap	577	1375	42	–	–	Liver abscess	Cholangitis

Case	Sex	Age	Disease	Real time sliding window's method	Operative time	Blood loss	Hospital stay	PL	BL	Other postoperative complications	Preoperative complications
9	F	75	BDC	+ Mini-lap	552	1284	90	–	–	Liver abscess	DM
10	F	74	PK	+ Mini-Lap	545	795	28	–	–	–	DM

PL: leakage of pancreatic juice; PvC: papilla vater carcinoma; BL: leakage of bile juice; BDC: bile duct cancer; DM: diabetes mellitus; PK: pancreatic cancer; Mini-Lap: mini-laparotomy.

Pancreatic leakage was the only one case of grade A by ISGPF classification. Two patients suffered from liver abscess and their hospital stay prolonged by 42 and 90 postoperative days, respectively. There were no cases that had bile leakage.

Table 1. Profiles and perioperative data of 10 patients who underwent PD with the Shuriken-shaped umbilicoplasty.

2. Surgical procedures

2.1. Shuriken-shaped umbilicoplasty with the sliding window's method

The patient was placed in the supine position with legs closed. Hybrid laparoscopic surgery was performed by the hand-assisted or the direct manipulation with a small open wound by the sliding window's method. Under general anesthesia, a Shuriken-shaped umbilical skin incision was made 6 cm horizontally, 4 cm longitudinally and 1.8 cm wide. The intermediate skin between outside and inside skin incision was removed. Subcutaneous tissue around the umbilicus and the upper abdominal subcutaneous region was dissected, and the upper abdominal minilaparotomy, from 8 to 12 cm, was performed (**Figures 1** and **2**). GelPort was used for the hand-assisted laparoscopic surgery.

After that, two of Kent retractors for the upper region and two of surgical arms for the lower region are placed at each bilateral side.

2.2. Real-time moving window's method for PD

The three operative fields were divided into the hepatic hilus region, pancreas head region, and SMA region (**Figure 3**). The four retractors were moved according to each operative region. For each operation of the hepatodudenal and common hepatic arterial regions, Kent retractor was pulled forward to the right or left upper by placing surgical gazes at the right subdiaphragmatic space. And then, for the paraduodenal approach of SMA or Treize'ligament, the right or left surgical arm was pulled to the right lower direction or the left lower direction after loosening the Kent retractor. For the pancreas head region, Kent retractor was pulled toward the middle upper after loosening the surgical arms.

The operative manipulations were done and were the same as those of the usual open PD.

Especially, the processing of IPDA was firstly made by paraduodenal approach under the concept of "artery first" before dealing with SMV.

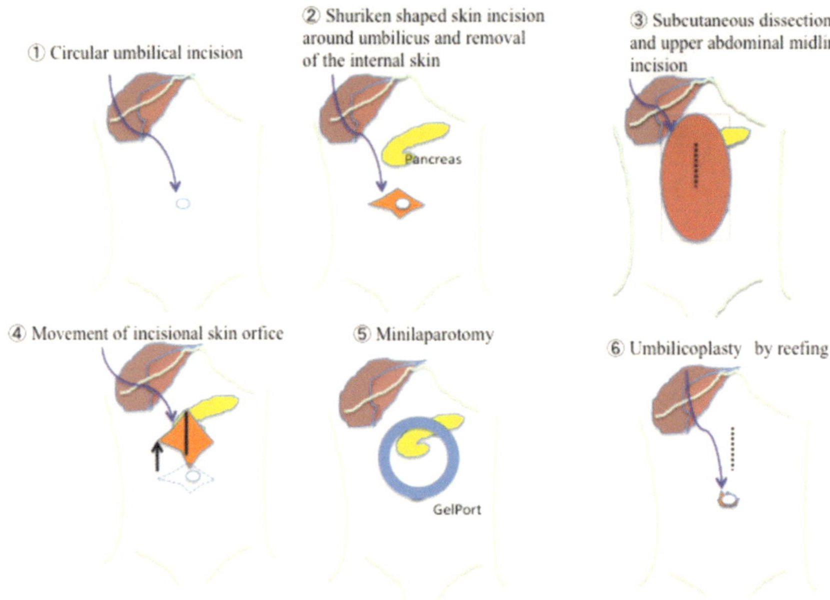

Figure 1. Schema of Shuriken-shaped umbilicoplasty with sliding window's method. The figure shows each step of our procedure by the laparotomy from ① to ⑤ and umbilicoplasty by reefing in ⑥.

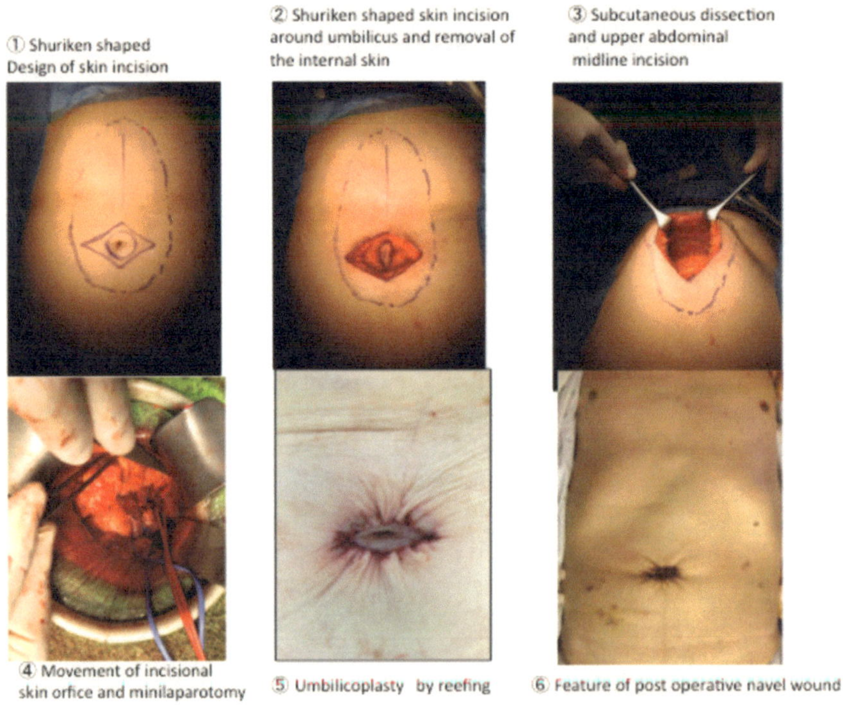

Figure 2. Operative photographs of Shuriken-shaped umbilicoplasty with sliding window's method. The figure also shows each step from ① to ⑥.

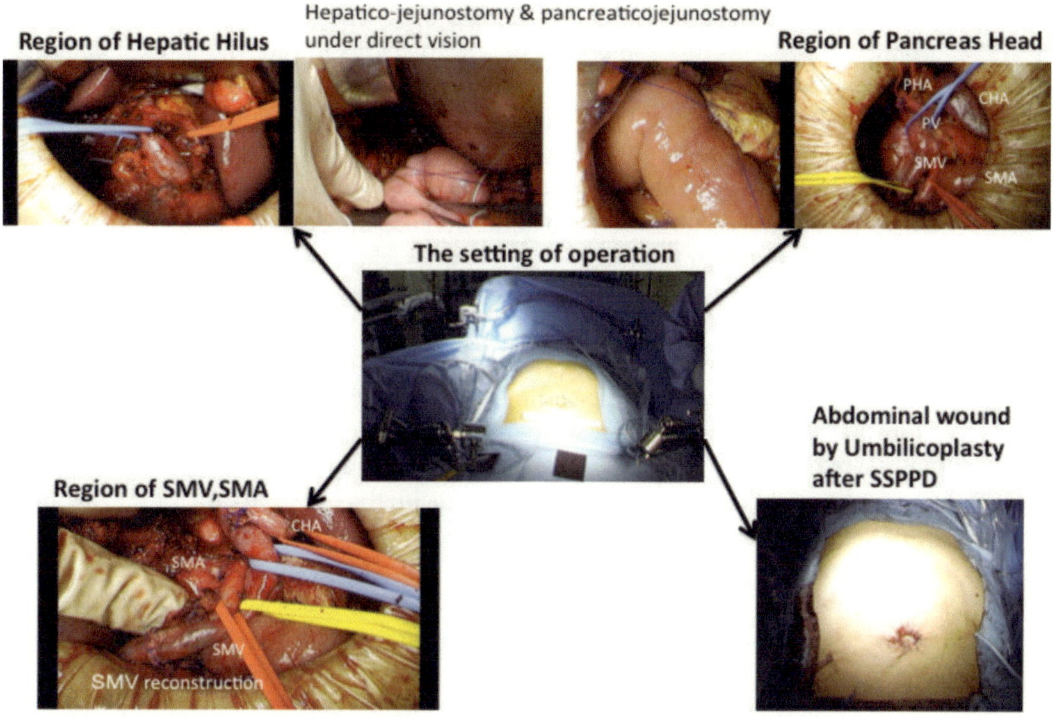

Figure 3. Schema of pancreatoduodenectomy by Shuriken-shaped umbilicoplasty with real-time sliding window's method using operative photographs. The center photograph shows the setting of operation using two Kent retractors and two surgical arms. The three operative fields, region of hepatic hilus, region of pancreas head, and region of SMA and SMV were exposed by real-time moving window's method by their retractors. The last photograph shows the 2-cm operative navel wound by umbilicoplasty and each of the three drains—Winslow`s drain, drain of post pancreaticojejunostomy, and subcutaneous drain.

The hepaticojejunostomy, the pancreaticojejunostomy, and the gastrojejunostomy were done under direct vision without laparoscopic manner. After the reconstruction, three closed drainage tubes were detained in the Winslow foramen, the posterior space of pancreaticojejunostomy, and subcutaneous space, respectively.

2.3. Pancreatojejunostomy by punctured stent slide guiding method (PSSGM)

2.3.1. The cutting and sealing of pancreas stump

A cause for PL is due to insufficient sealing of the pancreas stump. We cut the pancreas by using the SonoSurg or the bipolar forceps near the pancreatic duct. The pancreatic duct is cut by the surgical knife.

2.3.2. Anastomosis of duct to "seromuscular layer"

We consider that the major cause for PL is technical problems at the anastomosis in the PJ. The possible problems of PJ anastomosis are thought to be two reasons. One is a difference of caliber between the jejunal orifice and the pancreatic duct. The other is an inside out of jejunal mucosa in anastomosis of the duct to mucosa (**Figure 4**). These problems lead to PL and local infection around PJ anastomosis. Sometimes, those infections induce the arterial aneurism and its rupture and bleeding. As a solution, we devised the punctured stent slide guiding method. The first step in this method is a puncture of jejunum by a pancreatic stent adapted to the orifice of the pancreatic duct without any incineration of serosa of jejunum as shown in **Figures 5**① and **6A**. This surgical idea might prevent the difference of anastomotic orifice and not resist the healing of anastomosis because of the none of any destroy of fire by the surgical device. The second step is an anastomosis of the duct to jejunal seromuscular layer without the mucosa. This duct to seromuscular anastomosis might prevent the necrosis of mucosa by the ligating strings. These everting suturing by all around 8–10 needles are made by 6-0PDS doubly armed suture. Both the small orifice of the pancreatic duct and the jejunum are easily and simply anastamosed by each needle sliding on the pancreatic stent tube. After that, the third step is an anastomosis of the pancreatic parenchymal stump by the jejunal seromuscular layers with the Kakita method, utilizing a full, thick penetrating suture for tight stump adhesion. The last step is a resection of the pancreatic stent with the opposite side for the lost stent. The orifice after resection of stent is closed by suturing.

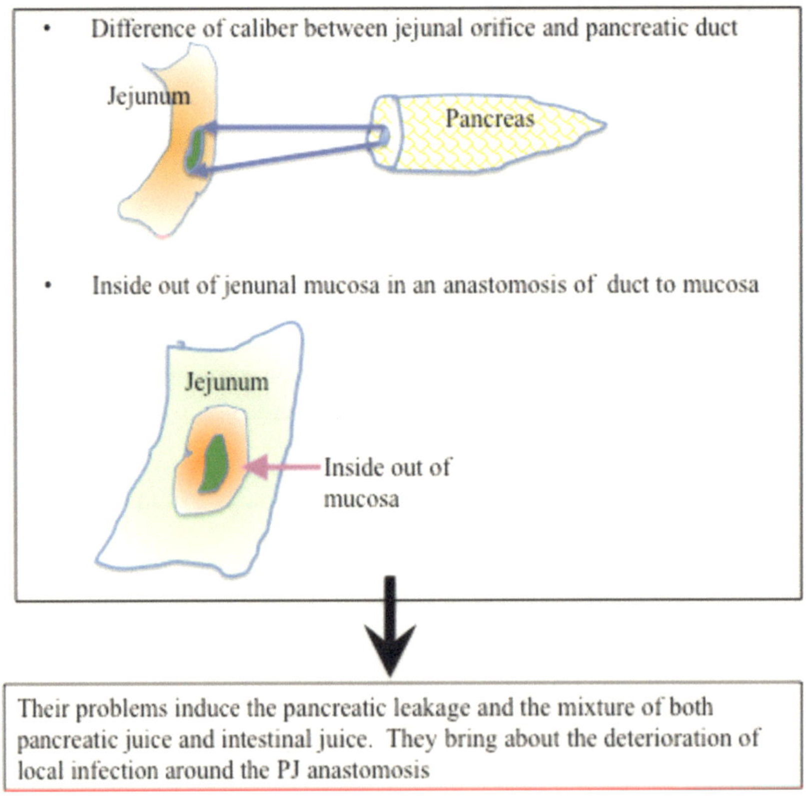

Figure 4. Ideas of technical causes of PL from anastomosis of duct to mucosa in pancreaticojejunostomy. The major technical cause is considered to be pancreaticojejunostomy of duct to mucosa. This origin will be induced by the two cause of the difference of caliber between jejunal orifice and pancreatic duct and the inside out of jejunal mucosa in an anastomosis of duct to mucosa.

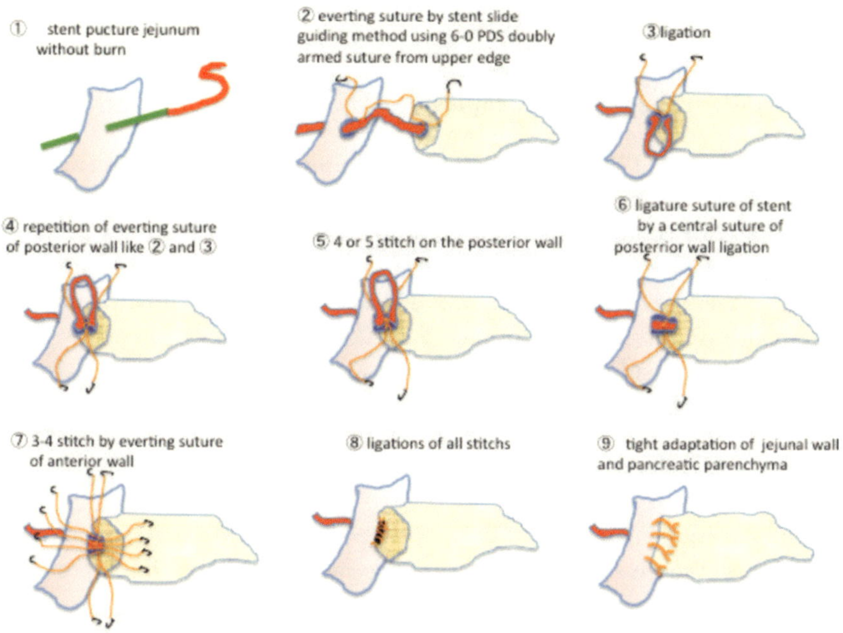

Figure 5. Schema of duct to seromuscular layer anastomosis by punctured stent slide guiding method (PSSGM). The first step of this device is a puncture of jejunum by a pancreatic stent adapted to the orifice of pancreatic duct without any incineration of serosa of jejunum like **Figure 5**①. After that, the everting suture of seromuscular layer to pancreatic duct by 6-0PDS double armed absorbed suture is started from upper edge using punctured stent slide guide. The posterior wall is anastomosed by the four or five stitches one by one according to the schema from ② to ⑥ The anterior wall is anastomosed by the consecutive three or four stitches by PSSGM. Finally, all stitches are ligated. The tight adaptation is the modified Kakita method.

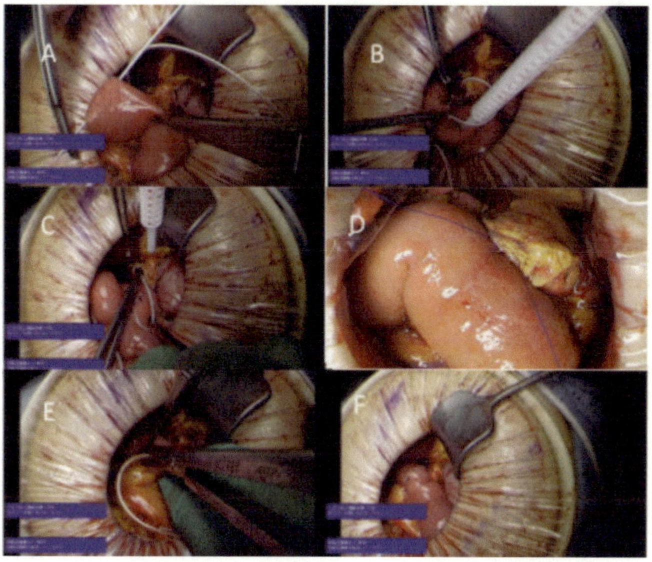

Figure 6. Operative photographs of pancreaticojejunostomy by punctured stent slide guiding method. Operative photographs showing the procedures of PSSGM according to the schema of **Figure 5**.

3. Patients and perioperative data

3.1. PD with Shuriken-shaped umbilicoplasty

We experienced 10 cases of PD by real-time moving window's method. Mean age was 72.6 ± 4.2 years old. Operative procedures were mentioned as described above. The pancreaticojejunostomy was done by our original stent slide guiding method. The patient's profile is demonstrated in **Figure 5**. Average of operative times was 528 ± 63 min. Average of operative blood was 795 ± 405 ml. Average of hospital stay was 33 ± 21 (17-90). Two patients suffered from liver abscess, and their hospital stay was prolonged by 42 and 90 postoperative days, respectively. There were no cases that had bile leakage. Pancreatic leakage was only one case of grade A by ISGPF classification (**Table 1**).

3.2. Pancreaticojejunostomy by punctured stent slide guiding method

Ten cases were operated using the Shuriken-shaped umbilicoplasty and one case by the usual open surgery. We divided the PD with PJ reconstruction into three groups from 2004 to 2015 in our center. There were 114 cases of PD with PJ reconstruction operated by the previous HPB surgeons in Group A from 2004 to 2013. There were 24 cases operated by present HPB surgeons from 2014 to 2015. Eleven cases in Group C were operated by the first author using PSSGM from 2014 to 2015. The 13 cases of Group B were operated by other surgeons without PSSGM. The PLs were compared among three groups according to the ISGPF criteria.

4. Changes in amylase level in the sump solution

The amylase level in the two sump solutions was measured (**Table 2**). The two drains of eight cases were removed within 5 days after operation without PL. The drains of the other two cases were removed 7 days after the operation. The one in two cases had a PL of grade A.

Levels of amylase in the sump solution of pancreatic anastomotic drain						Levels of amylase in the sump solution of winslow's drain					
Case	1POD	3POD	5POD	7POD	PF	Case	1POD	3POD	5POD	7POD	PF
1	142	47			0	1	137	45			
2	637	90	34		0	2	507	126	15		–
3	108	23	14		0	3	126	19	14		–
4	99	115	13	14	0	4	153	37	21	16	–
5	43	52	28		0	5	210	141	16		–
6	7192	2453	1777	254	GradeA	6	1735	368	344	129	Grade A
7	1034	83	18		0	7	539	281	14		–

Levels of amylase in the sump solution of pancreatic anastomotic drain						Levels of amylase in the sump solution of winslow's drain					
Case	1POD	3POD	5POD	7POD	PF	Case	1POD	3POD	5POD	7POD	PF
8	1228	180	99		0	8	2494	102	16		–
9	18	12	4		0	9	15	10	4		–
10	148	299			0	10	169	219			
11	78	38				11	125	134.8	55	72	
Av	975	308	248	134		Av	564	134	55	72	
SD	2105	716	618	169		SD	801	114	109	56	

The amylase level in the two drainage solutions of Winslow's foramen and posterior of PJ anastomosis was measured. All of the two drains in 8 cases were removed within 5 days after operation without PL. The drains of the other two cases were removed 7 days after operation. The one in two cases had grade A PL of ISGPF criteria.

Table 2. Changes of amylase in the sump solution after SSPPD with PSSGM.

4.1. Changes in the frequency of pancreatic leakage compared among the three distinguished periods from 2004 to 2015 in our hospital

Total frequency of PL was 39% in the 114 cases of PJ reconstruction of Group A from 2004 to 2015 (**Table 3**). Total frequency of PL of Group B and Group C was 31 and 9%, respectively, at the same period from 2014 to 2015. The frequency of grade C PL was 7.9% in Group A. Groups B and C had no grade C PL. Moreover, Group C had no grade B and grade C PL that underwent PSSGM.

Group	Number	ISGPF grade				Total (%)
		Grade 0	A(%)	B(%)	C(%)	Grade A–C
A (2004–2013)	114	60.5 (69)	5.2 (6)	26.3 (30)	7.9 (9)	39
B 2014.1.1–2015.10.31	13	69.2	15.3(2)	15.3(2)	0	31
C 2014.11.1–2015.10.31	11	91	9(1)	0	0	9

Total frequency of PL was 39% in the 114 cases of PJ reconstruction of Group A from 2004 to 2015. Total frequency of PL of Group B and Group C was 31 and 9%, respectively, at the same period from 2014 to 2015. The frequency of grade C PL was 7.9% in Group A. Group B and Group C had no grade C PL. Moreover, Group C had no grade B and grade C PL that underwent PSSGM.

Table 3. Changes in frequency of pancreatic leakage in our hospital for three distinguished periods from 2004 to 2015.

5. Discussion

In 1994, Gagner and Pomp [5, 6] first introduced LPPPD in an advanced laparoscopic surgical trial in an effort to reduce postoperative morbidity. Since then, however, there have been few reports from centers with experience performing this procedure, and the reported clinical outcomes of LPD have remained unsatisfactory over the last decade [7, 8]. Technical progress in LPD was achieved by several pioneering laparoscopic surgeons, including hand-assisted LPD [9, 10] as well as laparoscopically assisted [11, 12] and robot-assisted PD [13]. However, some surgeons have recently reported favorable outcomes [14–17]. LPD has not been accepted as a generalized surgical method for the resection of pancreatic head lesions. LPD includes technically difficult surgeries with high rates for mortality and morbidity.

Most of risky complications are leakages of pancreatic duct anastomosis and hepaticojejunostomy in the PD inspite of open or laparoscopic. Their reconstruction might be very stressful and fatigue for surgeons because of the limitations of laparoscopic approach and long operation.

In our operative procedure, the final main operative abdominal wound by Shuriken-shaped umbilicoplasty is almost 2 cm round around the navel except the three wounds for drainage tubes in our new device of operation. The length of subcutaneous upper abdominal incision is longer than that of the complete untinatectomy which was reported elsewhere. Although the opening window of abdomen using GelPort is small, the favorable operative window could be exposed by the real-time sliding window‘s method with two Kent retractors and two of surgical arms.

Otherwise, our techniques could bring their anastomosis under direct vision. Although our clinical research was very small number, the results of the only one case of pancreatic leakage of Grade A in ISGPF might be enough to verify the availability of our device. Moreover, all of surgical manipulations could be completely done under direct vision including ability to palpate the lesion and the vascular reconstructions as well as those of the open PD (OPD).

Therefore, our new device might be same as the OPD at the viewpoint of minimum invasive surgery and same as LPD at the viewpoint of cosmetic merit. However, that might be as same as the OPD at the viewpoint of safety.

In this chapter, we demonstrated the new device of PL by PSSGM. The causes for PL are shown in **Table 4**. We would consider that the origins of PL are divided into two parts, host's factor and surgeon‘s factor. The major cause for PL of PJ might be surgeon‘s technical problems. The PL from the anastomosis of the PJ and a cut stump of pancreas are the main origins, and we would consider that the difference of caliber of PJ anastomosis and the inside out of the jejunal mucosa are major obstacles. The only puncture by pancreatic stent to jejunum without burns must prevent from both the inside out of the jejunal mucosa and the difference of caliber of PJ anastomosis.The mixture of pancreatic juice and intestinal juice would deteriorate the PL and the local infection after the PL. Because the mixture of jejunal juice and pancreatice juice activate the inactivate pancreatic juice and activate pancreatic juice promote the PL. The above risk might be low in our new device. The other merit of our device is an easy anastomosis by the stent slide guiding method. If the pancreatic duct is small at the soft pancreas, the suture would be easy by handling of the needle using the guide of stent sliding. However, the comparison among three periods was retrospective and the surgeons also were various with the exception of Group C, the PL of Group C was low level in the frequency and the severity. Two major PJ reconstructions of Kakita method and Blumgart‘s technique have been reported [18–21]. Oda et al. reported that the rate of ISGPF grade B+C PF was 29/78 (37.2%) in the Kakita group and 16/78 (20.5%) in the Blumgart group ($P = 0.033$) [22]. The principal technique of these two methods is a tight adaptation of pancreatic parenchyma and duodenal seromusuclaris. Their device is not for the anastomosis of the pancreatic duct to mucosa. Our technique would be countermeasures against the difference of caliber of PJ anastomosis and the inside out of jejunal mucosa. Moreover, our device might prevent the mixture of pancreatic juice and jejunal juice, which deteriorate the local infection following PL. I performed this PJ anastomosis by PSSGM at the living related partial pancreas transplantation as a first case of enteric drainage in Japan and the heterotopic pancreas autotransplantation [23, 24]. This technique is thought to be useful for soft pancreas. Although the number of our studies about PL was very small, they included the retrospective data in the same period. Therefore, we confirm that our new device is theoretically useful and effective.

Host factor
1. DM, age, nutrition, obesity, general condition
2. Condition of pancreas
Soft pancreas, fibrosis, pancreatitis
Sugeon's factor
1. Technical problems
a. Type of surgical suture, skill of surgeon, management of stent
b. Surgical device of pancreatic resection
Dealing of pancreatic stump
Bleeding from pancreatic stump,
Lack of sealing of pancreatic stump
2. Differences of reconstruction method

Table 4. Causes for pancreatic leakage.

Many authors mentioned the necessity of learning periods for LPD. This complex procedure requires a relatively long training period to ensure technical proficiency.

Wang et al. [25] reported that based on the cumulative sum (CUSUM) and the risk-adjusted CUSUM analyses, the learning curve for LPD was grouped into three phases: phase I was the initial learning period, phase II represented the technical competence period, and phase III was regarded as the challenging period. There were no significant differences in terms of postoperative complications or the 30-day mortality among the three phases. More challenging cases were encountered in phase III. To attain technical competence for performing LPD, a minimum of 40 cases are required for laparoscopic surgeons with a degree of laparoscopic experience. Therefore, the acquisition of LPD might be not so easy, especially, in the center with a small amount of PD operations. Our device could be done by complete minilaparotomy so the usual HPB surgery might perform without the long learning period. Because the PJ and the HJ anastomosis could be done under direct vision as well as open surgery.

Of course, according to the learning curve, our operation could change from the complete minilaparotomy to the hybrid laparoscopic procedure or to complete LPD. Our procedure might be useful as a way of learning for LPD.

As other subjects, there is medical cost. Tan et al. reported that the mean total cost was higher in the total LPD (TLPD) group compared to the OPD group. When the total cost was broken down, TLPD was noted to result in significant increases in the cost of both surgery and anesthesia, but a decrease in the cost of admission evaluation. The higher cost of surgery and anesthesia in the TLPD group was due to the required surgical equipment and supplies and longer surgical time. The lower cost of admission evaluation in the TLPD group was due to a shorter hospital stay and reduced requirement for parenteral alimentation. From the thinking of learning cost, the cost of admission evaluation also must not decrease compared with OPD. Our operation could be done without any laparoscopic supplies.

6. Conclusions

In conclusion, the goal of minimal invasive surgery might be TLPD; however, there are several problems, for example, safety, complications, medical cost, and learning cost. Our PD by Shuriken-shaped umbilicoplasty with the real-time moving window's method might be a useful way for overcoming the above obstacles. Also, our new device of PJ reconstruction by PSSGM might be an easy and a useful device for preventing PL.

Abbreviations

PD	pancreaticoduodenectomy
LPD	laparoscopic pancreaticoduodenectomy
ISGPF	international study group on pancreatic fistula
PJ	pancreaticojejunostomy
PSSGM	punctured stent slide guiding method
PL	pancreatic leakage

Author details

Yoshinobu Sato[1,2]*, Yoshiaki Hara[1], Naruhiko Sawada[1], Shoji Shimada[1], Kenta Nakahara[1], Daisuke Takayanagi[1], Fumio Ishida[1], Shin-EI Kudo[1] and Junichi Tanaka[2]

*Address all correspondence to: kanishok@med.showa-u.ac.jp

1 Digestive Disease Center, Showa University, Yokohama Northern Hospital, Yokohama, Japan

2 Department of General and Digestive Surgery, Showa University, Fujigaoka Hospital, Fujigaoka, Japan

References

[1] Machado MA, Surjan RC, Basseres T, Silva IB, Makdissi FF. Laparoscopic pancreatoduodenectomy in 50 consecutive patients with no mortality: a single-center experience. J Laparoendosc Adv Surg Tech A. 2016 Apr 26 [Epub ahead of print].

[2] Nagakawa Y, Hosokawa Y, Sahara Y, Takishita C, Nakajima T, Hijikata Y, Tago T, Kasuya K, Tsuchida A. A novel "artery first" approach allowing safe resection in laparoscopic pancreaticoduodenectomy: the uncinate process first approach. Hepatogastroenterology. 2015 Jun;62(140):1037–1040.

[3] Doula C, Kostakis ID, Damaskos C, Machairas N, Vardakostas DV, Feretis T, Felekouras E. Comparison between minimally invasive and open pancreaticoduodenectomy: a systematic review. Surg Laparosc Endosc Percutan Tech. 2016 Feb;26(1):6–16.

[4] Sato Y, Sawada N, Shimada M, Takayanagi D, Mukai S, Shimada S, Kida H, Ishida F, Kudo S-E. Hybrid laparoscopic complete untinatectomy of pancreas by shuriken shaped umbilicoplasty with sliding window's method. Hepatogastoroenterology. 2014;61: 1486–1488.

[5] Gagner M, Pomp A. Laparoscopic pylorus-preserving pancreatoduodenectomy. Surg Endosc. 1994;8:408–410.

[6] Gagner M, Pomp A. Laparoscopic pancreatic resection: is it worthwhile? J Gastrointest Surg 1997;1:20–26.

[7] Cuschieri A. Laparoscopic surgery of the pancreas. J R Coll Surg Edinb. 1994;39:178–184.

[8] Kimura Y, Hirata K, Mukaiya M, Mizuguchi T, Koito K, Katsuramaki T. Hand-assisted laparoscopic pylorus-preserving pancreaticoduodenectomy for pancreas head disease. Am J Surg. 2005;189:734–737.

[9] Ammori BJ. Laparoscopic hand-assisted pancreaticoduodenectomy: initial UK experience. Surg Endosc. 2004;18:717–718.

[10] Masson B, Sa-cunha A, Laurent C. Laparoscopic pancreatectomy: report of 22 cases. Ann Chir. 2003;128:452–456.

[11] Staudacher C, Orsenigo E, Baccari P, Palo SD, Crippa S. Laparoscopic assisted duodenopancreatectomy. Surg Endosc. 2005;19:352–356.

[12] Giulianotti PC, Coratti A, Angelini M, Sbrana F, Cecconi S, Balestracci T, Caravaglios G. Robotics in general surgery: personal experience in a large community hospital. Arch Surg. 2003;138:777–784.

[13] Palanivelu C, Jani K, Senthilnathan P, Parthasarathi R, Rajapandian S, Madhankumar MV. Laparoscopic pancreaticoduodenectomy: technique and outcomes. J Am Coll Surg. 2007;205:222–223.

[14] Dulucq JL, Wintringer P, Mahajna A. Laparoscopic pancreatico duodenectomy for benign and malignant diseases. Surg Endosc. 2006;20:1045–1050.

[15] Zureikat AH, Breaux JA, Steel JL, Hughes SJ. Can laparoscopic pancreaticoduodenectomy be safely implemented? J Gastrointest Surg. 2011;15:1151–1157.

[16] Kendrick ML, Cusati D. Total laparoscopic pancreatico- duodenectomy; feasibility and outcome in an early experience. Arch Surg. 2010;145:19–23.

[17] Giulianotti PC, Sbrana F, Bianco FM, Elli EF, Shah G, Addeo P,Caravaglios G, Coratti A. Robot-assisted laparoscopicpancreatic surgery: single-surgeon experience. Surg Endosc. 2010;24:1646–1657.

[18] Kakita A, Yoshida M, Takahashi T. History of pancreaticojejunostomy in pancreaticoduodenectomy: development of a more reliable anastomosis technique. J Hepatobiliary Pancreat Surg. 2001;8:230–237.

[19] Grobmyer SR, Kooby D, Blumgart LH, Hochwald SN. Novel pancreaticojejunostomy with a low rate of anastomotic failure-related complications. J Am Coll Surg. 2010;210:54–59.

[20] Satoi S, Toyokawa H, Yanagimoto H, Yamamoto T, Hirooka S, Yui R, Yamaki S, Takahashi K, Matsui Y, Mergental H, Kwon AH. Is a nonstented duct-to-mucosa anastomosis using the modified Kakita method a safe procedure? Pancreas. 2010;39:165–170.

[21] Mishra PK, Saluja SS, Gupta M, Rajalingam R, Pattnaik P. Blumgart's technique of pancreaticojejunostomy: an appraisal. Dig Surg. 2011;28:281–287.

[22] Oda T, Hashimoto S, Miyamoto R, Shimomura O, Fukunaga K, Kohno K, Ohshiro Y, Akashi Y, Enomoto T, Ohkohchi N. The tight adaptation at pancreatic anastomosis without parenchymal laceration: an institutional experience in introducing and modifying the new procedure. World J Surg. 2015;39:2014–2022.

[23] Sato Y, Nakatsuka H, Yamamoto S, et al. Living related pancreas transplantation alone with enteric drainage in Japan: case report. Transplant Proc. 2008;40:2559–2561.

[24] Sato Y, Oya H, Yamamoto S, Kokai H, Miura K, Hatakeyama K. Heterotopic pancreas autotransplantation with spleen for uncontrollablehemorrhagic pseudocyst and disabling pain in chronic pancreatitis. Hepato-Gastroenterology. 2013;60:425–427.

[25] Wang M, Meng L, Cai Y, Li Y, Wang X, Zhang Z, Peng B. Learning curve for laparoscopic pancreaticoduodenectomy: a CUSUM analysis. J Gastrointest Surg. 2016;20:924–935.

Chapter 10

The Role of Vascular Resection in Pancreatic Cancer Treatment

Nikola Vladov, Ivelin Takorov and Tsonka Lukanova

Additional information is available at the end of the chapter

http://dx.doi.org/10.5772/66910

Abstract

Currently, porto-mesenteric vein resection is a standard procedure at high-volume pancreatic centers. Experience in vascular surgery is indispensable for a modern pancreatic surgeon. Nowadays, only arterial resections still are a controversial issue. Nevertheless, attempts at resection involving reconstruction of the main arteries such as the coeliac axis, hepatic artery, and superior mesenteric artery (SMA) have been reported, although in small case series. An overview of the historical and contemporary methods for surgical management of superior mesenteric/portal vein involvement as well as arterial involvement by pancreatic cancer is presented. We compare the data from the literature with our data based on the examination and long-term follow-up of more than 300 radical pancreatic resections. Seventy-two of the presented patients underwent pancreatic resection with simultaneous vascular resection—SMPV in 65 cases (44 with resection of the portal vein, 15 with resection of the superior mesenteric vein, 6 with resection of the porto-mesenterial confluence), arterial in 2 and partial resections of IVC in 5 cases. Combined vascular resections were done in three cases. Both groups PVR and PR showed similarly close results in complication rates, mortality, and morbidity. Three and 5 years survival rates were 42 and 38% in PD group and 28 and 19% in the PVR group. The vascular resection must be performed only upon carefully selected patients with data for presence of resectable tumors or tumors with borderline resectability from the preoperative imaging studies. The prompt management of pancreatic cancer with vascular involvement should involve multidisciplinary consultation in high-volume centers.

Keywords: pancreatic cancer, vascular resections, borderline resectability, venous reconstruction

1. Introduction

Nowadays, radical surgical treatment remains the only potentially curative treatment for patients with pancreatic cancer. Radical surgical resection followed by adjuvant chemotherapy can be performed in about 20% of all pancreatic ductal adenocarcinoma (PDAC) patients by the time of diagnosis and quite often is the only chance for long-term survival of the patients, with an average 5-year survival of 20–25% [1, 2]. More than 80 % of them are unresectable at the moment of diagnosis due to invasion of retroperitoneal tissue, portal vein (PV)/superior mesenteric vein (SMV), invasion of mesenteric artery, presence of liver or peritoneal metastases, or inability to sustain major surgical resection. As a result of the development of surgical techniques and technologies, extended operations, including vascular resections, have become more frequently performed in specialized centers [3]. This has led to a significant change in pancreatic surgery and has enlarged the border of resectability and ensured the possibility to achieve a curative surgical approach combined with neoadjuvant and adjuvant treatment strategies in patients with pancreatic cancer. Pancreatic carcinoma is characterized with high biological activity and early involvement of retroperitoneal tissue, lymph nodes, and peripancreatic blood vessels. The majority of pancreatic cancers are diagnosed at an advanced stage. Between 30 and 35% of them are classified as unresectablebecause of the isolated involvement of superior mesenteric/portal vein (**Figure 1**) [4]. For the first time the idea for resection of the portal vein for the sake of complete removal of the tumor was presented systematically by Fortner [5]. Currently, porto-mesenteric vein resection is a standard procedure at high-volume pancreatic centers. Experience in vascular surgery is indispensable for a modern pancreatic surgeon. Nowadays, only arterial resections are still a controversial issue. Nevertheless, attempts at resection involving reconstruction of the main arteries such as the coeliac axis, hepatic artery, and superior mesenteric artery (SMA) have been reported, although in small case series [6].

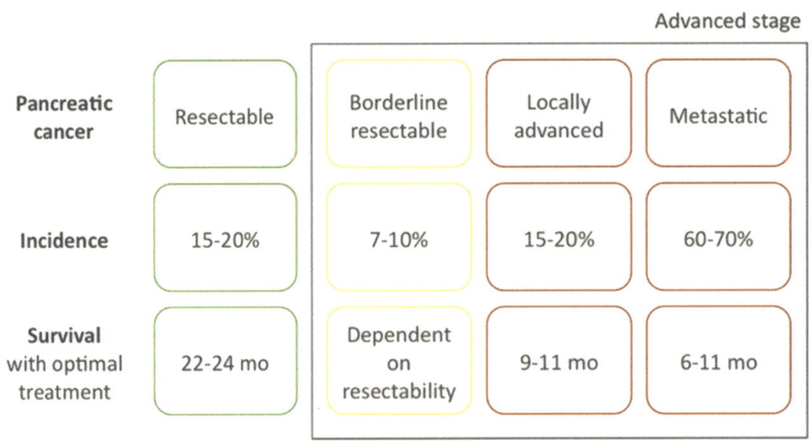

Figure 1. Resectability of pancreatic cancer patients at the time of initial diagnosis [4].

2. History

Moore et al. performed the first superior mesenteric vein (SMV) resection and reconstruction, thus making the base for the treatment of locally advanced pancreatic cancer with aggressive surgery [7]. Twelve years later (1963), Asade et al. published their results, followed by Fortner who first described a"regional pancreatectomy" involving total pancreatectomy, radical lymph node clearance, combined portal vein resection (Type 1), and/or combined arterial resection and reconstruction (Type 2) [6, 8]. These surgical interventions carried a greater morbidity and mortality than conventional surgery, so lately they were abandoned. Fuhrman et al. were the first to report that infiltration of the portal vein/SMV was not a function of the biological aggressiveness of the tumor but of the proximity of the tumor to the pancreatic head [9].

With the improvement of surgical technique, anesthesia, and critical care support, the interest in vascular resection in cases with isolated involvement of the portal vein (PV) and/or superior mesenteric vein (SMV) in locally advanced pancreatic cancer has gradually been renewed during the last decade (**Figure 2**) [3]. There are numerous reports on portal vein resection in locally advanced pancreatic cancer in the last decade, but still the results are conflicting [10–17]. Nowadays, it is accepted that the pancreatoduodenectomy with vein resection does not increase the postoperative risk, but there are still no reliable proofs that it significantly improves survival.

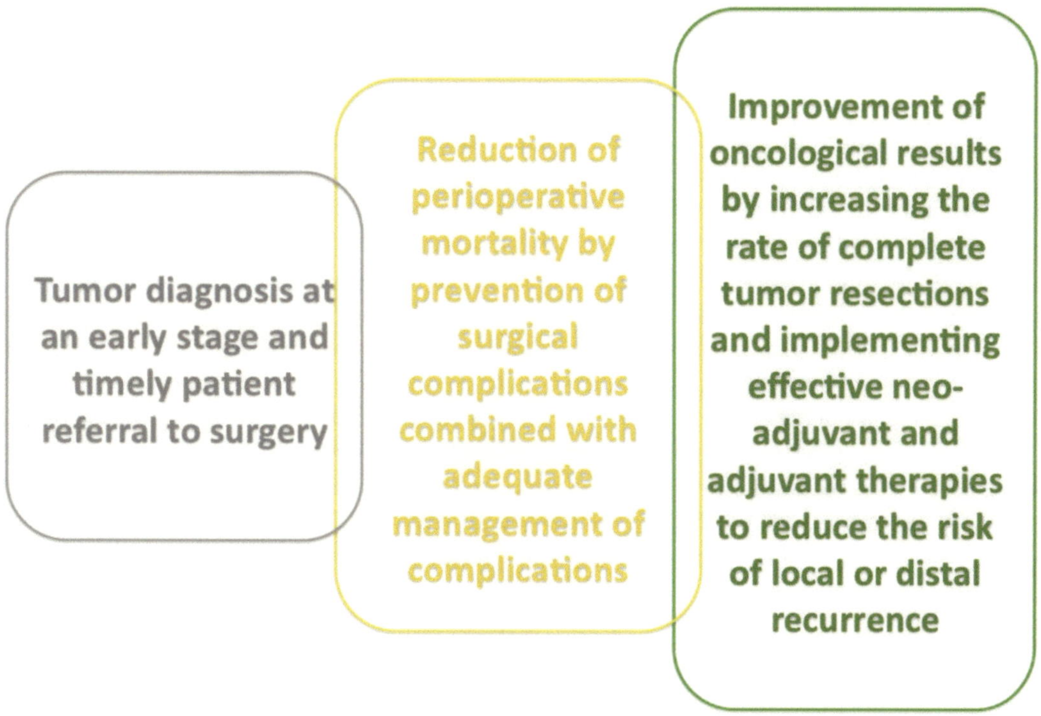

Figure 2. Improvement of surgical results for pancreatic cancer [3].

3. Rationale in vascular resections

3.1. Pro

Surgeons have gradually pushed the boundaries in surgical resection thanks to the advancements in oncology and critical care. Unfortunately, PDVR has not yet been generally accepted and applied as surgical management of patients with locally advanced adenocarcinoma of the head of the pancreas, despite of the growing evidence.

3.2. Cons

Pancreatic carcinoma is characterized with high biological activity and early involvement of retroperitoneal tissue, lymph nodes, and peripancreatic blood vessels. Vascular involvement is frequently combined with invasion in neural plexus so clear resection margin could not be achieved. Vascular resections especially arterial ones add an additional level of complexity to the usually difficult pancreatic surgery without clear impact on the long-term survival rates.

4. Indications for vascular resection

Extended surgical approaches, such as vascular and multivisceral resections, have become commonly performed in PDAC due to the improvement of surgical technique and intensive care, as well as the exact complications management [18].

Combined portal vein resection with pancreatectomy should be considered in order to achieve clear resection margins on the basis of preoperative imaging in cases suspectable of invasion of the portal vein rather than making the decision purely on operative findings. All patients should undergo contrast-enhanced tomography (CT) as routine preoperative work up. The development of multislice multidetector computed axial tomography allows imaging of the whole pancreas in peak contrast intensification. Additionally, the information from the CT may be processed for acquiring of three-dimensional images and visualization of different view planes. Spiral computed axial tomography with i.v. contrast and technique for thin sections may accurately assess the relations of tumor formation with low density to the celiac trunk, superior mesenteric artery, and superior mesenteric-portal vein confluence. Magnetic resonance imaging (MRI), endoscopic ultrasound scans (EUS), and laparoscopy should be performed on an individual patient basis depending on the multidisciplinary team (MDT) discussion. MRI is usually recommended when there is a suspicion of liver metastases present.

According to Ishikawa et al. and Nakao and coworker, the indications are limited to unilateral (<180°) segmental vascular involvement [19, 20]. Attention was especially paid to the exclusion of the cases with deep retroperitoneal invasion, defined by the absence of intact connective tissue between the tumor and the right lateral side of the superior mesenteric artery. Isolated arterial involvement is not accepted as an absolute contraindication. Endoscopic ultrasonography (EUS) at this stage is more reliable regarding detection of invasion in the porto-mesenteric system and is a standard procedure in the specialized medical centers. Tumors with simultaneous involvement of several blood vessels or massive retroperitoneal invasion are treated as resectable only in the case of sensitivity to neoadjuvant chemotherapy.

Preoperative evaluation of resectability should be based on a computed tomography (CT) scan with a pancreas-specific protocol, for example, a "hydropancreas" CT, according to these recommendations. Three grades of resectability can be defined for localized PDAC—"resectable," "borderline resectable," and "unresectable" [21]. A tumor is defined as resectable when no vascular attachment (no distortion of the venous structures and clearly preserved fat planes toward the arteries) is present. The resectability is accepted as borderline when distortion/narrowing/occlusion of the mesentericoportal veins with a technical possibility of reconstruction on the proximal and distal margin of the veins or a semicircumferential abutment (≤180°) of the superior mesenteric artery (SMA) or an attachment at the hepatic artery without the celiac axis is diagnosed—see below. The locally advanced, surgically unresectable tumors are defined as those with infiltration of celiac trunk and/or superior mesenteric artery or as tumors involving the superior mesenteric vein, portal vein, or their confluence. The term "encasement" indicates that the tumor is undistinguishable from the blood vessel for more than 180° of the circumference of the latter. A tumor is defined as unresectable when it presents with the presence of distant metastases, greater than 180° SMA encasement, any celiac abutment, unreconstructible SMV/portal vein, aortic/IVC invasion or encasement, or metastases to lymph nodes beyond the field of resection.

Despite the development of pancreatic imaging, distinguishing between the resectable (stage I and II) and locally advanced (stage III) disease may be difficult and these cases are named with the term "borderline resectability." Vascular resections are usually required in cases often described as with "borderline resectable" findings.

The definition of borderline resectable carcinoma according to an expert consensus statement from 2009 [22] includes short SMV/PV involvement with free proximal and distal venous segments, permitting secure reconstruction and SMA < 180° or short hepatic artery involvement with intact truncus coeliacus. The difference from the M. D. Anderson Group classification is in considering tumors, encasing or abutting (depending on the degree of tumor-vessel interface) the SMV/PV borderline but not resectable [23].

Effected vessel	AHPBA/SSAT/SSO/NCCN [1]	MD Anderson [2]	Alliance [3]
SMV/PV	Abutment, impingement, encasement of the SMV/PV or short segment venous occlusion	Occlusion	Tumor-vessel interface ≥180° of vessel wall circumference, and/or reconstructable occlusion
SMA	Abutment	Abutment	Tumor-vessel interface <180° of vessel wall circumference
HA	Abutment or short segment encasement	Abutment or short segment encasement	Reconstructable short segment interface of any degree between tumor and vessel wall
CA	Uninvolved	Abutment	Tumor-vessel interface <180° of vessel wall circumference

Table 1. CT criteria for borderline resectable pancreatic cancer.

The TVI-classification of Tran Cao et al. [24] considers the radiographic tumor-vein circumferential interface and its value as a predictive factor for concomitant vessel resection.

A consensus statement standardizing the definition of the term "borderline resectability" in accordance with the guidelines of the National Comprehensive Cancer Network (NCCN) as well as the definition of extended resections published by the International Study Group for Pancreatic Surgery (ISGPS) (**Table 1**) [21–23].

The approach should be different when borderline findings in venous and arterial vessel involvement are diagnosed. No neoadjuvant treatment is recommended in venous borderline resectability. Upfront surgery should be performed and, if the intraoperative finding matches the presumed borderline situation as defined above, completed as an en bloc tumor removal with venous replacement [21]. In contrast, palliative treatment should be regarded as the standard of care when suspected arterial borderline resectability is intraoperatively confirmed as a true arterial involvement. Stratification and recognition of the patients with borderline findings who do not benefit from extended resections could be done with the neoadjuvant treatment. Patients with a clear tumor progression under neoadjuvant treatment should be excluded from secondary exploration.

Vascular resection must be performed only upon carefully selected patients with data for presence of resectable tumors or tumors with borderline resectability from the preoperative computed axial tomography.

5. Arterial resections

Arterial resection is usually performed in cases of advanced tumors that infiltrate the retroperitoneal nerve plexus and are related with poor prognosis. Some studies doubted the question whether performing of arterial resection in patients with pancreatoduodenectomy is necessary because the procedure itself is a technical challenge. They confirmed that the arterial resection is possible, but there were not enough data in favor, and that is why it is applied in the context of randomized controlled trials (RCTs) [25].

Neoadjuvant treatment should be evaluated to achieve a better local tumor control in case of arterial tumor infiltration. It can be performed following different study protocols and is not standardized yet [26]. Following the restaging, patients should be subjected to surgical exploration as long as no signs of systemic tumor spread are visible. Further mobilization of the pancreatic head could be performed. First an incision of the peritoneal layer at the ligament of Treitz from the left side is made and then is continued with clearing of the tissue along the artery down to the origin from the aorta via this access. This preparation is used for confirmation or ruling out of the tumor infiltration, so that further needed procedures could be determined.

As a whole, arterial resections and reconstructions are limited to the common hepatic artery or resections (with or without any reconstruction) of the right or left hepatic artery in the presence of aberrant hepatic arterial anatomy. Segmental resections of the common hepatic artery may be considered in isolated involvement usually in the area of branching of

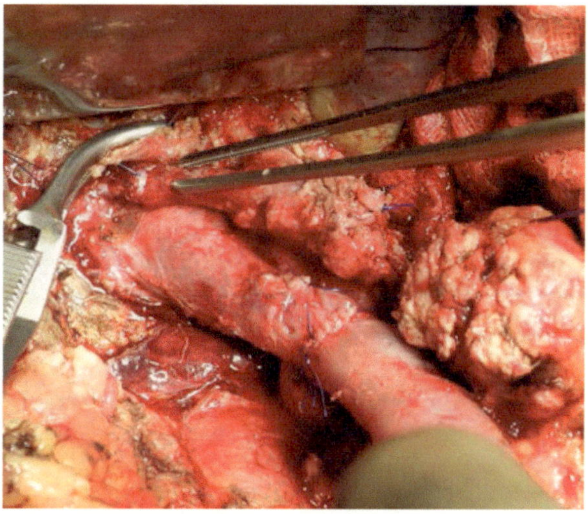

Figure 3. Combined resection of the common/proper hepatic artery with T-T anastomosis, along with segmental portal vein resection with T-T anastomosis.

gastroduodenal artery [6]. The transition between the common and proper hepatic artery is usually long enough and makes primary anastomosis possible, when the area of gastroduodenal artery is resected (**Figure 3**). The use of an interpositional graft from reversed saphenous vein is sometimes required. Due to the communication of the right and left hepatic artery inside the liver, ligation of the right hepatic artery is well tolerated, on providing that normal levels of the serum bilirubin and normal blood flow through the portal vein are maintained. Despite that, revascularization of these blood vessels is usually required

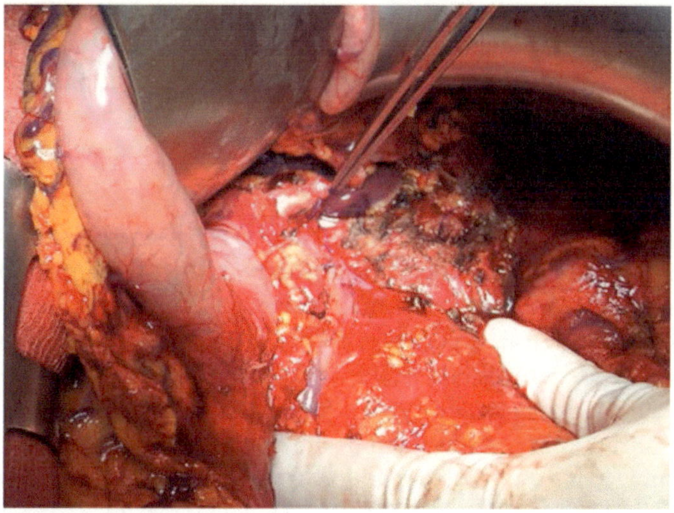

Figure 4. Distal spleno-pancreatectomy with resection of the celiac trunk and segmental resection of SMV. Ligated common hepatic artery is pointed by the forceps.

because the proximal hepatic duct receives almost all of its arterial blood flow from the right hepatic artery after interruption of the blood flow from the right gastric artery. The aberrant right hepatic artery may be infiltrated by the tumor, when the latter reaches the celiac trunk (upon early bifurcation and low position of the left hepatic artery) or when the artery branches from the superior mesenteric artery. Replaced right hepatic artery, branching from the superior mesenteric artery, in contrast to the accessory hepatic arteries, represents the only direct arterial branch toward the right lobe of the liver. When the right hepatic artery, branching from the superior mesenteric artery is infiltrated along the postero-lateral border of the head of pancreas, the pancreatoduodenal resection does not frequently require removal of these blood vessels, because the larger part of these tumors are localized more in front of the head of pancreas and uncinate process of pancreas. The whole common hepatic artery may rarely branch from the superior mesenteric artery (type IX), no identification of that anatomical variant and inattentive ligation of the hepatic artery requires performing of reconstruction.

A high rate of complete resection and favorable prognosis (estimated overall 5-year survival rate of 42%) could be observed in selected patients with distal pancreatectomy with en bloc coeliac axis resection for locally advanced pancreatic body cancer (**Figure 4**) [27, 28].

6. Venous resections

The tumor invasion in the porto-mesenteric system depends on the tumor localization and has no relation to the long-term survival and recurrence. This is not a prognostic factor, but it is an indicator of the biological aggressiveness of the tumor [9]. Invasion of the tumor process in the mesenteric portal blood vessels was considered as a contraindication for radical surgery until recently. Nowadays, this opinion has changed and vascular resections are considered justified if achievement of clear resection margins is possible. Radical resection may be performed in approximately 25—30% of the patients with preoperative diagnostic imaging data for invasion in the porto-mesenteric system [1]. Superior mesenteric/portal vein resections are quite well studied in clinical trials and large series demonstrate equivalence in short-term outcome and long-term survival of the pancreatoduodenectomies combined with venous resections.

Absence of dissemination of the process toward superior mesenteric artery and celiac trunk, which is the prerequisite for achieving of clear resection lines, is the main principle in resections of portal vein in the course of one duodenopancreatic resection [21]. The Japanese, as well as European and American experience, clearly demonstrate that positive resection lines are a prerequisite for recurrent lesions, as well as for lower survival. The level of infiltration of the tumor toward the porto-mesenteric vein is finally determined along the course of surgical operation by mobilization of the specimen from the surrounding tissues and its left repositioning to hang only from the growth. Resection of the vein and recovery of its integrity is the next step. It could be partial or segmental (**Figure 5**). Vein integrity is recovered by one of the following four methods:

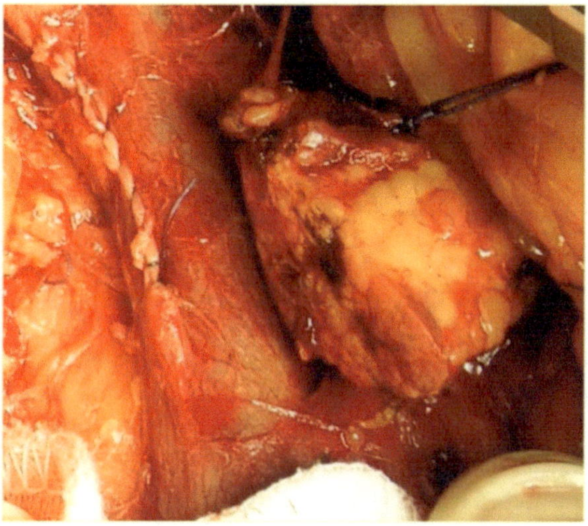

Figure 5. Partial tangential resection of the portal vein sutured longitudinally.

1. Partial tangential resection of no more than one-third of circumference of the vein with suture or placing of venous patch.
2. Segmental resection with termino-terminal veno-venous anastomosis.
3. Segmental resection with venous prosthesis from autologous vein.
4. Segmental resection with synthetic venous prosthesis.

The ISGPS proposes a classification of porto-mesenteric resections according to the type of venous reconstruction [21]:

Type 1: Partial excision of venous wall with a suture closure.

Type 2: Partial excision of venous wall with a patch closure.

Type 3: Segmental venous resection with termino-terminal anastomosis.

Type 4: Segmental venous resection with a conduit and at least two anastomoses.

More recent classification by Tseng et al. takes in general consideration the management of splenic vein along with the type of reconstruction [29]:

V1—Tangential resection with saphenous vein patch.

V2—Segmental resection with splenic vein ligation and primary anastomosis.

V3—Segmental resection with splenic vein ligation and interposition graft.

V4—Segmental resection without splenic vein ligation and primary anastomosis.

V5—Segmental resection without splenic vein ligation and interposition graft.

Shibata et al. divided SMV/PV resections into another four types being guided mainly from the localization of the resection line [30]:

1. Above and below the level of the splenic vein.

2. Above the level of the splenic vein.

3. Below the level of the splenic vein.

4. Tangential resection.

It seems that the management of the splenic vein plays a crucial role during the reconstruction of the SMV/PV confluence [31]. The classical technique of segmental venous resection includes transsection and ligation of the splenic vein. In technical aspect, this maneuver allows complete presentation of the superior mesenteric artery medially to the superior mesenteric vein, and elongation of the superior mesenteric vein and portal vein (because the latter blood vessels are not adducted by the splenic vein) for performing of primary venous anastomosis after segmental venous resection. The retroperitoneal dissection ends with cutting by sharp manner of soft tissues anteriorly to the aorta and on the right side of the so presented superior mesenteric artery. As a result of that the specimen remains fixed only to the superior mesenteric-portal vein confluence.

Extensive 2–3 cm segment of the superior mesenteric-portal vein confluence may be resected without any need for interposition of a venous graft, if the splenic vein is cut. The venous resection is always performed with occlusion of the incoming through superior mesenteric vein blood flow and heparinization before its interruption. Upper gastrointestinal tract bleeding could be observed due to the left-side portal hypertension after ligation of the splenic vein, inferior mesenteric vein, and left gastric veins. The mobilization of the neck of the pancreas frequently leads to ligation of the left gastric veins. If the blood flow of

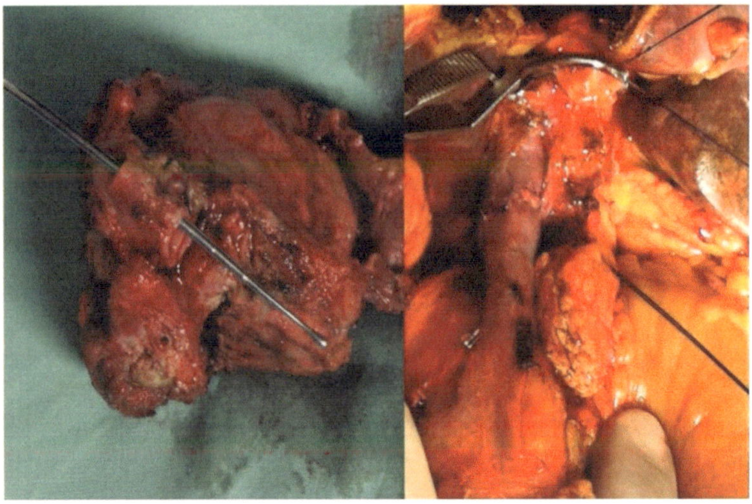

Figure 6. Segmental resection of portal vein with T-T venous anastomosis.

http://dx.doi.org/10.5772/66910

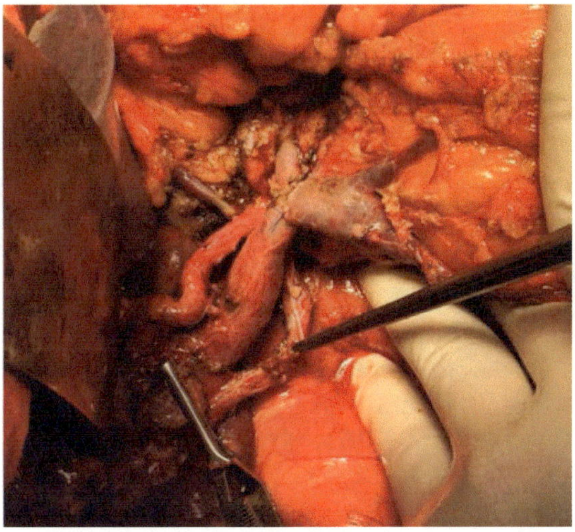

Figure 7. Segmental resection of SMV with T-T reconstruction. Replaced right hepatic artery is pointed by the forceps.

the inferior mesenteric vein runs into the segment of the superior mesenteric vein, which is to be resected, the former vein must also be cut. Upon running of superior mesenteric vein into the splenic vein a way of collateral venous flow is ensured (after interruption of the splenic vein) in retrograde direction and the cutting of splenic vein in this situation is usually well tolerated. Of course, it is recommendable the splenic-portal vein confluence to be preserved if possible, especially when ligation and cutting of inferior mesenteric vein is required. Preservation of the splenic vein is possible, only when the tumor invasion of the superior mesenteric vein or portal vein does not include the confluence with the splenic vein. Preservation of the splenic-superior mesenteric-portal vein confluence significantly limits the mobilization of the portal vein and preserves the primary anastomosis of superior mesenteric vein (following segmental resection of superior mesenteric vein), except in cases when the segmental resection is limited up to 2 cm or less. On account of the latter an interpositional graft should be placed after resection of the superior mesenteric vein with preservation of splenic vein in most of the patients.

Reconstruction of portal vein and superior mesenteric vein after Cattel-Braasch maneuver is usually possible without creating of considerable pressure on the venous anastomosis (**Figures 6** and **7**), at the same time the latter event could be avoided by implanting of a venous graft.

Segmental resection along a great extent of the porto-mesenteric vein makes impossible the reconstruction with termino-terminal anastomosis. In these cases a prosthesis (graft) is used, which may be an autologous one (most frequently internal jugular vein) or an artificial venous prosthesis.

Various types of autogenous veins have been used. Jugular, external iliac vein, great saphenous vein, left renal, and umbilical veins, as well as synthetic grafts could be used as substitutes for portal vein reconstruction. Fleming et al. reported that the superficial

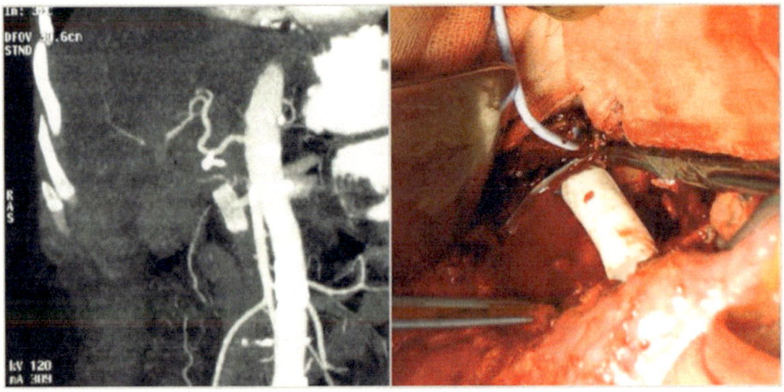

Figure 8. Large resection of the portal vein with PTFE prosthesis replacement.

femoral vein is an excellent size-matched conduit for reconstruction of the SMV or PV without serious complications associated with venous insufficiency in the leg [32]. The patency of reconstruction of the PV or SMV using superficial femoral vein (GSV) reported by Lee et al. was 88% at mean follow-up of 5 months with only a few patients developing mild lower leg edema. Chiba University's team [33] first reported the use of a left renal vein graft for reconstruction of the portal vein. No obvious left kidney dysfunction has been diagnosed after the removal of left renal vein graft [34]. This technique has the following advantages compared with other substitutes:

1. No additional skin incision because the vein is in the same operative field.

2. Usually harvesting takes only 5–10 min.

3. Vein size is often suitable for the portal vein to be reconstructed.

Chiba et al. reported a 100% patency rate in a cohort of 35 patients using a left renal vein graft for portal vein reconstruction, even at long-term follow-up. Suzuki et al. [34] also demonstrated that reconstruction of the inferior vena cava (IVC) or PV with the left renal vein is a durable and safe method without adverse effects on early and long-term renal function. Other veins with smaller diameters like external jugular vein also could be used. The vein is customized by cutting longitudinally and suturing it into a sheet or tube-like graft in order to overcome size discrepancy.

Its recommended synthetic grafts need to be avoided because many resections may involve contaminated bile and postoperative infectious complications could occur. On the other hand, the placement of autologous graft prolongs operative time, which is a prerequisite for postoperative complications. Use of artificial vascular prosthesis also bear risks from thrombosis, as well as infectious complications, which is the main reason for it not to be preferred by most of the medical specialists, although it decreases up to the minimum by the time of clamping of the portal blood flow and is completely justified in critical situation, according to us (**Figure 8**). No difference is observed regarding the hepatic function and hemodynamics of the portal blood flow in the postoperative period, compared to other patients.

Subacute or chronical thrombosis of the graft with the formation of collaterals are observed in long-term follow-up of patients with prosthesis of the porto-mesenteric vein. This process, however, is of minor clinical significance, because it does not influence the liver function or the pressure on the system of portal vein. Recently, a multicenter analysis reported of synthetic graft reconstruction after portal vein resection in pancreaticoduodenectomy. The overall graft patency rate after 36 procedures was 76%. Portal vein thrombosis within 30 days after surgery occurred in 9.1%. Based on the data obtained from this study, it may be recommended that synthetic graft should not to be selected as a portal vein substitute if an autogenous vein graft is available. Synthetic graft could be used as an intraoperative temporary portal vein shunt, followed by its removal after tumor excision combined with portal vein resection [35].

7. Operative techniques

Pancreaticoduodenectomy with or without vein resection should be performed in resectable cases. A classical Whipple procedure or a pylorus preserving pancreaticoduodenectomy (PPPD) could be carried out. The preferred access is trough bi-subcostal incision. The whole abdominal cavity is consecutively examined—the liver is palpated and intraoperative ultrasonography is performed for excluding metastatic lesions. The area around the celiac trunk is inspected for the presence of metastatic lymph nodes or local invasion. The parietal and visceral peritoneum are carefully examined for carcinosis. Mobilization of duodenum with Kocher maneuver ensures inspection of the head of pancreas and retroperitoneum in the area of the inferior vena cava. This is followed by dissection of the hepatoduodenal ligament. The suspected lesions are sent for express histological examination. Resectability is technically assessed based on the local status of the tumor and its relation to major blood vessels. If resectable, radical resection is undertaken. The type of the latter is determined by the anatomical localization of the process. If all resection margins are free of tumor invasion, the surgical operation is performed according to the standard approach, but if invasion is suspected, the course of operation may be changed by freeing the easier for dissection parts of the anatomical specimen at first, and proceeding to the most difficult for dissection areas at the end.

Vascular resections could be finished by primary closure of the vein, end-to-end anastomosis, or a segmental resection and reconstruction with interposition graft. Venous resections can be performed differently depending on the location and length of tumor adherence. In cases when the tumor infiltration reaches the vein from the right circumference and can be excised with a small patch and direct closure of the defect directly without a hemodynamically relevant stenosis, latero-tangential resection of the portal vein could be done [31, 36, 37].

The mesenteric root should be mobilized completely by resolving the attachment of the right hemicolon to the retroperitoneal adhesions in cases when tangential vein resection is not possible [38]. In such a way, a greater flexibility of the mesenteric vein is achieved and this almost always allows approximation of the distal and proximal resection margins of the vein without any critical tension. A vascular graft needs to be inserted when the resected venous length

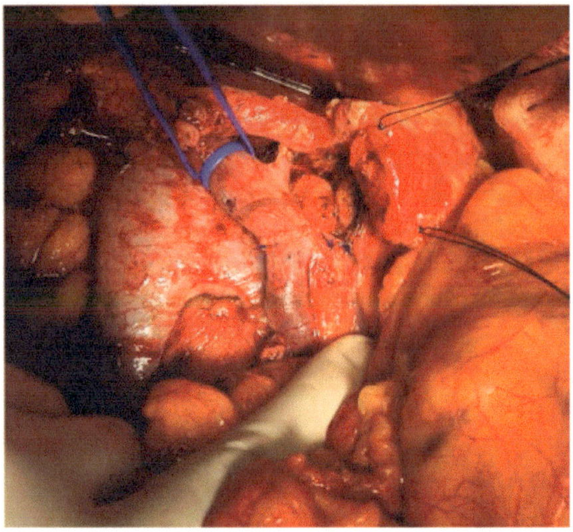

Figure 9. Resection of SMV/PV confluence with ligation of the splenic vein with preservation of the left gastric and inferior mesenteric veins.

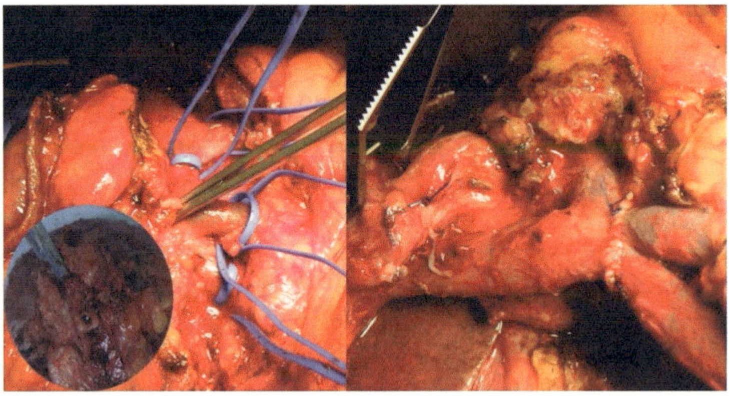

Figure 10. Resection of the proximal part of the superior mesenteric vein followed by difficult anastomosis between portal vein and trifurcation of the distal superior mesenteric vein.

cannot be bridged by the direct anastomosis. A study, including a series of 110 patients undergoing venous resection with different reconstruction techniques, revealed that no differences in surgical outcome were observed when different types of venous reconstruction (venorrhaphy, end-to-end anastomosis, or graft insertion) were performed [38].

Venous resection is also hampered by the need for preservation of the splenic vein, because this makes the direct approach to the most proximal 3–4 cm of the superior mesenteric artery much more difficult. Venous resection and reconstruction may be performed either before the separation of the specimen from the right lateral wall of the superior mesenteric artery, or after the accomplishment of the mesenteric dissection by separation of the superior mesenteric artery at first. Both techniques require significant pancreatic surgery experience and must be performed only by surgeons who have enough experience in vascular resections and reconstructions during pancreatoduodenal resections. The patency of the venous gastric drainage is a special aspect in venous resections that has to be respected in certain situations. The splenic vein can be closed during venous resection as the stomach is usually drained sufficiently via the coronary vein (if preserved) and collaterals via the short gastric veins (**Figure 9**).

A plan for reconstruction must be preliminarily drawn if the proximal part of superior mesenteric vein at the site where the three major veins join is involved. Major postoperative complications may result from the ligation of veins with no adequate collateral draining. Use of interpositional graft may become necessary for ensuring the possibility of lateral implantation of collaterals if reconstruction of more than one vein is needed. The first jejunal vein, which passes behind the superior mesenteric artery, could usually be ligated with no consequences. Despite that, every larger vein must at first be clamped for checking of presence of adequate collateral blood draining (**Figure 10**).

The temporary interruption of the portal blood flow could additionally damage the usually cholestatic liver. Data analysis shows a tendency for significant increase of the liver enzymes in patients with vascular resections, which is due to the clamping of the portal blood flow during the resection. However, this is observed only during the early postoperative period and does not influence liver function afterwards. The direct termino-terminal reconstruction requires fast performing of the anastomosis, independently from the clamping of the superior mesenteric vein. In cases of isolated involvement of superior mesenteric vein, the latter may be clamped proximally below the confluence with the splenic vein, which allows performing of anastomosis upon partially preserved portal blood flow through the splenic vein with intact inferior mesenteric vein. Portal blood flow is fully recovered through the created anastomosis after the specimen removal. Upon resection of the spleno-portal confluence, the splenic vein could be anastomized termino-laterally to the portal vein, while usually partial lateral clamping of the latter is performed. Avoidance of splanchnic stasis is exceptionally important upon performing of pancreatoduodenal resection combined with venous resection. The consequent intestinal and pancreatic edema hampers accomplishing of surgery and may have negative consequences regarding the digestive anastomosis.

Assessment of the specimen based on anatomical pathology is of considerable significance regarding size of the tumor, grade of invasion in the venous wall, as well as achievement of clear resection margins. Tumors' diameter is measured most precisely after its removal from the abdominal cavity. Resection lines are assessed during surgery with express histological examination after separation of 3–4 mm of the resection margin of pancreas. The presence of tumor cells in the vein, as well as growth of the process into the adventitia or media layer of venous wall reveals vascular infiltration.

8. Outcome

The overview of literature revealed that the resection and reconstruction of porto-mesenteric vein in case of pancreatoduodenal resection does not change the percentage of complications and mortality compared to the standard surgical operation. By excluding the first series with regional pancreatectomy, vein resection does not have prognostic significance regarding the survival. Large series with radical surgical resection showed that surgical morbidity and mortality rates are comparable to standard pancreatic head resections [38–40]. Comparable complication rates between standard pancreaticoduodenectomy (PD) and pancreaticoduodenectomy with vascular resection (PDVR) were reported by some studies [12, 13]. Tseng et al. from the MD Anderson Centre, found no survival difference in patients undergoing PD and PDVR [29]. Yekebas et al. found similar postoperative morbidity and mortality rates between PD and PDVR [41]. There are also studies that have reported increased morbidity with no survival benefit in PDVR [38]. The analysis of our data showed that the total level of complications in both groups of patients does not show statistical difference, while the present one is due mainly to patients with venous resection and interposition of artificial graft. In patients with vascular resection there is higher rate of early and late bleeding and a tendency for more frequent need for hemotransfusions. This is especially emphasized in patients with segmental resection and reconstruction with an artificial prosthesis. This fact is explained with the advanced stage of the disease, involving a larger portion of the vein and the more technically difficult destructive stage of surgical operation, related with higher volume of blood loss. The rate of relaparotomies in patients with vascular resections is not greater as compared to patients with no vascular resections. Regarding the porto-mesenteric invasion, the analysis of the literature and our experience leads to the following conclusions:

1. Involvement of superior mesenteric artery or celiac trunk usually means mesenteric nerve plexus involvement, which makes impossible the achievement of clear resection lines.

2. In portal and mesenteric venous resections there is no increase of the morbidity or mortality rates, compared to those of standard pancreatoduodenectomy.

3. The survival of patients with resection of portal vein does not differ significantly from that of patients with standard pancreatoduodenectomy.

Ishikawa et al. reported of 3-year survival in 59% of the cases with unilateral invasion and 18-month survival in patients with bilateral invasion of the process [19]. A systematic review by Siriwardena suggested that PDVR was associated with a high rate of nodal metastases and low survival rates [42]. There is also some evidence of better survival outcomes with PDVR over palliative treatment [36–38]. Recently, a meta-analysis by Zhou et al. [43] compared 19 studies and 661 patients with venous resections during PDAC with 2247 patients undergoing similar operation but without vessel resection. The surgical outcome of the two groups was comparable. No difference in overall survival between both patient groups was found, the 5-year survival rate being 12.3%—superior compared with palliative treatment. Bachellier et al. reported 22% and 2-year survival in 31 patients with pancreatoduodenectomy and resection of porto-mesenteric vein, which is close to the 24% reported for the conventional surgical

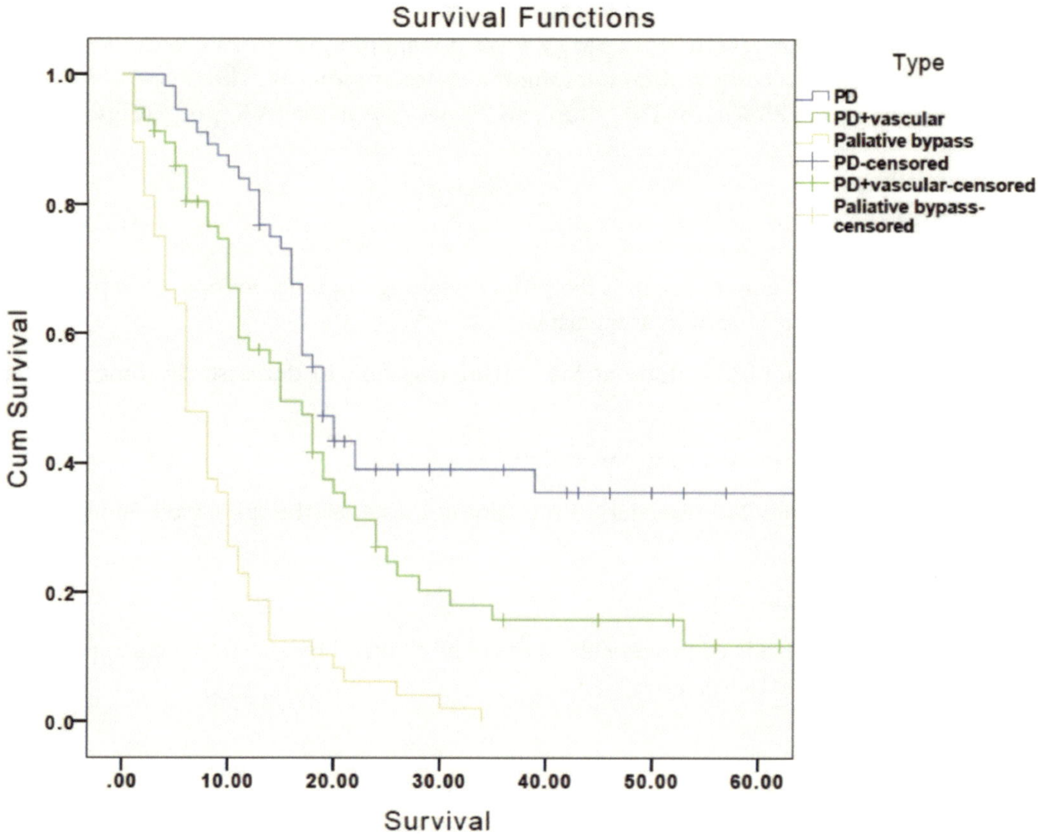

Figure 11. Survival rates depending on the type of intervention.

operation [35]. Nakagohri et al. reported absence of significant difference in the survival of 33 patients with porto-mesenteric venous resection compared to 48 conventional pancreatoduodenectomies (15 vs. 10 months; $p > 0.05$) [44]. Other researchers present similar results: Leach et al.—average survival of 20 vs. 22 months, Harrison et al.—average survival of 13 vs. 17 months, Tseng et al.—average survival of 23.43 vs. 26.5 months, and Hartel et al.—5-year survival of 22 vs. 24%. Moreover, in cases of resection of the vein and absence of histological verification of invasion, improvement of survival was observed, but these observations of Nakagohri and Hartel are still not confirmed and remain controversial [44].

Based on our experience with 356 patients with pancreatic cancer radically operated in our department for a 10-year period (2006–2016)—285 pancreatoduodenectomies and 71 distal pancreatectomies, we could point the level of combined vascular resections of 20.2%. Seventy-two of the presented patients underwent pancreatic resection with simultaneous vascular resection—SMPV in 65 cases (44 with resection of the portal vein, 15 with resection of the superior mesenteric vein, 6 with resection of the porto-mesenterial confluence), arterial in 2 and partial resections of IVC in five cases. Combined vascular resections were done in three cases. Twenty-eight segmental (21 end-to-end anastomosis and seven interposition grafts) and 37 partial wedge venous resections of SMPV were done. Both groups PVR and PR showed similarly close results in complication rates, mortality, and morbidity. Three- and 5-year survival rates were 42 and 38% in the PD group and 28 and 19% in the PVR group (**Figure 11**).

9. Tips and tricks

- CT with intravenous enhancement is the proper imaging modality for operative planning, MRI is better for searching of liver metastasis;
- Venous resection should be done at the end of resection to decrease the time of liver ischemia;
- Prolene 5/0 is the most used suture material;
- In cases with segmental resection direct anastomosis is the preferred method for reconstruction;
- Left renal vein is the ideal graft;
- Routine use of heparin is controversial—it could be changed by subcutaneous application of 40 mg enoxaparine twice daily.

10. Conclusions

At present, it is accepted that pancreatoduodenectomy with resection of the vein does not increase the postoperative risk and significantly improves survival compared with drainage procedures, this being supported by the results obtained from our study too. Most of the published series include mainly patients with exceptionally invasive tumors or patients, in which the infiltration of the vein is found lately during the operation with inability for discontinuing of the pancreatic resection. That is why the comparison of the results with standard pancreatectomy is not completely correct. Vascular resection must be performed only upon carefully selected patients with data for presence of resectable tumors or tumors with borderline resectability from the preoperative imaging studies. The prompt management of pancreatic cancer with vascular involvement should involve multidisciplinary consultation in high-volume centers.

Author details

Nikola Vladov*, Ivelin Takorov and Tsonka Lukanova

*Address all correspondence to: nvladov@yahoo.com

Department of HPB and Transplant Surgery, Military Medical Academy, Sofia, Bulgaria

References

[1] W. Hartwig, T. Hackert, U. Hinz et al., Pancreatic cancer surgery in the new millennium: better prediction of outcome. Annals of Surgery 2011, 254(2): 311–319.

[2] T. Schnelldorfer, A. Ware, M. Sarr et al., Long-termsurvival after pancreatoduodenectomy for pancreatic adenocarcinoma is cure possible. Annals of Surgery 2008, 247(3): 456–462.

[3] W. Hartwig, J. Werner, D. Jäger, J. Debus and MW Büchler, Improvement of surgical results for pancreatic cancer. Lancet Oncology 2013, 14: e476-85.

[4] V. Heinemann, M. Haas and S. Boeck, Neoadjuvant treatment of borderline resectable and non-resectable pancreatic cancer. Annals of Oncology 2013, 0: 1–8.

[5] J. Fortner, Regional resection of cancer of the pancreas: a newsurgical approach. Surgery 1973, 73(2): 307–320.

[6] N. Mollberg, N. Rahbari, M. Koch, W. Hartwig, Y. Hoeger, MW Büchler, J. Weitz, Arterial resection during pancreatectomy for pancreatic cancer: a systematic review and meta-analysis. Annals of Surgery 2011, 254: 882–893.

[7] G. Moore, Y. Sako, L. Thomas, Radical pancreaticoduodenectomy with resection and reanastomosis of the superior mesenteric vein. Surgery 1951, 30: 550–553.

[8] S. Asada, H. Itaya, K. Nakamura, T. Isohashi and S. Masuoka, Radical pancreatoduodenectomy and portal vein resection. Archives of Surgery 1963, 87:93–97.

[9] G. Fuhrman, S. Leach, Ch. Staley, J. Cusack, D. Evans et al., Rationale for En Bloc vein resection in the treatment of pancreatic adenocarcinoma adherent to the superior mesenteric-portal vein confluence. Annals of Surgery 1996, 223(2): 154–162.

[10] L. Harrison, D. Klimstra and M. Brennan, Isolated portal vein involvement in pancreatic adenocarcinoma: a contraindication for resection? Annals of Surgery 1996, 224(3): 242–348.

[11] M. Hartel, M. Niedergethmann, M. Farag-Soliman et al., Benefit of venous resection for ductal adenocarcinoma of the pancreatic head. European Journal of Surgery 2002, 168(12): 707–712.

[12] H. Riediger, F. Makowiec, E. Fischer, U. Adam and U. Hopt, Postoperative morbidity and long-term survival after pancreaticoduodenectomy with superior mesenterico-portal vein resection. Journal of Gastrointestinal Surgery 2006, 10(8): 1106–11.

[13] M. Ouaissi, C. Hubert, R. Verhelst et al., Vascular reconstruction during pancreatoduodenectomy for ductal adenocarcinoma of the pancreas improves resectability but does not achieve cure. World Journal of Surgery 2010, 34(11): 2648–2661.

[14] V. Banz, D. Croagh, C. Coldham et al., Factors influencing outcome in patients undergoing portal vein resection for adenocarcinoma of the pancreas. European Journal of Surgical Oncology 2012, 38(1): 72–79.

[15] Y. Murakami, K. Uemura, T. Sudo et al., Benefit of portal or superior mesenteric vein resection with adjuvant chemotherapy for patients with pancreatic head carcinoma. Journal of Surgical Oncology 2013, 107(4): 414–421.

[16] R. Ravikumar, C. Sabin, M. Hilal et al., Portal vein resection in borderline resectable pancreatic cancer: a United Kingdom multicenter study. Journal of the American College of Surgeons 2014, 218(3): 401–411.

[17] B. Kulemann, J. Hoeppner, U. Wittel et al., Perioperative and long-term outcome after standard pancreaticoduodenectomy, additional portal vein andmultivisceral resection for pancreatic head cancer. Journal of Gastrointestinal Surgery 2015, 19(3): 438–444.

[18] T. Hackert, C. Tjaden, and MW Buchler, Developments in pancreatic surgery during the past ten years. Zentralblatt fur Chirurgie 2014, 139(3): 292–300.

[19] O. Ishikawa, H. Ohigashi, S. Imaoka, T. Iwanaga et al., Preoperative indications for extended pancreatectomy for locally advanced pancreas cancer involving the portal vein. Annals of Surgery 1992, 215(3): 231–236.

[20] T. Kaneko, A. Nakao, S. Inoue, H. Takagi et al., Intraportal endovascular ultrasonography in the diagnosis of portal vein invasion by pancreatobiliary carcinoma. Annals of Surgery 1995, 222(6): 711–716.

[21] M. Bockhorn, F. G. Uzunoglu, M. Adham et al., Borderline resectable pancreatic cancer: a consensus statement by the International Study Group of Pancreatic Surgery (ISGPS). Surgery 2014, 155(6): 977–988.

[22] M. Callery, KJ Chang, E. Fishman, M. Talamonti, L. William Traverso et al., Pretreatment assessment of resectable and borderline resectable pancreatic cancer: expert consensus statement. Annals of Surgical Oncology 2009, 16(7): 1727–1733.

[23] G. Varadhachary, E. Tamm, J. Abbruzzese, H. Wang, J. Lee et al., Borderline resectable pancreatic cancer: definitions, management, and role of preoperative therapy. Annals of Surgical Oncology 2006, 13(8): 1035–1046.

[24] H. Tran Cao, A. Balachandran, H. Wang, Evans D et al., Radiographic tumor-vein interface as a predictor of intraoperative, pathologic, and oncologic outcomes in resectable and borderline resectable pancreatic cancer. Journal of Gastrointest Surg 2014, 18(2): 269–278.

[25] P. Bachellier, E. Rosso, I. Lucescu, D. Jaeck et al., Is the need for an arterial resection a contraindication to pancreatic resection for locally advanced pancreatic adenocarcinoma? A case-matched controlled study. Journal of Surgical Oncology 2011, 103: 75–84.

[26] D. Evans, P. Ritch, B. Erickson, Neoadjuvant therapy for localized pancraeatic cancer. Annals of Surgery 2015, 261–271.

[27] Y. Yamamoto, Y. Sakamoto, D. Ban, K. Shimada et al., Is celiac axis resection justified for T4 pancreatic body cancer? Surgery 2012, 151: 61–69.

[28] W. Pratt, Sh. Maithel, Ts. Vanounou, Clinical and economic validation of the International Study Group of Pancreatic Fistula (ISGPF) Classification Scheme. Annals of Surgery 2007, 245(3): 443–451.

[29] J. Tseng, Ch. Raut, J. Lee, JN Vauthey, E. Abdalla et al., Pancreaticoduodenectomy with vascular resection: margin status and survival duration. Journal of Gastorintest Surgery 2004, 8(8): 933–950.

[30] C. Shibata, M. Kobari, T. Tsuchiya, T. Yamazaki et al., Pancreatectomy combined with superior mesenteric-portal vein resection for adenocarcinoma in pancreas. World Journal of Surgery 2001,25: 1002–1005.

[31] M. Shoup, K. Conlon, D. Klimstra, and M. Brennan, Is extended resection for adenocarcinoma of the body or tail of the pancreas justified? Journal of Gastrointestinal Surgery 2003, 7(8); 946–952.

[32] J. Fleming, C. Barnett, G. Clagett, Superficial femoral vein as a conduit for portal vein reconstruction during pancreaticoduodenectomy. Arch Surg 2005; 140: 698–702.

[33] M. Miyazaki, H. Itoh, T. Kaiho et al. Portal vein reconstruction at the hepatic hilus using a left renal vein graft. J Am Coll Surg 1995, 180: 497–498.

[34] T. Suzuki, H. Yoshidome, F. Kimura, H. Shimizu et al. Renal function is well maintained after use of left renal vein graft for vascular reconstruction in hepatobiliary-pancreatic surgery. J Am Coll Surg 2006, 202:87–92.

[35] P. Bachellier, E. Rosso, P. Fuchshuber, P. Addeo, P. David, E. Oussoultzoglou et al. Use of a temporary intraoperative mesentericoportal shunt for pancreatic resection for locally advanced pancreatic cancer with portal vein occlusion and portal hypertension. Surgery 2014, 155: 449–456.

[36] J. Weitz, P. Kienle, J. Schmidt, H. Friess, and MW Buchler, Portal vein resection for advanced pancreatic head cancer. Journal of the American College of Surgeons 2007, 204(4): 712–716.

[37] A. Sasson, J. Hoffman, E. Ross et al. En bloc resection for locally advanced cancer of the pancreas: is it worthwhile? Journal of Gastrointestinal Surgery 2002, 6(2): 147–158.

[38] S. Muller, M. Hartel, A. Mehrabi et al. Vascular resection in pancreatic cancer surgery: survival determinants. Journal of Gastrointestinal Surgery 2009, 13(4): 784–792.

[39] P. Kim, A. Wei, E. Atenafu et al. Planned versus unplanned portal vein resections during pancreaticoduodenectomy for adenocarcinoma. British Journal of Surgery 2013, 100(10): 1349–1356.

[40] R. Martin II, C. Scoggins, V. Egnatashvili, C. Staley, K. McMasters and D. Kooby, Arterial and venous resection for pancreatic adenocarcinoma operative and longterm outcomes. Archives of Surgery 2009, 144(2): 154–159.

[41] E. Yekebas, D. Bogoevski, G. Cataldegirmen et al. En bloc vascular resection for locally advanced pancreaticmalignancies infiltrating major blood vessels: perioperative outcome and long-term survival in 136 patients. Annals of Surgery 2008, 247(2): 300–309.

[42] H. Siriwardana and A. Siriwardena, Systematic review of outcome of synchronous portal-superior mesenteric vein resection during pancreatectomy for cancer. British Journal of Surgery 2006, 93(6): 662–673.

[43] Y. Zhou, Z. Zhang, Y. Liu, B. Li and D. Xu, Pancreatectomy combined with superior mesenteric vein-portal vein resection for pancreatic cancer: a meta-analysis. World Journal of Surgery 2012, 36(4): 884–891.

[44] T. Nakagohri, T. Kinoshita, M. Konishi et al., Survival benefit of portal vein resection for pancreatic cancer. Am J Surg 2003, 186: 149–153.

Section 5

New Procedures in Diabetes

Chapter 11

Avoiding Immunosuppression for Islet Transplantation: Use of Protective Biomaterials

Michael Alexander, Huy Nguyen, Antonio Flores,
Shiri Li, Paul De Vos, Elliot Botvinick and
Jonathan Lakey

Additional information is available at the end of the chapter

http://dx.doi.org/10.5772/66492

Abstract

Islet transplantation, with the advent of the Edmonton protocol in 2000, has offered a significant alternative for long-lasting treatment of type 1 diabetes. However, the immunosuppression required for transplantation has the cytotoxic effect on pancreatic islets, and thus limiting the long-term efficacy of the transplant. Immediate loss of islets after transplant was also observed because of immediate blood-mediated inflammatory response (IBMIR), which kills islets transplanted in the liver through portal vein. There is also commonly a lack of microvascular blood supply to the transplanted islets. In this chapter, we will review the variety of technologies used to protect transplanted islets against toxicity of immunosuppression, immune rejection, and inflammatory response. We will evaluate the mechanisms of these technologies and their progress in solving the challenges to islet transplantation. The technologies include encapsulation of transplanted islets in various polymers, transplants in sites other than the liver, and creation of new prevascularized transplant site. These technologies offer several mechanisms to prevent immune rejection or immediate contact with cytotoxic inflammatory response, in addition to maintaining islet integrity. New transplant sites are also being developed to support the islets, by allowing establishment of microvasculature and innervation, prior to addition of the islets.

Keywords: cell encapsulation, type 1 diabetes, islet transplants, microcapsules, cell engineering

1. Introduction

Over 25 million people in the United States (USA) suffer from diabetes, with approximately 5% characterized as type 1 diabetes (T1DM). Diabetes is ranked as the seventh leading cause of death in the USA. T1DM is characterized by the autoimmune-mediated destruction of the β-cells of the pancreas, resulting in insulin deficiency [1]. The current method of treatment for T1DM is insulin injection to maintain blood glucose control, which treats the symptoms but not the underlying disease.

With the invention of the Edmonton protocol in 2000, islet transplantation has become an attractive treatment for T1DM. As a treatment option, islet transplantation meets the goal of treating the disease rather than the symptoms. The end goal of islet transplantation in patients is the elimination of exogenous insulin dependence, allowing for those with T1DM to return to normal lives without constant monitoring of their blood glucose levels. There have been a total of 677 islet transplant recipients from 2000 to 2010. The success of the treatment has improved as well, where 27% of recipients achieved 3 years of insulin independence before 2007. After 2007 that rate has increased to 44%. Compared to insulin injection regimen, islet transplantation resulted in significant reduction in episodes of hypoglycemia unawareness [2].

Islet transplantation faces two challenges from the host immune system: the rejection of the transplanted islets as foreign body and the existing autoimmunity against β-cells. Immunosuppressive drugs such as sirolimus and rapamycin used in the Edmonton protocol has toxic side effects on islets [3, 4]. As such, there is an impetus to move away from the use of immunosuppressive therapy and instead shift toward developing physical barriers against transplant rejection and autoimmunity.

Cell encapsulation to provide physical barrier has been tested in treating other diseases such as neurodegenerative diseases, pain, and epilepsy to name a few. So far, encapsulation has been used primarily to treat T1DM [5–9]. By providing a physical barrier to immune rejection, islet encapsulation has been shown to allow transplanted islet to function normally and avoid the use of immunosuppression [10, 11].

2. History of animal and human trials of islet encapsulation

The first encapsulated islet transplants occurred in 1980, where islets in an alginate hydrogel transplanted intraperitoneally into diabetic rats achieved normoglycemia for 3 weeks, compared to 8 weeks for nonencapsulated islets [12]. Currently, there are a number of achievements in encapsulating islets seen in small and large animal studies, as well as in early phase clinical trials. A syngeneic transplant of nonobese diabetic (NOD) into prediabetic islets diabetic NOD recipients, using 5% agarose encapsulating 1500–2000 islet equivalents (IEq), showed that intraperitoneal implantation as well as omental pouch transplants demonstrated prolonged euglycemia for a period of 100 days compared to 8 days for unencapsulated islet transplants [13]. This study was repeated in 2006, where the same period of normoglycemia was observed in transplant recipients. In addition, when the devices were removed after 400 days, viable

http://dx.doi.org/10.5772/66492

islets were recovered with a small percentage of necrotic cells [14]. Aside from agarose, polyethylene glycol-poly lactic-co-glycolic acid (PEG-PLGA) has been used to encapsulate 500–600 IEq islets for syngeneic transplant into streptozotocin (STZ) induced diabetic BALB/c mice, where over half of the recipients achieved normal glucose levels for up to 100 days [15].

Results in large animal studies have mostly mirrored that of the small animal trials. Diabetic canine recipients, receiving 15,000–20,000 IEq islets/kg in alginate microcapsule into the intraperitoneal cavity, were able to maintain normoglycemia without insulin injection for up to 110 days, with c-peptide detectable in the blood for more than 1 year [16]. In 2010, allogeneic transplant in nonhuman primate was tested using subcutaneous and kidney capsule transplants of alginate micro and macroencapsulated islets, at a dose of 30,000 IEQ/kg. In this study, normoglycemia was observed for 28 weeks [17]. In a xenotransplant study of neonatal porcine islets into diabetic cynomolgus monkey, 10,000 IEq/kg of alginate encapsulated islets resulted in more than 40% reduction in injectable insulin dose compared to preimplantation [18].

The first human clinical trial of encapsulated islets transplant in T1DM was reported in 1994. In a type 1 diabetes patient, a postoperative kidney transplant maintained on low dose immunosuppression initially received 10,000 IEQ/kg of cadaver human islets encapsulated in an alginate microcapsule followed by a repeat infusion of 5000 IEQ/kg 6 months later. The patient's insulin requirements were reduced to 1–2 insulin units per day, and eventually he was able to discontinue all exogenous insulin after 9 months [19]. In 2006, human cadaveric islets (400,000–600,000 IEQ) were encapsulated into sodium alginate beads and placed intraperitoneally into two diabetic patients. The patients showed improved daily glucose levels and a decline in daily exogenous insulin intake. However, neither patient became insulin independent [20].

Living Cell Technologies Ltd. an Australia company has achieved the best outcomes for encapsulated islet transplants. The company, which owns a pathogen-free pig farm in New Zealand, performed xenotransplantation of alginate encapsulated fetal pig islets in several human clinical trials. The most significant achievement has been in the reduction of hypoglycemic episodes to around 40%. Several patients achieved improvements in daily glucose levels and a reduction in exogenous insulin dosing, while two patients became insulin independent after 4 months [21, 22].

Unfortunately, there is a lack of consistency in the human clinical results. For example, a human clinical trial by Tuch et al. used alginate encapsulated human islets and tracked the presence of plasma C-peptide levels for up to 2.5 years, ultimately resulting in no change in insulin requirements for the recipients [23]. While these early phase clinical trials aim to ensure safety and determine optimal islet dose, most of the trial patients do not achieve sustainable insulin independence.

3. Biomaterials used for islet encapsulation

One of the important steps to bring islet encapsulation into widespread clinical use is to develop a standard for the type of biomaterial used and the dose of islets to be infused.

The type of biomaterial has also been shown to affect graft survival. A test of several encapsulation methods using alginate with or without poly L-lysine (PLL) as well as with high guluronic (G) or mannuronic (M) acid in mouse recipients showed that significant results were achieved with PLL-free high M microcapsules, showing sustained normoglycemia for 8 weeks [24]. Likewise, improved capsule integrity and graft function could be achieved by altering the concentration of alginate in their xenotransplants into diabetic Lewis rats [25].

Currently, the most common employed method for islet encapsulation involves alginate microcapsules [24, 26, 27]. The original device was developed over three decades ago as capillary fibers in a culture-coated medium [28], shaped as arterial-venous shunts into diabetic canines. These devices showed promising results with several canines achieving reduced insulin requirements [29, 30]. Vascular shunts are limited by the volume and number of islets that can be contained within the fibers. Elongation of the fibers resulted in increased fibrosis, leading to abandonment of this device as the higher dose of islets needed for human recipients would require such large fibers that resulted in a large amount of fibrosis [31]. Other macroscale devices have seen less use due to their increased immunogenicity as well as the larger diffusion parameters required for oxygen and nutrients to reach the cell.

Nanoencapsulation has an advantage compared to other techniques because of its more efficient diffusion capability. With a better surface area to volume ratio, this means that nanoencapsulation can improve insulin response time to blood glucose levels, offering the protection of encapsulation without compromising tissue function due to the physical barrier. PEG has been used for nanoencapsulation devices and can be cross-linked through exposure to UV or visible light. This characteristic also allows for a reduction in the amount of damage done to the capsule's inner cells normally achieved by other cross-linking methods. On the other hand, PEG biocompatibility still leaves much to be desired compared to other hydrogels, and complete protection from cytokines is still not achieved [32]. Despite these concerns, some success has been attained with these gels [33].

By far the most common encapsulation device is a microscale vehicle. These capsules have mechanical stability, optimal surface area to volume ratio, and have enhanced immunologic profiles [26, 33]. Microscale device is also easily made using standard droplet-based encapsulators that produces consistent size and shape of the resulting capsules [34, 35], as shown in **Figure 1**.

Microcapsules can also be easily made using materials other than alginate. The most common synthetic chemicals used for microcapsule production are poly ethylene oxide, poly acrylic acid, poly vinyl alcohol, polyphosphazene, and polypeptides and their derivatives. Natural occurring hydrogels include gelatin, fibrin, agarose, hyaluronate, chitosan, and alginate [36, 37]. Poly glycolic and lactic acid polymers continue to be the most commonly used synthetic materials used in medical devices.

Regardless of the materials used, capsule materials still face the fundamental flaw of being foreign materials. Thus there will always be the possibility they will elicit a greater immune response, eventually leading to fibrosis and loss of the encased cells. As such, it is important to ensure that the materials are nontoxic and purified prior to microcapsule production.

http://dx.doi.org/10.5772/66492

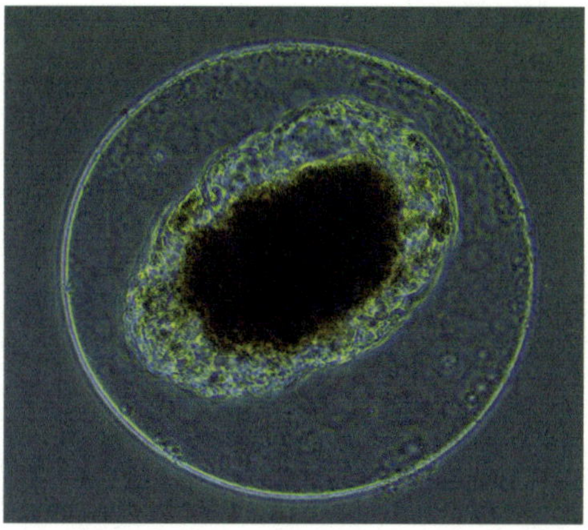

Figure 1. Porcine islet encapsulated in alginate. Isolated juvenile porcine islets (from 22 to 24 days old pigs, matured for 7 days) were encapsulated in 2.5% low viscosity mannuronate (Pro-Nova UPLVM) alginate (Novamatrix) using an electrostatic gas-driven encapsulator (Nisco Engineering AG).

Because of their tolerability, biologically derived materials have been of interest for islet encapsulation. One possible material is collagen, a naturally derived polymer that is the most widely used in medical devices today. However, collagen gels exhibit poor strength, which are expensive and have high variability of purity, making standardization of the process a problem [37]. Comparatively, alginate has excellent biocompatibility, hydrophilic properties, easy gelation process, stable architecture, and relatively low cost. Alginate is polysaccharide derived from seaweed, which can be highly purified to prevent foreign body response [38]. Impure alginate has been implicated in islet cell necrosis and recruitment of inflammatory mediators [39].

Alginate is a polymer of 1-4 linked β-D-mannuronic acid (M) and 1-4 linked α-L-guluronic acid (G). This polysaccharide can contain varying concentrations of M and G carbohydrates, which provides a variety of molecular weight, stability, permeability, and immunogenicity. High G alginates form gels, which are smaller and stronger than high M alginates [38]. High-M alginate was often avoided when immunosuppression was the desired outcome, because mannuronic acid tends to provoke both innate and antibody-mediated immune response, independent of the type of cation used for cross-linking (Ca^{2+} or Ba^{2+}). High-M also triggers macrophages to secrete pro-inflammatory cytokines including IL-1, IL-6, and TNF-α through interactions with the monocyte CD14 receptor [39]. However, recent studies seem to contradict these earlier findings, reporting a higher amount of cellular adhesion to high-G alginate capsules when compared to high-M alginate [40, 41]. It is likely that the observed difference in the immune response depends not on the identity of the alginate material, but instead on the quality of the alginate purification method [42, 43].

Using surface modification, poly-methyl co-guanidine-cellulose sulfate/poly l-lysine-sodium alginate (PMCG)-CS/PLL was used for syngeneic transplant into T1DM canine recipients [44]. Their study reported normoglycemia in the canines for approximately 160 days, with one canine achieving euglycemia for 214 days [45].

Alginate converts into a gel form by ionic cross-linking with bivalent cations such as calcium, magnesium, and more commonly barium [46]. Cross-linking establish a mesh of porous material that allows bidirectional flow of materials, including oxygen, nutrients, and hormones (especially insulin). However, hydrogel polymerization does not result in uniform pore size, while internal permeability tends to vary between batches [38].

An increase in the degree of cross-linking results in gels that have superior mechanical strength but inversely reduces the size of the pores available for diffusion. It is possible to artificially organize the islets in alginate gels into clusters mimicking natural islets [47].

Surface modification using polycations and anions can change the permeability and mechanical strength of alginate, but the polarity tends to increase the immune response. Common molecules used for this purpose include: poly-d-lysine (PDL), polyethylene glycol (PEG), poly-L-ornithine (PLO), and poly-L-lysine (PLL). This effect can be counteracted by adding another layer of alginate to prevent direct contact with a polar surface [38], or by modifying the alginate [48].

Capsule fibrosis was the most significant problem encountered when utilizing alginate capsules [23, 49–51]. Theoretically, immune isolation is achieved by encapsulation of the cells, but some levels of immune rejection and foreign body response still occur. Also, while oxygen and nutrients are able to freely diffuse across a matrix, studies have shown that at the time of explant, histology showed a necrotic core in the encapsulated islets without evidence of fibrosis. This suggests inadequate oxygen diffusion into the center of the encapsulated islets [52].

The results demonstrated by these prior studies suggest that there are key points to be considered during engineering of the encapsulation vehicle. The raw and the purified capsule material must be nontoxic, while the purification method needs to be reproducible across batches. The polymerization of the capsule material needs to be noncytotoxic to the islets. If there is any degradation of the material, it must follow physiological tissue growth and its products must not adversely affect the coated cells or human body. For clinical application, it would be important for the capsule engineering to be easily scalable, while maintaining good manufacturing practices (GMP) adherence to satisfy regulatory standards.

4. Improvement on islet encapsulation engineering

4.1. Co-encapsulation

Co-encapsulation is the process of adding additional molecules to the capsule to enhance the performance of the encapsulated islets. Encapsulation of islets along with dexamethasone, a corticosteroid serving as local immune suppression, can improve islet survival in mice recipients compared to those islets alone [53]. In another study, co-encapsulation of mouse monocyte macrophage cells and hamster kidney cells with ibuprofen improved the encapsulated cell survival both *in vitro* and *in vivo* [54].

While encapsulation protects the cells inside from large molecules such as antibodies as well as direct cellular contact, smaller molecules such as pro-inflammatory cytokines can still diffuse across most hydrogel gradients due to their smaller molecular weight. To achieve this, an attempt at islet encapsulation with a silicon nanopore membrane found observed cytokine protection and islet viability for over 6 hours, with the islets remaining responsive to glucose levels [55]. Thus, protection from these cytokines may promote capsule survival. In an *in vitro* study performed by Leung, capsules with anti-TNF alpha were able to remove active TNF-α, a pro-inflammatory cytokine from a culture medium, which resulted in better encapsulated cell survival [56].

4.2. Protection against hypoxia

In order to improve oxygen supply to the cell, access to a rich vascular bed is essential. Addition of the angiogenic factor, fibroblast growth factor 1 (FGF-1), into capsule was able to affect a continuous FGF-1 release for a 1-month period *in vitro* [57]. In another study, encapsulation of solid peroxide within polydimethylsiloxane resulted in sustained oxygen release from the matrix for approximately 6 weeks [58].

Extracellular matrix components, derived from laminin, have been shown to improve islet human islet function for encapsulated islet transplants. These extracellular matrix components are also found in native islets located in the pancreas prior to islet isolation. In this case, a variety of laminin-derived peptides or collagen were co-encapsulated with human islets and islet function was measured *in vitro*. Islet viability and insulin response to glucose were improved by the addition of laminin-derived peptide or collagen [59].

4.3. Prevascularization

Prevascularization of islet implant consists of establishing a well-vascularized matrix or scaffold, by implanting the scaffold, then encouraging angiogenesis that leads to scaffold penetration by microcapillaries. Angiogenesis is promoted by addition of fibrin at the time of scaffold implant. Islets were then added to the scaffold after a certain duration that has been shown to allow significant vascularization, as shown in **Figure 2**. This method was shown to improve subcutaneous islet efficacy in restoring normoglycemia when compared to subcutaneous transplants of islets alone [60].

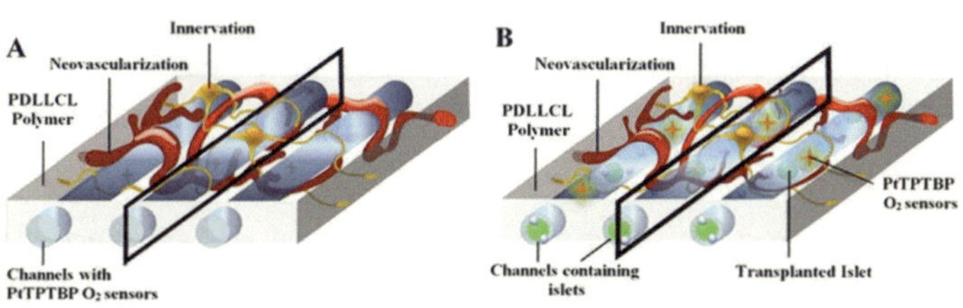

Figure 2. Prevascularized scaffold for islet transplant. Device is implanted subcutaneously 28 days before the introduction of the β-cell clusters during which the foreign body response and neovascularization are completed (A). The device contains polyethylene rods with high hydrophobicity to avoid cell adhesion. Upon removal of the rods, the islets can be infused (B).

4.4. Toward GMP standard

One of the key issues facing the engineering of encapsulating material for islet transplantation would be to define standards for the materials. The standards required contain the choice of raw material, the purification method and quality control of the purification, the shape of the device used for encasing the islets, and the quality of the encased islets. The lack of such standards is likely to account for the current variability in the results reported in the literature on the encapsulated islet transplant.

As an example of the standard necessary for clinical translation of the encapsulation technology, commercially available alginates used to create islet capsules have been found to contain pathogen-associated molecular patterns (PAMPS). PAMP such as peptidoglycan, lipoteichoic acid, and flagellin among other proteins, endotoxins, and polyphenols [61] can trigger recognition by the innate immune system. PAMPS are recognized by toll-like receptors (TLRs) and pattern-recognition receptors (PRRs) [61, 62], leading to pericapsular fibrotic overgrowth (PFO) [63] as the immune system attempts to isolate the graft. PFO severely hinders graft survival by preventing diffusion of nutrients and waste.

In addition to cellular adhesion and PFO, death of encapsulated islets may also be caused by chemokines and cytokines that are small enough to pass through the permeable capsules [64]. TLRs, upon recognition and binding of PAMPS to the receptor surface, initiate an intracellular signaling cascade ultimately resulting in the secretion of a host of inflammatory cytokines attributed to translocation of the NF-κB (nuclear factor kappa-light-chain-enhancer of activated B cells) into the nucleus [65].

Before alginate can be used for clinical transplantation, it will need further development in the GMP manufacturing and purification of the raw materials, to ensure a low amount of PAMP detectable by the recipient's immune system. In addition, the production of the encapsulated islets, including the islet isolation and the encapsulation process, needs to achieve a threshold of standard of quality to ensure a consistent and reliable result, to make it possible to compare the effect of the variety of encapsulation techniques and improvements.

5. Conclusion

In this chapter, we have covered the variety of options used to protect transplanted islets physically against both transplant rejection and autoimmune assault on β-cells. The technologies covered include the variety of encapsulation devices, materials, and addition of supportive materials to improve islet function and survivability.

A key step toward translating biomaterial encapsulation of islets toward clinical trial would be to develop a standard of quality that has to be met by the raw encapsulation material, the islets, and the encapsulation process. This will eventually lead to a process that can be scaled up and to adhere to GMP quality requirements. The current variability of results in the literature on encapsulated islet transplants as T1DM treatment can likely be explained by the lack of such standard, making it impossible to reliably compare multiple encapsulation technologies.

http://dx.doi.org/10.5772/66492

The results in the literature on the encapsulation of islets for the treatment of T1DM showed that it is a promising technology that can revolutionize the treatment paradigm for diabetics. Although significant advances have occurred, there are several obstacles that must be addressed before achieving widespread use of this technology.

Author details

Michael Alexander[1], Huy Nguyen[1], Antonio Flores[1], Shiri Li[1,], Paul De Vos[2], Elliot Botvinick[3] and Jonathan Lakey[1]*

*Address all correspondence to: jlakey@uci.edu

1 Department of Surgery, University of California Irvine, Orange, CA, USA

2 Department of Pathology and Medical Biology, University Medical Center Groningen, Groningen, Netherlands

3 Department of Biomedical Engineering, University of California Irvine, Irvine, CA, USA

References

[1] American Diabetes Association. Diagnosis and classification of diabetes mellitus. Diabetes Care. 2004; 1:s5–s10.

[2] Barton FB, Rickels MR, Alejandro R, Hering BJ, et al. Improvement in outcomes of clinical islet transplantation. Diabetes Care. 2012; 35:1436–1445.

[3] Hafiz MM, Faradji RN, Froud T, et al. Immunosuppression and procedure-related complications in 26 patients with type 1 diabetes mellitus receiving allogeneic islet cell transplantation. Transplantation. 2005; 80:1718–1728.

[4] Niclauss N, Bosco D, Morel P, et al. Rapamycin impairs proliferation of transplant islet beta cells. Transplantation. 2011; 91:714–722.

[5] Bachoud-Levi A, Deglon N, Nguyen JP, et al. Neuroprotective gene therapy for Huntington's disease using a polymer encapsulated BHK cell line engineered to secrete human CNTF. Hum Gen Ther. 2000; 11:1723–1729.

[6] Jeon Y. Cell based therapy for the management of chronic pain. Korean J Anesthesiol. 2011; 60:3–7.

[7] Eriksdotter-Jonhagen M, Linderoth B, Lind G, et al. Encapsulated cell biodelivery of nerve growth factor to the basal forebrain in patients with Alzheimer's disease. Dement Geriatr Congn Disord. 2012; 33:18–28.

[8] Fernandez M, Barcia E, Fernandez-Carballido A, et al. Controlled release of rasagiline mesylate promotes neuroprotection in a rotenone-induced advanced model of Parkinson's disease. Int J Pharm. 2012; 438:266–278.

[9] Huber A, Padrun V, Deglon N, et al. Grafts of adenosine-releasing cells suppress seizures in kindling epilepsy. Proc Natl Acad Sci USA. 2012; 98:7611–7616.

[10] Hearing B, Ricordi C. Islet transplantation for patients with type 1 diabetes: results, research priorities, and reasons for optimism. Graft. 1999; 2:12–27.

[11] Shapiro AM, Nanji SA, Lakey JR. Clinical islet transplant: current and future directions toward tolerance. Immunol Rev. 2003; 196:219–236.

[12] Lim F, Sun AM. Microencapsulated islets as bioartificial pancreas. Science. 1980; 210:908.

[13] Kobayashi Y, Aomatsu H, Iwata T, et al. Indefinite islet protection from autoimmune destruction in nonobese diabetic mice by agarose microencapsulation without immunosuppression. Transplantation. 2003; 75:619–625.

[14] Kobayashi T, Aomatsu Y, Iwata H, et al. Survival of microencapsulated islets at 400 days posttransplantation in the omental pouch of NOD mice. Cell Transplant. 2006; 15:359–365.

[15] Dong H, Fahmy TM, Metcalfe SM, et al. Immuno-isolation of pancreatic islets allografts using pegylated nanotherapy leads to long-term normoglycemia in full MHC mismatch recipient mice. PLoS One. 2012; 7:e50625.

[16] Soon-Shiong P, Feldman E, Nelson R, et al. Long-term reversal of diabetes by the injection of immunoprotected islets. Proc Natl Acad Sci USA. 1993; 90:5843–5847.

[17] Dufrane D, Goebbels RM, Gianello P. Alginate macroencapsulation of pig islets allows correction of streptozotocin-induced diabetes in primates up to 6 months without immunosuppression. Transplantation. 2010; 90:1054–1062.

[18] Elliott RB, Escobar L, Tan PL, et al.. Intraperitoneal alginate-encapsulated neonatal porcine islets in a placebo-controlled study with 16 diabetic cynomolgus primates. Transplant Proc. 2005; 37:3505–3508.

[19] Soon-Shiong RE, Heintz N, Merideth QX, et al. Insulin independence in a type 1 diabetic patient after encapsulated islet transplantation. Lancet. 1994; 343:950–951.

[20] Calafiore R, Basta G, Luca G, et al. Microencapsulated pancreatic islet allografts into non immunosuppressed patients with type 1 diabetes: first two cases. Diabetes Care. 2006; 29:1137–1139.

[21] Elliott RB, Escobar L, Tan PL, et al. Live encapsulated porcine islets from a type 1 diabetic patient 9.5 yr after xenotransplantation. Xenotransplantation. 2007; 14:157–161.

[22] Elliot RB, Garkavenko O, Tan P, et al. Transplantation of microencapsulated neonatal porcine islets in patients with type 1 diabetes: safety and efficacy. In: American Diabetes Association: 70th Scientific Sessions; June 25–29 2010; Orlando, Florida, USA. 2010.

[23] Tuch BE, Keogh GW, Williams LJ, et al. Safety and viability of microencapsulated human islets transplanted into diabetic humans. Diabetes Care. 2009; 32:1887–1889.

[24] King A, Lau J, Nordin A, et al. The effect of capsule composition in the reversal of hyperglycemia in diabetic mice transplanted with microencapsulated allogeneic islets. Diabetes Technol Ther. 2003; 5:653–663.

[25] Lanza RP, Jackson R, Sullivan A, et al. Xenotransplantation of cells using biodegradable microcapsules. Transplantation. 1999; 67:1105–1111.

[26] Krishnamurthy NV, Gimi B. Encapsulated cell grafts to treat cellular deficiencies and dysfunction. Crit Rev Biomed Eng. 2011; 39:473–491.

[27] Khanna O, Larson JC, Moya ML, et al. Generation of alginate microsphere for biomedical applications. J Vis Exp. 2012; 66:e3388.

[28] Chick WL, Like AA, Lauris V. 8-cell culture on synthetic capillaries: an artificial endocrine pancreas. Science. 1975; 187:847–849.

[29] Maki T, Otzu I, O'Neil JJ, et al. Treatment of diabetes by xenogeneic islets without immunosuppression. Use of a vascularized bioartificial pancreas. Diabetes. 1996; 45:342–347.

[30] Maki CS, Ubhi H, Sanchez-Farpon SJ, et al. Successful treatment of diabetes with the biohybrid artificial pancreas in dogs. Transplantation. 1991; 51:43–51.

[31] Lanza RP, Borland KM, Lodge P, et al. Treatment of severely diabetic, pancreatectomized dogs using a diffusion-based hybrid pancreas. Diabetes. 1992; 41:886–889.

[32] Jang JY, Lee DY, Park SJ, Byun Y. Immune reactions of lymphocytes and macrophages against PEG-grafted pancreatic islets. Biomaterials. 2004; 25:3663–3669.

[33] Borg DJ, Bonifacio E. The use of biomaterials in islet transplantation. Curr Diab Rep. 2011; 11:434–444.

[34] Fiszman GL, Karara AL, Finocchiaro LM, et al. A laboratory scale device for microencapsulation of genetically engineered cells into alginate beads. Electron J Biotechnol. 2002; 5:23–24.

[35] Sun AM. Microencapsulation of pancreatic islet cells: a bioartificial endocrine pancreas. Methods Enzymol. 1988; 137:575–580.

[36] Nicodemus G, Bryant S. Cell encapsulation in biodegradable hydrogels for tissue engineering applications. Tissue Eng Part B Rev. 2008; 14:149–165.

[37] Lee K, Mooney D. Hydrogels for tissue engineering. Chem Rev. 2000; 101:1869–1879.

[38] O'Sullivan ES, Johnson AS, Omer A, et al. Rat islet cell aggregates are superior to islets for transplantation in microcapsules. Diabetologia. 2010; 53:937–945.

[39] Otterlei M, Ostgaard K, Skjak-Braek G, et al. Induction of cytokine production from human monocytes stimulated with alginate. J Immunother. 1991; 10:286–291.

[40] Tam SK, Bilodeau S, Dusseault J, et al. Biocompatibility and physicochemical characteristics of alginate-polycation microcapsules. Acta Biomaterialia. 2011; 7:1683–1692.

[41] Duvivier-Kali VF, Omer A, Parent RJ, et al. Complete protection of islets against allorejection and autoimmunity by a simple barium-alginate membrane. Diabetes. 2001; 50:1698–1705.

[42] Omer A, Duvivier-Kali V, Fernandes J, et al. Long-term normoglycemia in rats receiving transplants with encapsulated islets. Transplantation. 2005; 79:52–58.

[43] de Vos P, de Haan BJ, Wolters GH, et al. Improved biocompatibility but limited graft survival after purification of alginate for microencapsulation of pancreatic islets. Diabetologia. 1997; 40:262–270.

[44] Wang T, Lacik I, Brissova M, et al. An encapsulation system for the immunoisolation of pancreatic islets. Nat Biotechnol. 1997; 15:358–362.

[45] Wang T, Adcock J, Kuhtreiber W, et al. Successful allotransplantation of encapsulated islets in pancreatectomized canines for diabetic management without the use of immunosuppression. Transplantation. 2008; 85:331–337.

[46] King S, Dorian R, Storrs R. Requirements for encapsulation technology and the challenges for transplantation of islets of langerhans. Graft. 2001; 4:491–499.

[47] Li N, et al. Engineering islet for improved performance by optimized reaggregation in alginate gel beads. Biotechnol Appl Biochem. 2016[23]. DOI: 10.1002/bab1489

[48] Bygd H, Bratlie K. The effect of chemically modified alginates on macrophage phenotype and biomolecule transport. J Biomed Mater Res A. 2016; 104:1707–1719.

[49] Suzuki K, Bonner-Weis S, Trivedi N, et al. Function and survival of macroencapsulated syngeneic islets transplanted into streptozocin-diabetic mice. Transplantation. 1998; 66:21–28.

[50] Tze WJ, Cheung SC, Tai J, Ye H. Assessment of the in vivo function of pig islets encapsulated in uncoated alginate microsphere. Transplant Proc. 1998; 30:477–478.

[51] Duvivier-Kali VF, Omer A, Lopez-Avalos MD, et al. Survival of microencapsulated adult pig islets in mice in spite of an antibody response. Am J Transplant. 2004; 12:1991–2000.

[52] de Vos P, Van Straaten JF, Nieuwenhuizen AG, et al. Why do microencapsulated islet grafts fail in the absence of fibrotic overgrowth? Diabetes. 1999; 48:1381–1388.

[53] Bunger CM, Tiefenbach B, Jahnkea A, et al. Deletion of the tissue response against alginate-PLL capsules by temporary release of co-encapsulated steroids. Biomaterials. 2005; 26:2353–2360.

[54] Baruch L, Benny O, Gilbert A, Ukobnik O. Alginate PLL cell encapsulation system co-entrapping PLGA-microspheres for the continuous release of anti-inflammatory drugs. Biomedical Microdevices. 2009; 11:1103–1113.

[55] Song S, et al. Silicon nanopore membrane (SNM) for islet encapsulation and immunoisolation under convective transport. Sci Rep. 2016; 6:23679.

[56] Leung A, Lawrie G, Nielson LK, Trau M. Synthesis and characterization of alginate/poly-L-ornitihine/alginate microcapsules for local immunosuppression. J Microencapsul. 2008; 25:387–398.

[57] Khanna O, Moya EC, Opara EC, Brey EM. Synthesis of multilayered alginate microcapsules for the sustained release of fibroblast growth factor-1. J Biomed Mater Res A. 2010; 95:632–640.

[58] Pedraza E, Coronel MM, Fraker CA, et al. Preventing hypoxia-induced cell death in beta cells and islets via hydrolytically activated, oxygen-generating biomaterials. Proc Natl Acad Sci USA. 2012; 109:4245–4250.

[59] Llacua A, de Haan BJ, Smink SA, de Vos P. Extracellular matrix components supporting human islet function in alginate-based immunoprotective microcapsules for treatment of diabetes. J Biomed Mater Res A. 2016; 104:1788–1796.

[60] Smink AM, Hertsig DT, Schwab L, et al. A retrievable, efficacious polymeric scaffold for subcutaneous transplantation of rat pancreatic islets. Ann Surg. 2016.

[61] Paredes Juarez GA, Spasojevic M, Faas MM, de Vos P. Immunological and technical considerations in application of alginate-based microencapsulation systems. Front Bioeng Biotechnol. 2014; 2:26.

[62] Kumar S, Ingle H, Prasad DV, Kumar H. Recognition of bacterial infection by innate immune sensors. Crit Rev Microbiol. 2013; 39:229–246.

[63] Mallett AG, Korbutt GS. Alginate modification improves long-term survival and function of transplanted encapsulated islets. Tissue Eng Part A. 2009; 15:1301–1309.

[64] de Vos P, van Hoogmoed CG, de Haan BJ, Busscher HJ. Tissue responses against immunoisolating alginate-PLL capsules in the immediate posttransplant period. J Biomed Mater Res A. 2002; 62:430–437.

[65] Pearl JI, Ma T, Irani AR, et al. Role of the toll-like receptor pathway in the recognition of orthopedic implant wear-debris particles. Biomaterials. 2011; 32:5535–5542.